# ECG Workout

**Exercises in Arrhythmia Interpretation**

FIFTH EDITION

# ECG Workout

## Exercises in Arrhythmia Interpretation

### FIFTH EDITION

**JANE HUFF,** RN, CCRN

Education Coordinator, Critical Care Unit
Arrhythmia Instructor
Advanced Cardiac Life Support (ACLS) Instructor
White County Medical Center
Searcy, Arkansas

Guest Faculty, Physician Assistant Program
Harding University
Searcy, Arkansas

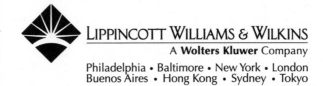

LIPPINCOTT WILLIAMS & WILKINS
A **Wolters Kluwer** Company
Philadelphia • Baltimore • New York • London
Buenos Aires • Hong Kong • Sydney • Tokyo

## Staff

**Executive Publisher**
Judith A. Schilling McCann, RN, MSN

**Senior Acquisitions Editor**
Margaret Zuccarini

**Editorial Director**
H. Nancy Holmes

**Clinical Director**
Joan M. Robinson, RN, MSN

**Senior Art Director**
Arlene Putterman

**Art Director**
Elaine Kasmer

**Editorial Project Manager**
William Welsh

**Copy Editor**
Stacey Ann Follin

**Illustrator**
Joseph John Clark, Judy Newhouse

**Digital Composition Services**
Diane Paluba (manager), Joyce Rossi Biletz,
Donna S. Morris

**Manufacturing**
Patricia K. Dorshaw (manager), Beth J. Welsh

**Editorial Assistants**
Megan L. Aldinger, Karen J. Kirk, Linda K. Ruhf

**Indexer**
Barbara Hodgson

ECGWO011005 — 040307

---

**Library of Congress Cataloging-in-Publication Data**

Huff, Jane, RN.
  ECG workout : exercises in arrhythmia interpretation / Jane Huff. — 5th ed.
    p. ; cm.
    1. Arrhythmia — Diagnosis — Problems, exercises, etc.  2. Electrocardiography — Interpretation — Problems, exercises, etc.  I. Title.
    [DNLM: 1. Arrhythmia — diagnosis — Problems and Exercises.  2. Electrocardiography — Problems and Exercises. WG 18.2 H889e 2006]
RC685.A65H84 2006
616.1'2807547'076 — dc22
ISBN13 978-0-7817-8230-2
ISBN10 0-7817-8230-9 (alk. paper)                          2005019444

# Contents

# Reviewers

**Sonia Astle,** RN, MS, CCRN, CCNS
Clinical Nurse Specialist, Critical Care
Inova Fairfax Hospital
Falls Church, Va.

**Ginger S. Braun,** RN, MSN, CCRN
Cardiovascular Clinical Nurse Specialist
Hoag Hospital
Newport Beach, Calif.

**Janice M. Judy,** RN, MSN
Instructor
University of Nebraska Medical Center
Scottsbluff

**Margaret A. Lantz,** RN, MS, CCRN
Assistant Director, Intensive Care Unit/Neuro Stepdown Unit
Hinsdale (Ill.) Hospital

**Michael P. Nozdrovicky,** RN, MA, NP, CCRN
Clinical Nurse Manager, Medical Intensive Care/Collaborative
  Medicine Associates
Mount Sinai Medical Center
New York

**Beth Oliver,** MS, RN
Clinical Nurse Manager, Cardiac Stepdown Unit
Mount Sinai Medical Center
New York

**Gayla P. Smith,** RN, MS, CCRN
Cardiovascular Clinical Nurse Specialist
Hoag Hospital
Newport Beach, Calif.

# Preface

*ECG Workout: Exercises in Arrhythmia Interpretation,* Fifth Edition, was written to assist physicians, nurses, medical and nursing students, paramedics, emergency medical technicians, telemetry technicians, and other allied health personnel in acquiring the knowledge and skills essential for identifying basic arrhythmias. The text can also be used as a reference for electrocardiogram (ECG) review for those already knowledgeable in ECG interpretation.

The text is written simply and illustrated with drawings, figures, tables, and ECG tracings. Each chapter is designed to build on the knowledge base from the previous chapters so the beginning student can quickly understand and grasp the basic concepts of electrocardiography. A great effort has been made not only to provide ECG tracings of good quality but also to provide a sufficient number and variety of ECG practice strips so the learner feels confident in arrhythmia interpretation. There are 567 practice strips — more than any book on the market.

Chapter 1 provides a discussion of basic anatomy and physiology of the heart. The electrical basis of electrocardiology is discussed in Chapter 2. The components of the ECG tracing (waveforms, intervals, segments, and complexes) are described in Chapter 3. This chapter also includes practice tracings on waveform identification. Cardiac monitors, lead systems, lead placement, ECG artifacts, and troubleshooting monitor problems are discussed in Chapter 4. A step-by-step guide to rhythm strip analysis is provided in Chapter 5, in addition to practice tracings on rhythm strip analysis. The individual arrhythmia chapters (Chapters 6 through 9) include a description of each arrhythmia, arrhythmia examples, causes, and management protocols. Current Advanced Cardiac Life Support guidelines are incorporated into each arrhythmia chapter as applicable to the rhythm discussion. Each arrhythmia chapter also includes 95 to 100 practice strips for self-evaluation. Chapter 10 presents a general discussion of cardiac pacemakers (types, indications, function, pacemaker terminology, malfunctions, and pacemaker analysis), along with practice tracings. Chapter 11 includes a posttest of mixed rhythm strips that can be used as a self-evaluation tool or for testing purposes.

The text has been updated, including text expansion and the revision or addition of tables, figures, and rhythm strips. Other important additions to the 5th edition include color, summary tables of identifying ECG features for each rhythm after each arrhythmia chapter, arrhythmia flash cards, and a glossary and index section.

The ECG tracings are actual strips from patients. Above each rhythm strip are 3-second indicators for rapid rate calculation. For precise rate calculation, an ECG conversion table for heart rate is printed after the index. For convenience, a removable version is also attached inside the back cover. **The heart rates for regular rhythms listed in the answer keys were determined by the precise rate calculation method and will not always coincide with the rapid rate calculation method.** Rate calculation methods are discussed in Chapter 5.

The author and publisher have made every attempt to check the content, especially drug dosages and management protocols, for accuracy. Medicine is continually changing, and the reader has the responsibility to keep informed of local care protocols and changes in emergency care procedures.

*This book is dedicated to
the twins, Isabella and Reece.*

# 1 Anatomy and physiology of the heart

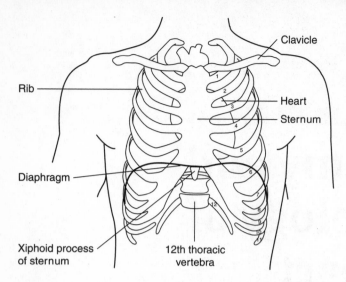

**Figure 1-1.** Thoracic projection of the boundaries of the heart on the chest wall.

# Description and location of the heart

The heart is a hollow, four-chambered muscular organ, which lies in the mediastinal cavity between the right and left lung, just behind the body of the sternum, and in front of the spinal column (Figure 1-1). The upper heart border (the *base*) is located at about the level of the second intercostal space. The lower heart border (the *apex*) terminates in a blunt point at the level of the fifth intercostal space, left midclavicular line. There, the apex can be palpated during ventricular contraction. This physical examination landmark is referred to as the *point of maximal impulse* (PMI) and is an indicator of the heart's position within the thorax. The heart's position isn't straight up and down, however; it's rotated toward the left so that the right side of the heart lies toward the front anteriorly. Thus, when viewed from the front of the body, the heart appears to be lying sideways. About two-thirds of the heart lies to the left of the body's midline, and one-third extends to the right. The average adult heart is cone shaped and is about 5″ long, 3½″ wide, and 2½″ thick (about the size of a normal-sized fist). The adult male heart averages 300 g in weight; the adult female heart is about 250 g. Heart size and weight are influenced by age, weight, body build, frequency of exercise, and heart disease.

# Function of the heart

The heart is a muscular organ that functions primarily as a pump to propel sufficient blood through the vascular system to meet the needs of the body. The heart is capable of adjusting its pump performance to meet various metabolic demands. As demands increase, the heart responds by accelerating its rate to increase cardiac output. As demands decrease, the heart slows its rate, resulting in a reduction in cardiac output. The heart has several unique properties: It can withstand continual activity without developing muscle fatigue and it's capable of generating electrical impulses that stimulate the heart to beat.

## Heart surfaces

There are four main heart surfaces to consider when discussing the heart: anterior, posterior, inferior, and lateral (Figure 1-2). A simplified concept of the heart surfaces is listed as follows:

- anterior – the front
- posterior – the back
- inferior – the bottom
- lateral – the side.

## Structure of the heart wall

The heart wall is arranged in three layers (Figure 1-3):

- the pericardium – the outermost layer
- the myocardium – the middle muscular layer
- the endocardium – the inner layer.

The pericardium is a saclike structure that encases the heart. The pericardium consists of an outer tough, inelastic, fibrous sac (the *fibrous pericardium*) and an inner thin, two-layered, fluid-secreting membrane (the *serous pericardium*). The outer fibrous pericardium comes in direct contact with the covering of the lung, the pleura, and is attached to the center of the diaphragm inferiorly, to the sternum anteriorly, and to the esophagus, trachea, and main

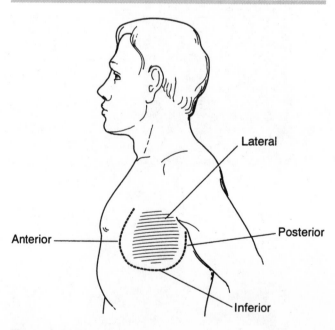

**Figure 1-2.** Heart surfaces.

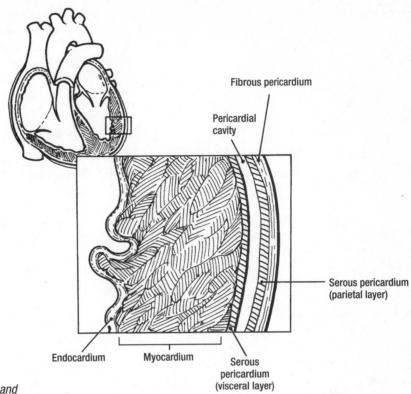

**Figure 1-3.** Heart wall. (From Bullock, B.L., and Rosendahl, P.P. *Pathophysiology: Adaptations and Alterations in Function,* 3rd ed. Philadelphia: Lippincott, 1992.)

bronchi posteriorly. This position anchors the heart to the chest and prevents it from shifting about. The moist serous pericardium is a continuous membrane that doubles back on itself to form two layers: the parietal layer, which lines the inside of the fibrous pericardium, and the visceral layer (also called *epicardium*), which lines the outer surface of the myocardium. Between the two layers of the serous pericardium is the pericardial space or cavity, which is usually filled with 10 to 30 ml of thin, clear, serous fluid secreted by the serous layers. The primary function of the pericardial fluid is to provide lubrication, preventing friction as the heart beats. Large accumulations of blood or fluid in the pericardial space can lead to cardiac tamponade, impeding ventricular filling and the heart's ability to contract.

The *myocardium* is the thick, middle, muscular layer that makes up the bulk of the heart wall. This layer is composed primarily of cardiac muscle cells and is responsible for the heart's ability to contract. The thickness of the myocardium varies from one heart chamber to another. The approximate wall thickness of the chambers are as follows: right atrium, 2 mm; left atrium, 3 mm; right ventricle, 3 to 5 mm; left ventricle, 13 to 15 mm. Chamber thickness is related to the amount of resistance the muscle must overcome to pump blood out of the chamber.

The *endocardium* is a smooth, thin layer of tissue that lines the heart chambers and valves. The smooth inner surface allows blood to flow more easily through the heart.

## Circulatory system

The human body requires a circulatory system to provide a continuous flow of blood to each cell. The circulatory system is a closed system consisting of heart chambers and blood vessels. Blood is continuously pumped in a circular route from the heart, to the arteries, through capillaries, into veins, and back to the heart.

The circulatory system consists of two separate circuits, the *systemic circuit* and the *pulmonary circuit*. The systemic circuit is a large circuit and includes the left side of the heart and vessels, which carry blood to the body and back to the right heart. The pulmonary circuit is a small circuit and includes the right side of the heart and vessels, which carry blood to the lungs and back to the left heart. The two circuits are designed so that blood flow is pumped from one circuit to the other.

## Heart chambers

The interior of the heart consists of four hollow chambers (Figure 1-4). The two upper chambers, the right atrium and the left atrium, are divided by a wall called the *interatrial septum*. The two lower chambers, the right ventricle and the left ventricle, are divided by a thicker wall called the *interventricular septum*. The two septa divide the heart into two pumping systems—the right side of the heart and the

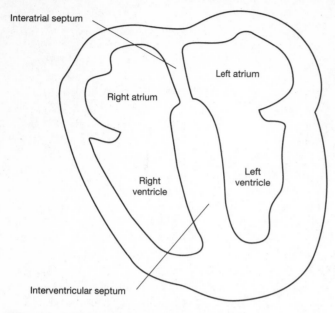

Figure 1-4. Chambers of the heart.

left side of the heart. The right side of the heart pumps venous (deoxygenated) blood into the lungs. The left side of the heart pumps arterial (oxygenated) blood into the systemic circulation.

The thickness of the walls in each chamber is related to the workload performed by that chamber. Both atria are low-pressure chambers serving as blood-collecting reservoirs for the ventricles. They add a small amount of force to the moving blood. Therefore, their walls are relatively thin. The right ventricular wall is thicker than the walls of the atria, but

much thinner than that of the left ventricle. The right ventricular chamber pumps blood a fairly short distance to the lungs against a relatively low resistance to flow. The left ventricle has the thickest wall because it must eject blood through the aorta to all parts of the body against a much greater resistance to flow.

## Heart valves

There are four valves in the heart: the *tricuspid valve,* separating the right atrium from the right ventricle; the *pulmonic valve,* separating the right ventricle from the pulmonary arteries; the *mitral valve,* separating the left atrium from the left ventricle; and the *aortic valve,* separating the left ventricle from the aorta (Figure 1-5). The primary function of the valves is to allow blood flow in one direction through the heart's chambers and prevent a backflow of blood (regurgitation). Changes in chamber pressure govern the opening and closing of the heart valves.

The tricuspid and mitral valves separate the atria from the ventricles and are referred to as the *atrioventricular (AV) valves.* The tricuspid valve orifice is larger (about 11 cm in circumference) and has three valve cusps or leaflets. The mitral valve is about 9 cm in circumference and has two valve leaflets. Both valves are encircled by tough, fibrous rings (valve rings). The leaflets of the AV valves are attached to thin strands of fibrous cords called *chordae tendineae* ("heart strings") (Figure 1-6). The chordae tendineae are then attached to papillary muscles, which arise from the walls and floor of the ventricles. Chordae tendineae and papillary muscles work together as anchors to prevent the leaflets from bulging back into the atria during ventricular con-

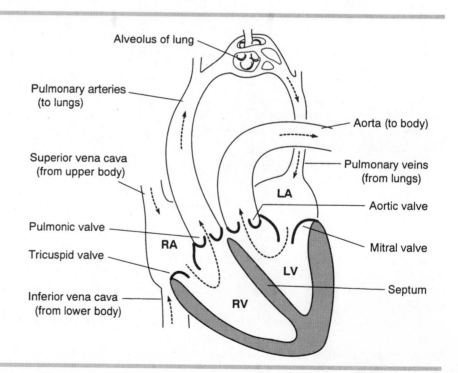

Figure 1-5. Chambers, valves, blood flow.
*RA,* right atrium: *RV,* right ventricle;
*LA,* left atrium; *LV,* left ventricle.

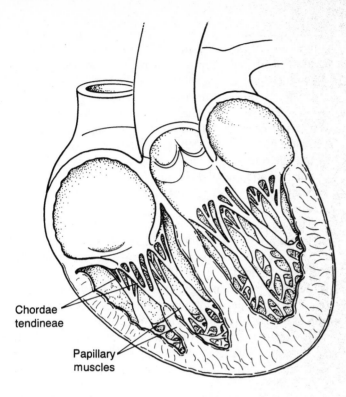

**Chordae tendineae**

**Papillary muscles**

**Figure 1-6.** Papillary muscles and chordae tendineae.

traction. Dysfunction of the chordae tendineae or papillary muscles can cause incomplete closure of the AV valves, resulting in a regurgitation murmur. As the atria fill with blood, pressure in the atria exceeds that of the ventricles, forcing the AV valves open and allowing blood to flow passively from the atria into the ventricles. During ventricular filling (diastole) when the AV valves are open, the valve leaflets, the chordae tendineae, and the papillary muscles form a funnel, promoting blood flow into the ventricles. Toward the end of ventricular diastole, the two atria contract, pumping the remaining blood into the ventricles. Contraction of the atria during the final phase of diastole to complete ventricular filling is called the *atrial kick*. The ventricles are 70% filled before the atria contract. The atrial kick adds an additional 30% to ventricular capacity. In normal heart rhythms the atria contract before the ventricles. The atrial kick is lost in those arrhythmias that have asynchronous contraction between the atria and the ventricles. Loss of the atrial kick decreases cardiac output and may lead to heart failure. At the end of diastole the increased pressure in the ventricles, compared with lessening pressure in the atria, helps to close the AV valves. During ventricular contraction (systole), the valve cusps are prevented from bulging back into the atria by contraction of the papillary muscles and tension in the chordae tendineae. Thus, blood is prevented from flowing backward into the atria despite the high ventricular pressures. Closure of the AV valves constitutes the first heart sound ($S_1$).

The aortic and pulmonic valves, or *semilunar valves*, are each composed of three half-moon shaped cusps of about equal size (7.5 to 8.5 cm). The pulmonic valve is located just inside the orifice of the pulmonary artery, and the aortic valve lies just inside the orifice of the aorta. The aortic cusps are thicker than the pulmonic cusps; both are thicker than the AV cusps. Like that of the AV valves, the rim of the semilunar valves is supported by valve rings. During ventricular systole, the cusps are thrust open as blood flows from an area of greater pressure in the ventricles to an area of lesser pressure in the aorta and pulmonary artery. The semilunar valves close as the pressure in the outflow arteries exceeds that of the ventricles. Backflow into the ventricles is prevented because of the cusps' strength, shape, and ability to form a tight seal. Closure of the semilunar valves constitutes the second heart sound ($S_2$).

## Blood flow through the heart and lungs

Blood flow through the heart and lungs is traditionally described by tracing the flow as blood returns from the systemic veins to the right side of the heart, to the pulmonary circuit, back to the left side of the heart, and out to the arterial vessels of the systemic circuit (Figure 1-5). The right atrium receives venous blood from the superior vena cava, the inferior vena cava, and the coronary sinus. The superior vena cava returns venous blood from the head, upper extremities, and the chest wall. The inferior vena cava returns venous blood from the trunk, abdominal organs, and lower extremities. The coronary sinus returns venous blood from the myocardium.

As the right atrium fills with blood, the pressure in the chamber increases. When pressure in the right atrium exceeds that of the right ventricle, the tricuspid valve opens, allowing blood to flow into the right ventricle. As the right ventricle fills with blood, pressure in that chamber increases, forcing the tricuspid valve shut and the pulmonic valve open, ejecting blood into the pulmonary arteries and on to the lungs. In the lungs, the blood picks up oxygen and releases carbon dioxide.

Pulmonary veins return the oxygenated blood from the lungs to the left atrium. As the left atrium fills with blood, the pressure in the chamber increases. When the pressure in the left atrium exceeds that of the right ventricle, the mitral valve opens allowing blood to flow into the left ventricle. As the left ventricle fills with blood, pressure in that chamber increases, forcing the mitral valve shut and the aortic valve open, ejecting blood into the aorta and systemic circuit where the blood releases oxygen to the cells and picks up carbon dioxide.

Although blood flow can be traced from the right side of the heart to the left side of the heart, right-sided events and left-sided events occur simultaneously. At the same time the right atrium receives venous blood from the body, the left atrium receives oxygenated blood from the lungs. Increased pressures in the filled atria force the tricuspid and mitral valves open, allowing blood to enter both ventricles. Increased pressure in the filled ventricles forces both AV valves shut and the pulmonic and aortic valves open. The ventricles contract simultaneously, ejecting blood through the pulmonary artery into the pulmonary circulation and through the aortic valve into the systemic circulation.

## Coronary circulation

The blood supply to the heart is provided by the right and left coronary arteries, which arise from the aorta just above and behind the aortic valve (Figure 1-7). They extend over the epicardial surface of the heart and branch several times. These arteries plunge inward through the myocardial wall and undergo further branching. There is much individual variation in the pattern of coronary artery branching. A discussion of the most common pattern follows.

The right coronary artery supplies blood to the right atrium, the right ventricle, the inferior wall of the left ventricle, the posterior one-third of the interventricular septum and, in 90% of the population, the posterior wall of the left ventricle. It supplies the SA node in 55% of the population, the AV node and bundle of His in 90% of the population, and the posterior fascicle of the left bundle branch.

The left coronary artery has a short main stem, the left main coronary artery, which branches into the left anterior descending and the left circumflex arteries. The left an-

terior descending artery supplies blood to the anterior-lateral wall of the left ventricle, the anterior two-thirds of the interventricular septum, the majority of the right bundle branch, the anterior fascicle of the left bundle branch, and a portion of the posterior fascicle of the left bundle branch. The left circumflex supplies blood to the left atrium, the anterior-lateral and posterior-lateral walls of the left ventricle and, in 10% of the population, the posterior wall of the left ventricle. It supplies the SA node in 45% of the population and the AV node and bundle of His in 10% of the population. Table 1-1 summarizes the coronary artery circulation.

The coronary artery that gives rise to the posterior descending artery is usually considered the dominant coronary artery. The posterior descending artery is commonly the terminal branch of the right coronary artery. When this is the case, the patient is said to have a right-dominant system. When the posterior descending branch is a continuation of the left circumflex artery, the patient is said to have a left-dominant system. Right dominance occurs in 85% to 90% of the population, even though the left coronary artery is of wider caliber and perfuses the largest proportion of the myocardium.

The right and left coronary artery branches are interconnected by an extensive network of small arteries that provide the potential for cross flow from one artery to the other. These small arteries are commonly called *collateral vessels* or *collateral circulation*. Collateral circulation exists at birth and apparently grows in size along with the rest

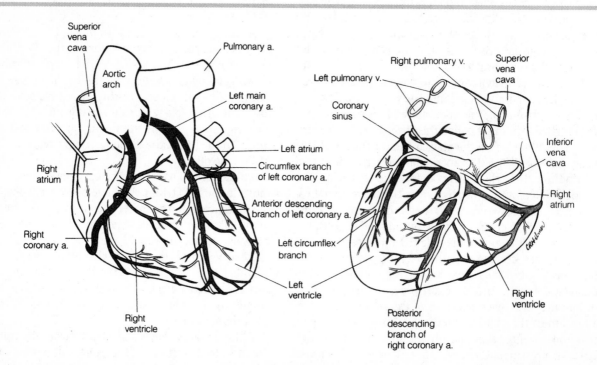

**Figure 1-7.** Coronary blood supply. (From Porth, C.M.: *Pathophysiology: Concepts of Altered Health States,* 3rd ed. Philadelphia: Lippincott, 1990.)

Table 1-1.
## Coronary artery circulation

| Coronary artery and its branches | Myocardium supplied | Conduction system supplied |
|---|---|---|
| **Right coronary artery** | Right atrium<br>Right ventricle<br>Inferior wall of left ventricle<br>Posterior wall of left ventricle (90%)*<br>Posterior one-third of interventricular septum | Sinoatrial (SA) node (55%)*<br>Atrioventricular (AV) node and bundle of His (90%)*<br>Posterior fascicle of left bundle branch |
| **Left coronary artery**<br>  Anterior descending branch | Anterolateral wall of left ventricle<br>Anterior two-thirds of interventricular septum | Majority of right bundle branch<br>Anterior fascicle of left bundle branch<br>Portion of posterior fascicle of left bundle branch |
|   Circumflex branch | Left atrium<br>Anterolateral wall of left ventricle<br>Posterolateral wall of left ventricle<br>Posterior wall of left ventricle (10%)* | SA node (45%)*<br>AV node and bundle of His (10%)* |

\* = of population

of the coronary circulation. If a blockage occurs in a major coronary artery, the collateral vessels enlarge and provide additional blood flow to those areas of reduced blood supply. However, blood flow through the collateral vessels isn't sufficient to meet the total needs of the myocardium in most cases.

In other vascular beds of the body, arterial blood flow reaches a peak during ventricular contraction (systole). However, myocardial blood flow is greater during ventricular diastole (when the ventricular muscle mass is relaxed) than it is during systole (when the heart's blood vessels are compressed).

The blood that has passed through the capillaries of the myocardium is drained by branches of the cardiac veins whose path runs parallel to those of the coronary arteries. Some of these veins empty directly into the right atrium and right ventricle, but the majority feed into the coronary sinus, which empties into the right atrium.

## Cardiac innervation

The heart is under the control of the autonomic nervous system (Figure 1-8), a control center that regulates functions of the body that are involuntary, or not under conscious control, such as heart rate and blood pressure. The autonomic nervous system is located in the medulla oblongata, a part of the brain stem. There are two major divisions of the autonomic nervous system: the *sympathetic nervous system* and the *parasympathetic nervous system*. The sympathetic nervous system prepares the body to function under stress (fight-or-flight response). The parasympathetic nervous system regulates the calmer functions (rest-and-digest response).

Automatic regulation of cardiac function requires sensory receptors, afferent (sensory) pathways, an integration center, efferent (motor) pathways, and motor receptors. Nerve impulses are carried from the sensory receptors to the brain by means of the afferent pathways. The medulla (the integration center) interprets the sensory information

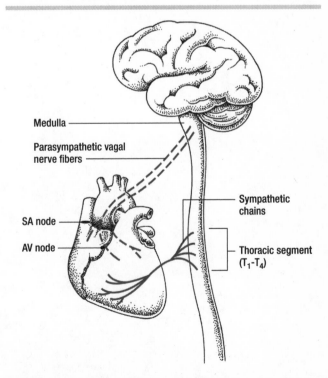

**Figure 1-8.** Autonomic nervous system innervation of the heart by parasympathetic vagal nerve fibers and sympathetic chains.

received, determines what action (if any) to take, and relays that information along the efferent pathways to the appropriate parasympathetic or sympathetic receptor site, which then transmits the information to the heart and blood vessels.

The sympathetic (accelerator) nervous system innervates the heart through nerve fibers arising from the thoracic segment of the spinal cord. Stimulation of the sympathetic nervous system results in the release of norepinephrine, which increases heart rate, speeds conduction through the AV node, and increases the force of ventricular contraction.

The parasympathetic (inhibitory) nervous system innervates the heart through vagal nerve fibers, which originate in the medulla oblongata. Stimulation of the parasympathetic nervous system results in the release of acetylcholine, which decreases heart rate, slows conduction through the AV node, and causes a small decrease in the force of ventricular contraction (there is minimal parasympathetic innervation of the ventricles). Normally, a balance is maintained between the inhibitory effects of the parasympathetic fibers and the excitatory effects of the sympathetic fibers.

Painful impulses originating within the heart are relayed via sensory nerve fibers to the nerve cell bodies located in the T1 through T4 segment of the thoracic spine. Cardiac pain tends to be referred to skin or skeletal muscles that share nerve supplies from the same or adjacent spinal segments. Therefore, cardiac pain is commonly referred to areas innervated by thoracic segments T1 through T4, such as the epigastric area, anterior chest wall, sternum, jaw, shoulders, scapula, arms, wrists, and hands.

# 2 Electrophysiology

## Cardiac cells

The heart is composed of cardiac muscle (myocardium), which is made up of thousands of cardiac cells. Cardiac cells are long and narrow, and many of them are branched. They interconnect with branches of adjacent cells forming an anastomosing network of cells. At the junctions where the branches join together is a specialized cellular membrane of low electrical resistance, which permits rapid conduction of electrical impulses from one cell to another throughout the cell network. Stimulation of one cardiac cell initiates stimulation of adjacent cells and ultimately leads to cell contraction.

There are two basic cardiac cell groups: the *pacemaker cells* and the *myocardial cells*. The pacemaker cells are specialized cells of the electrical conduction system responsible for generation of electrical impulses. The myocardial (working or mechanical) cells consist of contractile protein filaments called *actin* and *myosin*. When these cells are stimulated, the filaments shorten and slide together, causing myocardial cell contraction.

Cardiac cells have four primary cell characteristics:

■ automaticity – the ability of the pacemaker cells to generate their own electrical impulses spontaneously; this characteristic is specific to the pacemaker cells.

■ excitability – the ability of the cardiac cells to respond to an impulse; this characteristic is shared by all cardiac cells.

■ conductivity – the ability of cardiac cells to receive an electrical impulse and transmit it to other cardiac cells; this characteristic is shared by all cardiac cells.

■ contractility – the ability of the myocardial cells to shorten and cause muscle contraction; this characteristic is specific to myocardial cells.

Only one of these characteristics, contractility, is considered a mechanical function of the heart. The other three characteristics are electrical functions of the heart.

## Depolarization and repolarization

Cardiac cells are surrounded and filled with an electrolyte solution. An *electrolyte* is a substance whose molecules dissociate into charged particles (ions) when placed in water, producing positively and negatively charged ions. An ion with a positive charge is called a *cation*. An ion with a negative charge is called an *anion*. Potassium ($K^+$) is the primary intracellular ion and sodium ($Na^+$) the primary extracellular ion.

Normally, there is an ionic difference on the two sides (intracellular and extracellular) of the cardiac cell. In the resting cardiac cell, the inside of the cell is more negative than the outside as a result of the number and types of ions inside the cell. The constant movement of ions across the cardiac cell membrane continuously changes the electrical charge inside the cell, resulting in periods of stimulation (depolarization) and periods of rest (repolarization). The dis-

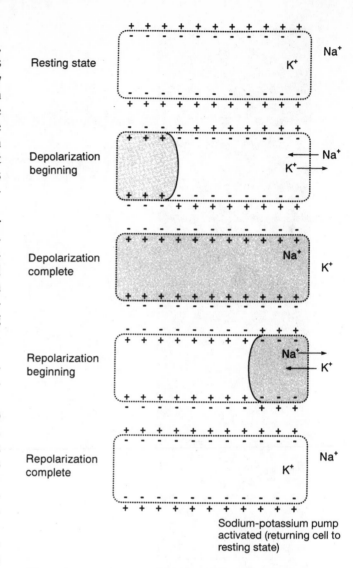

**Figure 2-1.** Depolarization and repolarization of a cardiac cell.

tribution of ions on either side of the membrane is determined by several factors:

■ **Membrane channels (pores)** – The cell membrane has openings through which ions pass back and forth between the extracellular and intracellular spaces. Some channels are always open; others can be opened or closed; still others can be selective, allowing one kind of ion to pass through and excluding all others. Membrane channels open and close in response to a stimulus (electrical, mechanical, or chemical).

■ **Concentration gradient** – Particles in solution move, or diffuse, from areas of higher concentration to areas of lower concentration. In the case of uncharged particles, movement proceeds until the particles are uniformly distributed within the solution.

■ **Electrical gradient** – Charged particles also diffuse, but the diffusion of charged particles is influenced not only by the concentration gradient but also by an electrical gradient. Like charges repel; opposite charges attract. Therefore, positively charged particles tend to flow toward negatively charged particles; negatively charged particles, toward positively charged particles.

■ **Sodium-potassium pump** – The sodium-potassium pump is a mechanism that actively transports ions across the cell membrane against its electrochemical gradient.

Pacemaker cells are able to generate and conduct electrical impulses that result in stimulation of the cardiac cell (depolarization), myocardial muscle contraction, and cardiac cell recovery (repolarization). These electrical impulses are the result of a brief—but rapid—flow of ions (primarily sodium and potassium) back and forth across the semipermeable cardiac cell membrane (Figure 2-1).

In the resting myocardial cell (the polarized state), the electric discharge inside the cell is more negative while the extracellular charge is more positive. During this time, no electrical activity is occuring and a straight line (isoelectric line) is recorded on the ECG. (Figure 2-5)

Once a cell is stimulated, the membrane permeability changes. Potassium begins to leave the cell, increasing cell permeability to sodium. Sodium rushes into the cell, causing the inside of the cell to become more positive than negative (cell is depolarized). The depolarization process proceeds from the innermost layer of the heart to the outer-

most layer. Muscle contraction follows depolarization. Therefore, depolarization is not the same as contraction. Depolarization is an electrical event that results in muscle contraction (a mechanical event).

After depolarization, there is an excess of sodium inside the cell and an excess of potassium outside the cell. The sodium-potassium pump is activated to actively transport sodium out of the cell and move potassium back into the cell, causing the inside of the cell to become more negative than positive (cell is repolarized). The repolarization process proceeds from the outermost layer of the heart to the innermost layer.

Depolarization of one cardiac cell acts as a stimulus on adjacent cells and causes them to depolarize. Propagation of the electrical impulses from cell to cell produces an electric current that can be detected by skin electrodes and recorded as waves or deflections onto a graph paper called the *ECG*.

## Electrical conduction system of the heart

The heart is supplied with an electrical conduction system that generates and conducts electrical impulses along specialized pathways to the atria and ventricles, causing them to contract (Figure 2-2). The system consists of the sino-

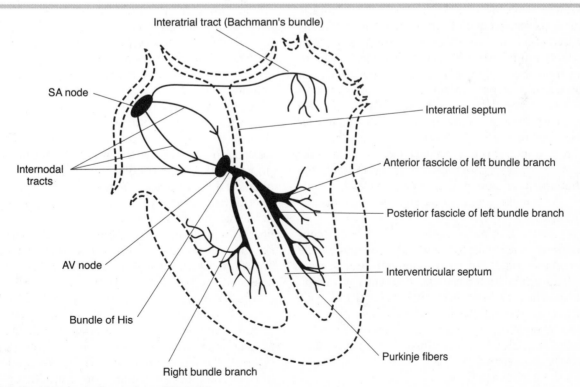

**Figure 2-2.** Electrical conduction system of the heart.

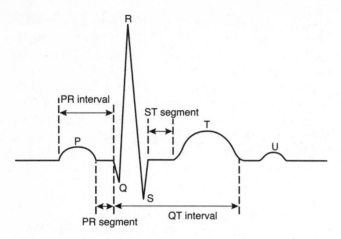

**Figure 2-3.** Relationship of the electrical conduction system to the ECG.

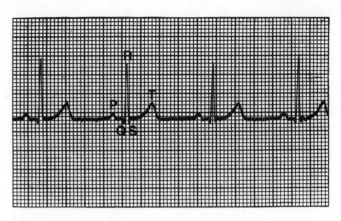

**Figure 2-4.** The cardiac cycle.

atrial (SA) node, the interatrial tract (Bachmann's bundle), the internodal tracts, the atrioventricular (AV) node, the bundle of His, the right and left bundle branches, and the Purkinje fibers.

The SA node is located in the wall of the upper right atrium near the inlet of the superior vena cava. Specialized electrical cells, called pacemaker cells, in the SA node discharge impulses at a rate of 60 to 100 beats/minute in rhythmic fashion.

Pacemaker cells are located at other sites along the conduction system, but the SA node is normally in control and is called the pacemaker of the heart because it possesses the highest level of automaticity (its inherent firing rate is greater than that of the other pacemaker sites). Pacemaker cells located in the upper and lower regions of the AV node can function as a secondary pacemaker at a rate of 40 to 60 beats/minute, whereas ventricular pacemaker cells fire at a rate of 30 to 40 beats/minute or less. If the SA node fails to generate electrical impulses at its normal rate or the conduction of these impulses is interrupted (blocked), pacemaker cells in other sites can assume control as pacemaker of the heart, but usually at a much slower rate. In general, the farther away the impulse originates from the SA node, the slower the rate.

As the electrical impulse leaves the SA node, it's conducted through the left atria by way of Bachmann's bundle and through the right atria via the internodal tracts, causing electrical stimulation (depolarization) and contraction of the atria. The impulse is then conducted to the AV node located in the lower right atrium near the interatrial septum. The AV node relays the electrical impulses from the atria to the ventricles. It provides the only normal conduction pathway between the atria and the ventricles. The AV node has three main functions:

- to slow conduction of the electrical impulse through the AV node to allow time for the atria to contract and empty its contents into the ventricles (atrial kick) before the ventricles contract. This delay in the AV node is represented on the ECG tracing as the flat line of the PR interval.
- to serve as a backup pacemaker if the SA node fails, at a rate of 40 to 60 beats/minute.
- to block some of the impulses from being conducted to the ventricles when the atrial rate is rapid, thus protecting the ventricles from dangerously fast rates.

After the delay in the AV node, the impulse moves rapidly through the bundle of His. The bundle of His divides into two important conducting pathways called the *right bundle branch* and the *left bundle branch.* The right bundle branch conducts the electrical impulse to the right ventricle. The left bundle branch divides into two divisions: the *anterior fascicle,* which carries the electrical impulse to the anterior wall of the left ventricle, and the *posterior fascicle,* which carries the electrical impulse to the posterior wall of the left ventricle. Both bundle branches terminate in a network of conduction fibers called *Purkinje fibers.* These fibers make up an elaborate web that penetrates and becomes continuous with the ventricular muscle mass. The Purkinje fibers carry the electrical impulse directly to the contractile cells of the ventricle. The term *His-Purkinje system* refers to the bundle of His, bundle branches, and the Purkinje fibers. Conduction of the electrical impulse through this system is the fastest of any tissue in the conduction system. The ventricles are capable of serving as a backup pacemaker at a rate of 30 to 40 beats/minute (sometimes less).

The heart's electrical activity is represented on the monitor or ECG tracing by three basic waveforms: the P wave, the QRS complex, and the T wave (Figure 2-3). Between the waveforms are the following segments and intervals: the PR interval, the PR segment, the ST segment, and the QT interval. A U wave is sometimes present. Although the letters themselves have no special significance, each component represents a particular event in the depolarization-repolarization cycle. The *P wave* depicts atrial depolarization, or the spread of the impulse from the SA node throughout the atria. The *PR interval* represents the time from the onset of atrial depolarization to the onset of ventricular depolarization. The *PR segment,* a part of the PR interval, is the short isoelectric line between the end of the P wave to the beginning of the QRS complex. It's used as a baseline to evaluate elevation or depression of the ST segment. The *QRS complex* depicts ventricular depolarization, or the spread of the impulse throughout the ventricles. The *ST segment* represents the end of ventricular depolarization and the beginning of ventricular repolarization. The *T wave* represents the latter phase of ventricular repolarization. The *U wave* (which isn't always present) is thought to represent further repolarization of the ventricles. The *QT interval* represents both ventricular depolarization and repolarization.

## The cardiac cycle

A cardiac cycle consists of one heartbeat or one PQRST sequence. It represents a sequence of atrial contraction and relaxation followed by ventricular contraction and relaxation. The basic cycle repeats itself again and again (Figure 2-4). Regularity of the cardiac rhythm can be assessed by measuring from one heartbeat to the next (from one R wave to the next R wave, also called the *R-R interval*). Between cardiac cycles the monitor or ECG recorder returns to the isoelectric line (baseline), the flat line in the ECG during which electrical activity is absent (Figure 2-5). Any waveform above the isoelectric line is considered a positive (up-

right) deflection and any waveform below this line a negative (downward) deflection. A deflection having both a positive and negative component is called a *biphasic deflection.* This basic concept can be applied to the P wave, the QRS complex, and the T-wave deflections.

## Waveforms and current flow

A monitor lead or ECG lead provides a view of the heart's electrical activity between two points or poles (a positive pole and a negative pole). The direction in which the electric current flows determine how the waveforms appear on the ECG tracing (Figure 2-6). An electric current flowing toward the positive pole will produce a positive deflection; an electric current traveling toward the negative pole, a negative deflection. Current flowing away from the poles will produce a biphasic (both positive and negative) deflection. Biphasic deflections may be equally positive and negative, more negative than positive, or more positive than negative (depending on the angle of current flow to the pole). This explains why QRS complexes can have different shapes and sizes.

The size of the wave deflection depends on the magnitude of the electrical current flowing toward the individual pole. The magnitude of the electrical current is determined by how much voltage is generated by depolarization of a particular portion of the heart. The QRS complex is normally larger than the P wave because depolarization of the larger muscle mass of the ventricles generates more voltage than does depolarization of the smaller muscle mass of the atria.

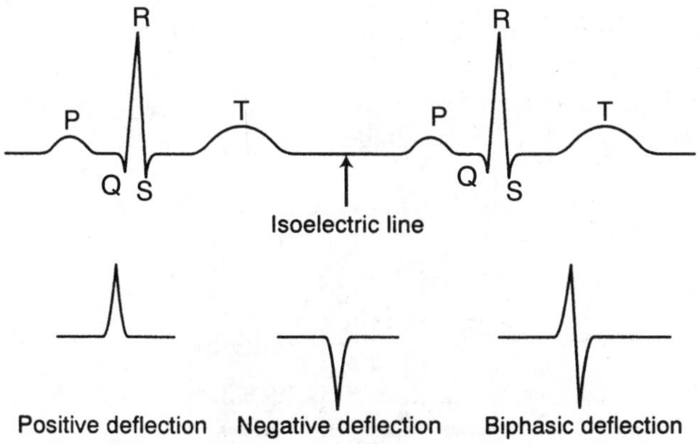

**Figure 2-5.** Relationship between waveforms and the isoelectric line.

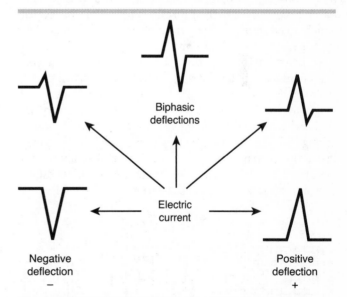

**Figure 2-6.** Relationship between current flow and waveform deflections.

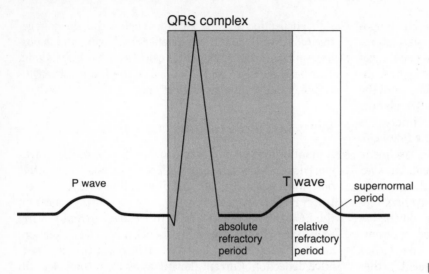

**Figure 2-7.** Refractory and supernormal periods.

## Refractory and supernormal periods of the cardiac cycle

There is a period of time in the cardiac cycle during which the cardiac cells may be refractory, or unable to respond, to a stimulus. Refractoriness is divided into three phases (Figure 2-7):

■ **Absolute refractory period** – During this period the cells absolutely can't respond to a stimulus. This period extends from the onset of the QRS complex to the peak of the T wave. During this time, the cardiac cells have depolarized and are in the process of repolarizing. Because the cardiac cells haven't repolarized to their threshold potential (the level at which a cell must be repolarized before it can be depolarized again) they can't be stimulated to depolarize.

■ **Relative refractory period** – During this period the cardiac cells have repolarized sufficiently to respond to a strong stimulus. This period begins at the peak of the T wave and ends with the end of the T wave. The relative refractory period is also called the *vulnerable period of repolarization*. A strong stimulus occurring during the vulnerable period may usurp the primary pacemaker of the heart (usually the SA node) and take over pacemaker control. An example might be a premature ventricular contraction (PVC) that falls dur-

ing the vulnerable period and takes over control of the heart in the form of ventricular tachycardia.

■ **Supernormal period** – During this period the cardiac cells will respond to a weaker than normal stimulus. This period occurs near the end of the T wave, just before the cells have completely repolarized.

## ECG graph paper

The PQRST sequence is recorded on special graph paper made up of horizontal and vertical lines (Figure 2-8). The horizontal lines measure the duration of the waveforms in seconds of time. Each small square measured horizontally represents 0.04 second in time. The width of the QRS complex in Figure 2-9 extends across for 2 squares and represents 0.08 second (0.04 second × 2 squares). The vertical lines measure the voltage or amplitude of the waveform in millimeters (mm). Each small square measured vertically represents 1 mm in height. The height of the QRS complex in Figure 2-9 extends upward from baseline 16 small squares and represents 16 mm voltage (1 mm × 16 squares).

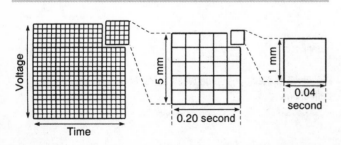

**Figure 2-8.** Electrocardiographic paper.

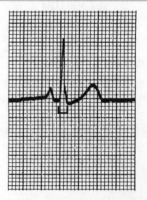

**Figure 2-9.** QRS width: 0.08 second; QRS height: 16 mm.

# 3 Waveforms, intervals, segments, and complexes

Much of the information that the ECG tracing provides is obtained from the examination of the three principal waveforms (the P wave, the QRS complex, and the T wave) and their associated intervals and segments. Assessment of this data provides the facts necessary for an accurate cardiac rhythm interpretation.

## P wave

The first deflection of the cardiac cycle, the P wave, is caused by depolarization of the atria. The waveform begins as the deflection leaves baseline and ends when the deflection returns to baseline (Figure 3-1). The normal P wave is smooth and rounded. Because there is a relatively small amount of atrial muscle mass to depolarize, only low voltages are normally produced. The amplitude of the P wave shouldn't exceed 2.5 mm and its duration shouldn't be greater than 0.10 second. The P wave is normally positive in lead II. There should be one P wave preceding each QRS complex. More than one P wave before a QRS complex indicates a conduction disturbance, such as that which occurs in second- and third-degree heart block. A normal P wave indicates that the electrical impulse responsible for the P wave originated in the sinus node and that normal depolarization of the right and left atria has occurred.

Normal P waves are smooth and round, positive in lead II, no more than 2.5 mm in height, and no more than 0.10 second in width, with one P wave to each QRS complex

A P wave that's abnormal is caused by either an abnormal sinus P wave or an ectopic P wave. An abnormal sinus P wave occurs when the electrical impulse leaves the SA node and travels through abnormal atrial tissue, resulting in P waves of greater amplitude or width. Enlargement of the right atrium produces an abnormally tall, peaked P wave. The abnormal P wave in right atrial enlargement (RAE) is sometimes referred to as *p pulmonale* because the atrial enlargement that it signifies is common with severe pulmonary disease (for example, chronic obstructive pulmonary disease, status asthmaticus, acute pulmonary embolism, and acute pulmonary edema). It's also common with congenital heart disease. Enlargement of the left atrium produces a P wave that's wide and notched. The term *p mitrate* is sometimes used to describe the abnormal P waves seen in left atrial enlargement (LAE) because they were first described in patients with rheumatic mitral valve disease. LAE is seen with mitral and aortic valvular disease, hypertension, coronary artery disease, and cardiomyopathies. An ectopic P wave is a P wave that arises from a site other than the SA node. These P waves will be abnormal in size, shape, or direction (small and pointed or inverted) or the P wave may be absent.

Abnormal P waves are typically tall and peaked (abnormal sinus P wave resulting from RAE), wide and notched (abnormal sinus P wave resulting from LAE), small and pointed (ectopic P wave), inverted (ectopic P wave), and absent (ectopic P wave).

Examples of P waves are shown in Figure 3-2.

## PR interval

The PR interval (sometimes abbreviated PRI) represents the time from the onset of atrial depolarization to the onset of ventricular depolarization. The PR interval (Figure 3-3) includes a P wave and the short, isoelectric line (PR segment) that follows it. The PR interval is measured from the beginning of the P wave as it leaves baseline to the beginning of the QRS complex. The duration of the normal PR interval is 0.12 to 0.20 second. A normal PR interval indicates that the period of time from the onset of atrial depolarization (P wave) to the onset of ventricular depolarization (QRS complex) is normal.

The PR interval may be shorter than normal if the electrical impulse is conducted from the atria to the ventricles through an accessory conduction pathway that bypasses the AV node, depolarizing the ventricles earlier than usual. One example of such a bypass channel is known as *Wolff-Parkinson-White (WPW) syndrome*. A short PR interval may also occur if the impulse originates in an ectopic pacemaker site in the AV node. The PR interval may be longer than normal if the electrical impulse is abnormally delayed traveling through the AV node. Prolonged PR intervals are seen in first-degree AV block and hypothyroidism and in those taking certain drugs (for example, digitalis, beta-blockers, or calcium channel blockers). A long PR interval is also associated with aging and may be the first sign of underlying conduction system disease. Examples of PR intervals are shown in Figure 3-4.

## QRS complex

The QRS complex (Figure 3-5) consists of the Q, R, and S waves and represents the conduction of the electrical impulse from the bundle of His throughout the ventricular myocardium (ventricular depolarization). The QRS complex is the largest complex on the ECG because it represents depolarization of a larger muscle mass.

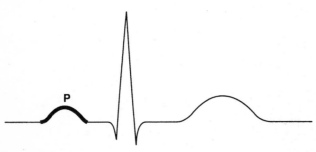

**Figure 3-1.** The P wave.

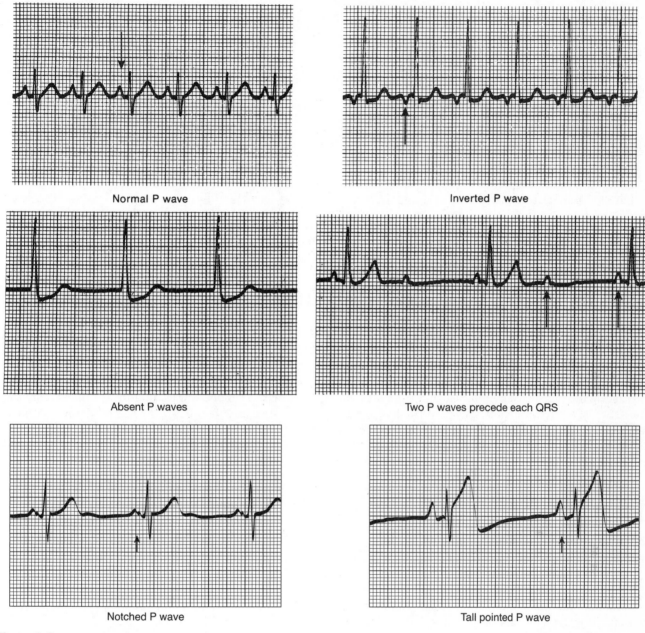

**Figure 3-2.** P wave examples.

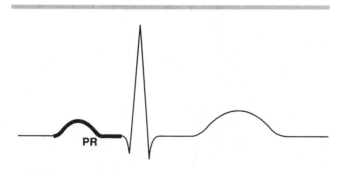

**Figure 3-3.** The PR interval.

The QRS complex is measured from the beginning of the QRS complex (as the first wave of the complex leaves baseline) to the end of the QRS complex (when the last wave of the complex begins to level out into the ST segment). The point where the QRS complex ends is called the *J point*. Finding the beginning of the QRS complex usually isn't difficult. However, finding the end of the QRS complex is at times a challenge because of elevation or depression of the ST segment. Remember, the QRS complex ends as soon as the straight line of the ST segment begins, even though the straight line may be above or below baseline.

The normal QRS complex is predominantly positive in lead II, with a duration of 0.10 second or less. The abnor-

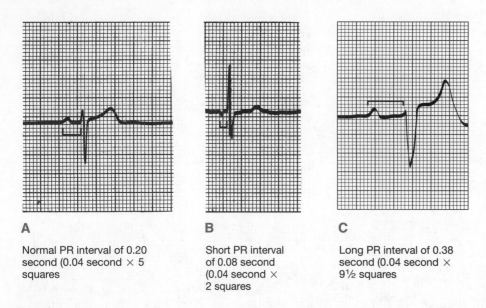

**A**

Normal PR interval of 0.20 second (0.04 second × 5 squares

**B**

Short PR interval of 0.08 second (0.04 second × 2 squares

**C**

Long PR interval of 0.38 second (0.04 second × 9½ squares

**Figure 3-4.** PR interval examples.

mal QRS complex is wide, with a duration of 0.12 second or more. There are wide limits to the amplitude of the R wave in the QRS complex, but it generally ranges from 2 to 15 mm, depending on the lead. A normal QRS complex indicates that the electrical impulse has been conducted normally from the bundle of His to the Purkinje network through the right and left bundle branches and that normal depolarization of the right and left ventricles has occurred.

As mentioned previously, the QRS complex is composed of three wave deflections: the Q wave, the R wave, and the S wave. The R wave is a positive waveform; the Q wave, a negative waveform that precedes the R wave; and the S wave, a negative waveform that follows the R wave. Although the term *QRS complex* is used, many variations exist in the configuration of the QRS complex, and you may not always see all three QRS complex waveforms (Figure 3-6). Whatever the variation, the complex is still called the QRS complex. For example you might see a QRS complex with a Q and an R wave but no S wave (Figure 3-6 D), an R and S wave without a Q wave (Figure 3-6 F), or an R wave without a Q or an

S wave (Figure 3-6 A). If the entire complex is negative (Figure 3-6 I), it's termed a *QS complex* (not a negative R wave because R waves are always positive). It's also possible to have more than one R wave (Figure 3-6 J) and more than one S wave (Figure 3-6 M). The second R wave is called *R*

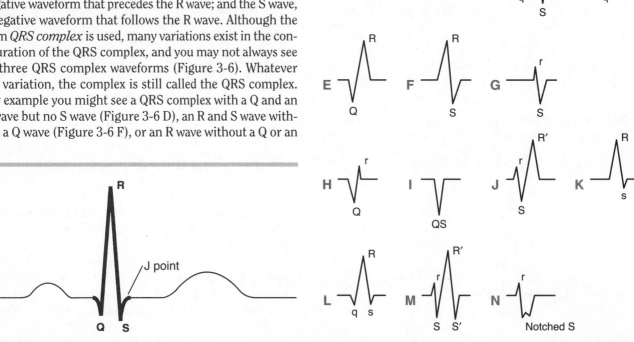

**Figure 3-6.** QRS variations.

**Figure 3-5.** The QRS complex.

*prime* and is written R´. The second S wave is called *S prime* and is written S´. To be labeled separately, a wave must cross the baseline. A wave that changes direction but doesn't cross the baseline is called a *notch* (Figure 3-6 B and 3-6 N).

Capital letters are used to designate waves of large amplitude (5 mm or more) and lowercase letters are used to designate waves of small amplitude (less than 5 mm). This allows you to visualize a complex mentioned in a textbook when illustrations aren't available. For example, if a complex is described in a text as having an rS waveform, the reader can easily picture a complex with a small r wave and a big S wave.

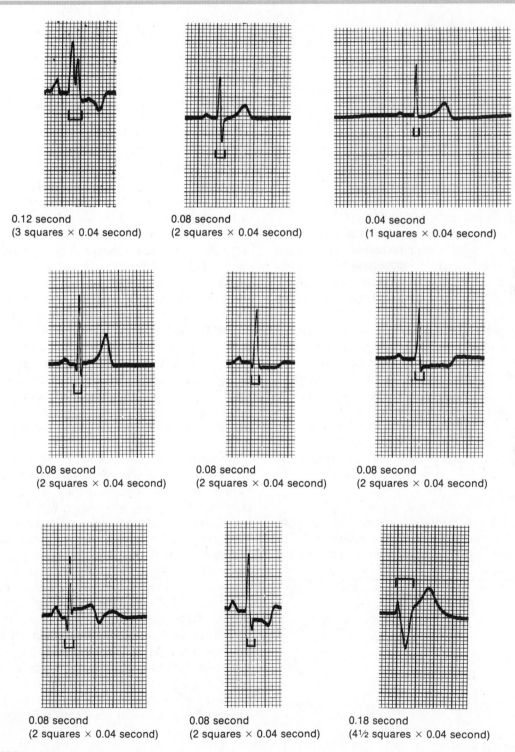

0.12 second
(3 squares × 0.04 second)

0.08 second
(2 squares × 0.04 second)

0.04 second
(1 squares × 0.04 second)

0.08 second
(2 squares × 0.04 second)

0.08 second
(2 squares × 0.04 second)

0.08 second
(2 squares × 0.04 second)

0.08 second
(2 squares × 0.04 second)

0.08 second
(2 squares × 0.04 second)

0.18 second
(4½ squares × 0.04 second)

**Figure 3-7.** QRS examples.

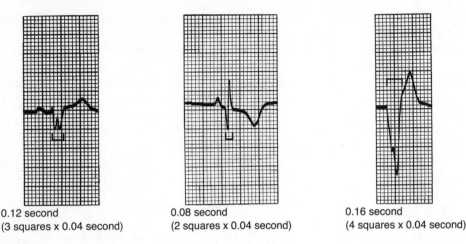

| 0.12 second | 0.08 second | 0.16 second |
| (3 squares x 0.04 second) | (2 squares x 0.04 second) | (4 squares x 0.04 second) |

**Figure 3-7.** *(continued)*

An abnormally wide QRS complex may result from:
■ a block in the conduction of impulses through the right or left bundle branch (bundle-branch block)
■ an electrical impulse that has arrived early (as with premature beats) at the bundle branches before repolarization is complete, allowing the electrical impulse to initiate depolarization of the ventricles earlier than usual, resulting in abnormal (aberrant) ventricular conduction and causing a wide QRS complex
■ an electrical impulse that has been conducted from the atria to the ventricles through an abnormal accessory conduction pathway that bypasses the AV node, allowing the electrical impulse to initiate depolarization of the ventricles earlier than usual, resulting in abnormal (aberrant) ventricular conduction and causing a wide QRS complex
■ an electrical impulse that has originated in an ectopic site in the ventricles.

Examples of QRS complexes are shown in Figure 3-7.

## ST segment

The ST segment represents the end of ventricular depolarization and the beginning of ventricular repolarization. The ST segment begins with the end of the QRS complex and

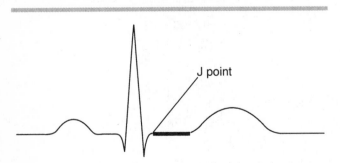

**Figure 3-8.** The ST segment.

ends with the onset of the T wave (Figure 3-8). The normal ST segment is flat (isoelectric). The point marking the end of the QRS complex and the beginning of the ST segment is called the *J point.* The ST segment is considered elevated if the segment is above baseline and depressed if the segment is below baseline. The PR segment is normally used as a baseline reference to evaluate the degree of displacement of the ST segment from the isoelectric line. To determine the degree of displacement, measure at a point 0.04 second (1 small square) past the J point. ST segment elevation or depression is considered significant if the displacement is more than 1 mm (1 small square) and is seen in two or more leads facing the same area of the heart. If elevated, the ST segment may be horizontal (straight across), convex (arched upward), or concave (arched inward). If depressed, the ST segment may be horizontal, downsloping, or sagging.

An elevated ST segment is an ECG sign of myocardial injury, as seen in an acute myocardial infarction. Other causes of ST segment elevation include coronary vasospasm (Prinzmetal's angina), pericarditis, ventricular aneurysm, hyperkalemia, and early repolarization (a normal variant). Early repolarization is a variant of myocardial repolarization seen in healthy people (common in young individuals) that produces ST segment elevation closely mimicking that of an acute myocardial infarction or acute pericarditis.

A depressed ST segment is an ECG sign of myocardial ischemia. Although ST segment depression is typically associated with myocardial ischemia, other common causes include left and right ventricular hypertrophy, left and right bundle-branch block, hypokalemia, and drug effects (for example, digitalis). Digitalis causes a sagging ST segment depression, with a characteristic "scooped-out" appearance. Examples of ST segments are shown in Figure 3-9.

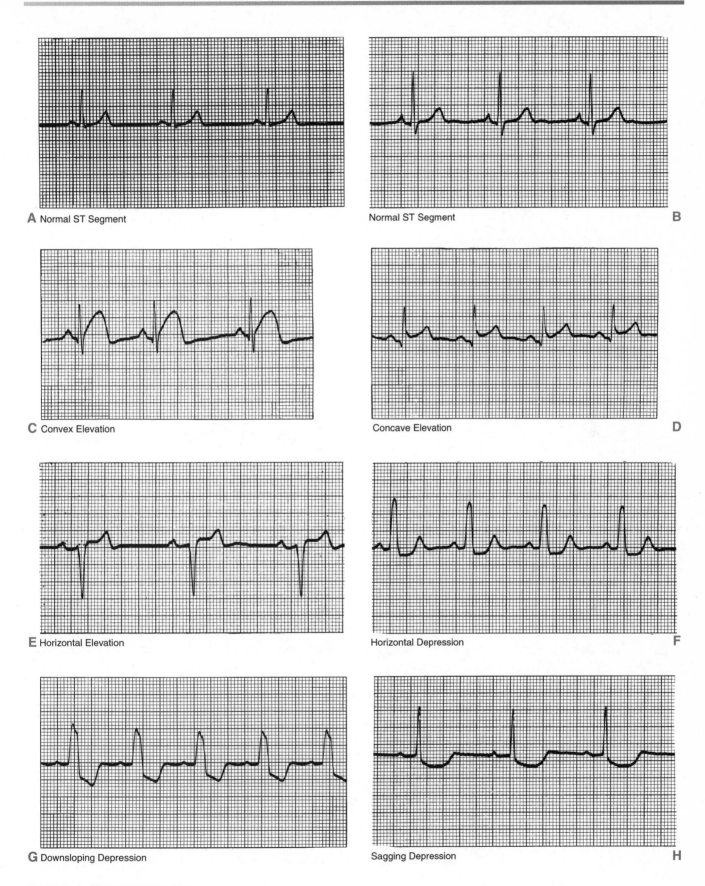

A Normal ST Segment

B Normal ST Segment

C Convex Elevation

D Concave Elevation

E Horizontal Elevation

F Horizontal Depression

G Downsloping Depression

H Sagging Depression

**Figure 3-9.** ST segment samples.

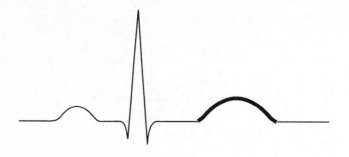

**Figure 3-10.** The T wave.

## T wave

The T wave represents the latter phase of ventricular repolarization. The normal T wave begins as the deflection gradually slopes upward from the ST segment and ends when the waveform returns to baseline (Figure 3-10). Normal T waves are rounded, asymmetrical (the peak is closer to the end of the wave than to the beginning), and positive in lead II, with an amplitude less than 5 mm. The T wave always follows the QRS complex (repolarization always follows depolarization).

Abnormal T waves tend to be symmetrical and may be abnormally tall or low, flattened, biphasic, or inverted. Ab-

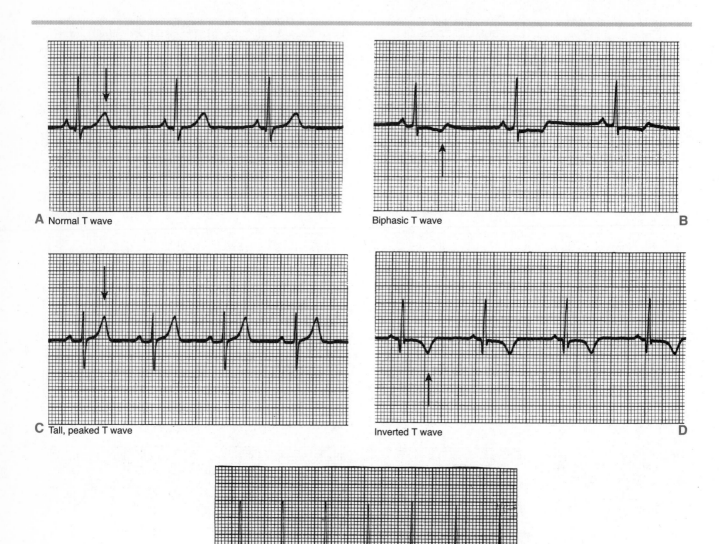

**A** Normal T wave

**B** Biphasic T wave

**C** Tall, peaked T wave

**D** Inverted T wave

**E** Flat T wave

**Figure 3-11.** T wave examples.

normal T waves are seen in myocardial ischemia, myocardial infarction, pericarditis, hyperkalemia, ventricular enlargement, bundle-branch block, subarachnoid hemorrhage, and the administration of certain drugs (for example, quinidine or procainamide). Examples of T waves are shown in Figure 3-11.

## QT Interval

The QT interval represents the time between the onset of ventricular depolarization and the end of ventricular repolarization. The QT interval is measured from the beginning of the QRS complex to the end of the T wave (Figure 3-12). The length of the QT interval normally varies according to age, sex, and particularly heart rate. As the heart rate in-

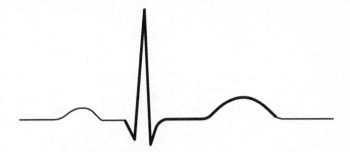

**Figure 3-12.** QT interval.

creases, the QT interval decreases; as the heart rate decreases, the QT interval increases. Therefore, the QT interval can be

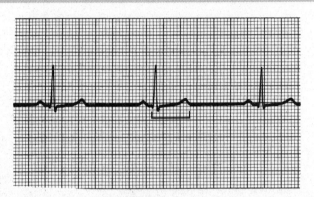

A  1. Number of small squares between R waves = 31. Half of 31 = 15.
   2. Number of small squares in QT interval = 11
   3. Compare the difference: QT interval is less than half the R-R interval (11 small squares are less than 15 small squares); QT interval is normal for this heart rate.
   4. Duration of QT interval: 11 squares × 0.04 sec = 0.44 second

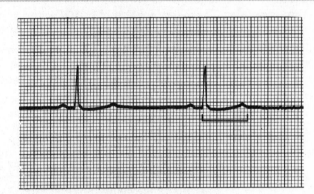

B  1. Number of small squares between R waves = 38. Half of 38 = 19.
   2. Number of small squares in QT interval = 13.
   3. Compare the difference: QT interval is less than half the R-R interval (13 small squares are less than 19 small squares); QT interval is normal for this heart rate.
   4. Duration of QT interval: 13 small squares × 0.04 second = 0.52 second.

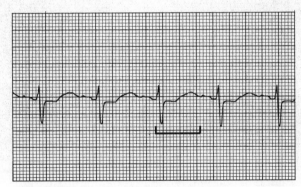

C  1. Number of small squares between R waves = 18. Half of 18 = 9.
   2. Number of small squares in QT interval = 13.
   3. Compare the difference: QT interval is more than half the R-R interval (13 small squares are more than 9 small squares); QT interval is prolonged for this heart rate.
   4. Duration of QT interval: 13 squares × 0.04 second = 0.52 second.

**Figure 3-13.** QT interval examples.

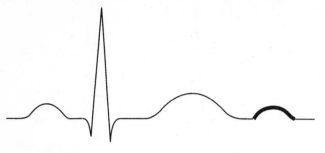

**Figure 3-14.** The U wave.

measured more accurately if it's corrected for heart rate (QT rate corrected, or QTc). Generally speaking, the normal QT interval should be less than half the distance between two consecutive R waves (called the *R-R interval*) when the rhythm is regular. The determination of the QT interval should be made in a lead where the T wave is most prominent and shouldn't include the U wave. Also, accurate measurement of the QT interval can be done only when the rhythm is regular for at least two cardiac cycles before the measurement.

To determine if the QT interval is normal or abnormal according to the patient's heart rate:

- Count the number of small boxes between two consecutive R waves (R-R interval) and divide by two.
- Count the number of small boxes in the QT interval.
- Compare the difference. If the QT interval (in small boxes) measures less than half the R-R interval (in small boxes), it's probably normal. If the QT interval measures the same as half the R-R interval, it's considered borderline. If the QT interval measures longer than half the R-R interval, it's prolonged.
- Multiply the number of small squares in the QT interval by 0.04 second to determine the duration of the QT interval.

A normal QT interval indicates that ventricular depolarization and repolarization has occurred within a normal amount of time. A short QT interval represents an increase in the rate of repolarization of the ventricles and is insignificant. A prolonged QT interval represents a delay in ventricular repolarization. A prolonged QT interval lengthens the relative refractory period (the vulnerable period) of the cardiac cycle, allowing more time for an ectopic focus to take control and putting the ventricles at risk for life-threatening dysrhythmias such as torsades de pointes

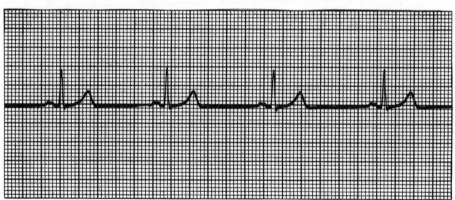

ECG without U wave

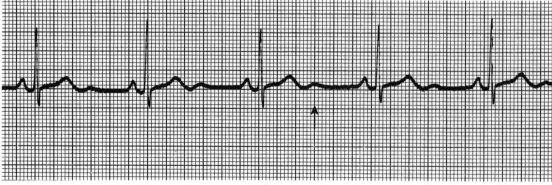

ECG with U wave

**Figure 3-15.** U wave examples.

(discussed in Chapter 9). Some causes of a prolonged QT interval include electrolyte imbalances (for example, hypokalemia, hypomagnesemia, and hypocalcemia), hypothermia, bradyarrhythmias, liquid protein diets, myocardial ischemia, antiarrhythmics, psychotropic agents (for example, phenothiazines and tricyclic antidepressants), and hereditary long-QT-interval syndrome. It can also occur without a known cause (idiopathic). Examples of QT intervals are shown in Figure 3-13.

## U wave

The U wave is a small, rounded, wave deflection sometimes seen after the T wave (Figure 3-14). Neither its presence nor its absence is considered abnormal. U waves represent the last phase of ventricular repolarization.

The waveform begins as the deflection leaves baseline and ends when the deflection returns to baseline. Normal U waves are small, rounded, and symmetrical; positive in lead II; and usually less than 2 mm in amplitude (always smaller than the preceding T wave). The U wave can best be seen when the heart rate is slow.

Some causes of abnormally large U waves include hypokalemia, cardiomyopathy, left ventricular enlargement, and the administration of certain drugs (such as digitalis, quinidine, and procainamide). A prominent U wave is also indicative of delayed ventricular repolarization and (like a prolonged QT interval) predisposes the individual to development of a specific type of ventricular tachycardia called *torsades de pointes* (discussed in Chapter 9).

A large U wave may sometimes be mistaken for a P wave. In most cases, however, close inspection of both waveforms will help differentiate the U wave from the P wave. Examples of U waves are shown in Figure 3-15.

# Waveform practice: Labeling waves

For each of the following rhythm strips (strips 3-1 through 3-14) label the P, Q, R, S, T, and U waves. Some of the strips may not have all of these waveforms. Check your answers with the answer key in the back of the book.

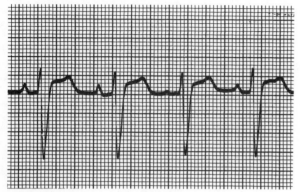

**Strip 3-1.**

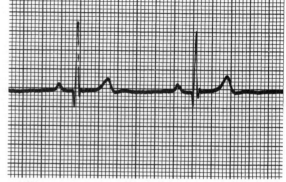

**Strip 3-2.**

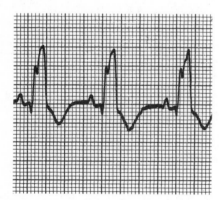

**Strip 3-3.**

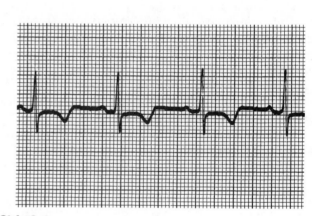

**Strip 3-4.**

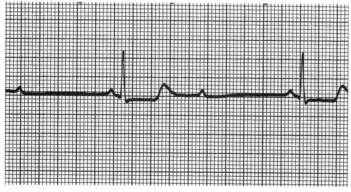

**Strip 3-5.**

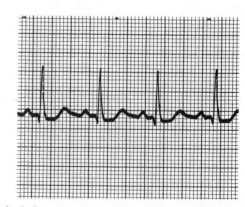

**Strip 3-6.**

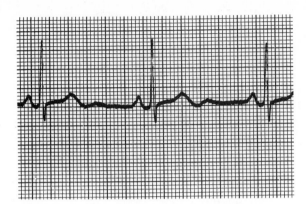

**Strip 3-7.**

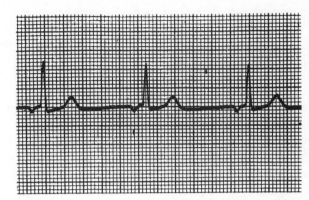

**Strip 3-8.**

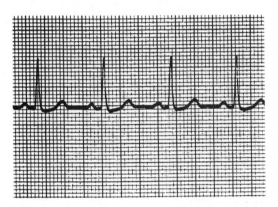

**Strip 3-9.**

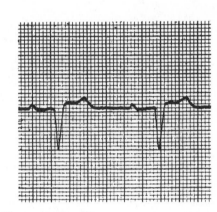

**Strip 3-10.**

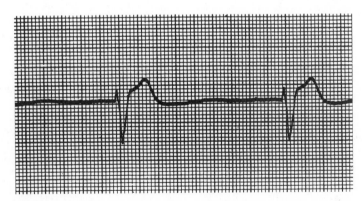

**Strip 3-11.**

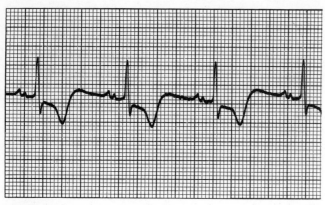

Strip 3-12.

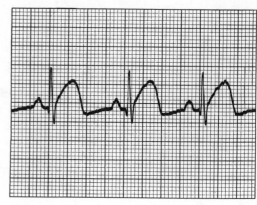

Strip 3-13.

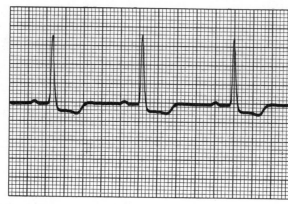

Strip 3-14.

# 4 Cardiac monitors

## Purpose of ECG monitoring

The electrocardiogram (ECG) is a recording of the electrical activity of the heart. The ECG records two basic electrical processes:

■ **Depolarization** – the spread of the electrical stimulus through the heart muscle producing the P wave from the atria and the QRS complex from the ventricles.

■ **Repolarization** – the return of the stimulated muscle to the resting state, producing the ST segment, the T wave, and the U wave.

The depolarization-repolarization process produces electrical currents that are transmitted to the surface of the body. This electrical activity is detected by electrodes attached to the skin. After the electric current is detected, it's amplified, displayed on a monitor screen (oscilloscope), and recorded on ECG graph paper as waves and complexes. The waveforms can then be analyzed in a systematic manner and the "cardiac rhythm" identified.

Bedside monitoring allows continuous observation of the heart's electrical activity and is used to identify arrhythmias (disturbances in rate, rhythm, or conduction), evaluate pacemaker function, and evaluate the response to medications (for example, antiarrhythmics). Continuous cardiac monitoring is useful in monitoring patients in critical care units, cardiac stepdown units, surgery suites, outpatient surgery departments, emergency departments, postanesthesia recovery units, and so forth.

## Types of bedside monitoring

There are two types of bedside monitoring: hardwire and telemetry. With hardwire monitoring, conductive gel pads (electrodes) are placed on the patient's chest and attached to a lead-cable system, which is then connected to a bedside monitor. With telemetry (wireless monitoring), electrode pads are attached to the patient's chest and the leads connected to a portable monitor transmitter.

### Hardwire monitoring

Hardwire monitoring uses either a five-leadwire system or a three-leadwire system.

With the *five-leadwire system* (Figure 4-1), five electrode pads and five leadwires are used. One electrode is placed below the right clavicle (2nd interspace, right midclavicular line), one below the left clavicle (2nd interspace, left midclavicular line), one on the right lower rib cage (8th interspace, right midclavicular line), one on the left lower rib cage (8th interspace, left midclavicular line), and one in a chest lead position ($V_1$ to $V_6$). The six chest lead positions (Figure 4-2) include:

■ $V_1$ – 4th intercostal space, right sternal border
■ $V_2$ – 4th intercostal space, left sternal border
■ $V_3$ – midway between $V_2$ and $V_4$
■ $V_4$ – 5th intercostal space, left midclavicular line
■ $V_5$ – 5th intercostal space, left anterior axillary line
■ $V_6$ – 5th intercostal space, left midaxillary line.

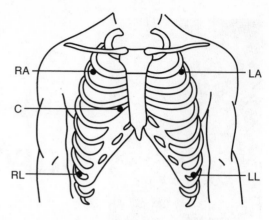

**Figure 4-1.** Hardwire monitoring — Five leadwire system. This illustration shows you where to place the electrodes and attach leadwires using a five-leadwire system. The leadwires are color-coded as follows:

■ white — right arm (RA)
■ black — left arm (LA)
■ green — right leg (RL)
■ red — left leg (LL)
■ brown — chest (C).

  Leads placed in the arm and leg positions as shown allow you to view leads I, II, III, aVR, aVL, and aVF. To view chest leads $V_1$–$V_6$, the chest lead must be placed in the specific chest lead position desired. In this example, the brown chest lead is in $V_1$ position.

The right arm (RA) lead is attached to the electrode pad below the right clavicle; the left arm (LA) lead, to the electrode pad below the left clavicle; the right leg (RL) lead, to the electrode pad on the right lower rib cage; the left leg (LL) lead, to the electrode pad on the left lower rib cage; and the chest lead, to the chest electrode pad.

With the five-leadwire system for hardwire monitoring you can continuously monitor two leads using a lead selector on the monitor. Leads placed in the arm and leg positions as shown in Figure 4-1 allow you to view leads I, II, III, $AV_R$, $AV_L$, and $AV_F$. To view chest leads $V_1$ to $V_6$, the chest lead must be placed in the specific chest lead position de-

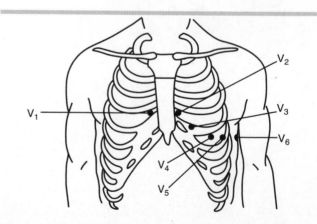

**Figure 4-2.** Chest lead positions.

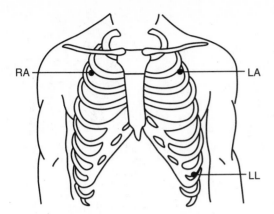

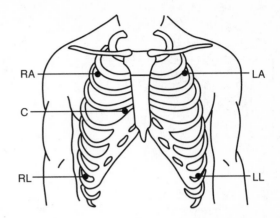

**Figure 4-3.** Hardwire monitoring—Three-leadwire system. This illustration shows you where to place the electrodes and attach leadwires using a three-leadwire system. The lead wires are color-coded as follows:

- white—right arm (RA)
- black—left arm (LA)
- red—left leg (LL).

Leads placed in this position will allow you to monitor leads I, II, or III using the lead selector on the monitor.

**Figure 4-5.** Telemetry monitoring—Five-leadwire system. This illustration shows you where to place the electrodes and attach leadwires using a five-leadwire system. The leadwires are color-coded as follows:

- white—right arm (RA)
- black—left arm (LA)
- green—right leg (RL)
- red—left leg (LL)
- brown—chest (C).

With the 5 leadwire system for telemetry monitoring you can monitor any one of the 12 leads using a lead selector on the monitor. Leads placed in the conventional limb positions allow you to view leads I, II, III, aVR, aVL, and aVF. To view chest leads $V_1$–$V_6$ the chest lead must be placed in the specific chest lead desired.

sired. Generally, a limb lead (usually I, II, or III) and a chest lead (usually $V_1$ or $V_6$) are chosen to be monitored.

With the *three-leadwire system* (Figure 4-3), three electrode pads and three leadwires are used. One electrode pad is placed below the right clavicle (2nd interspace, right midclavicular line), one below the left clavicle (2nd interspace, left midclavicular line), and one on the left lower rib cage (8th interspace, left midclavicular line). The RA lead is attached to the electrode pad below the right clavicle, the LA lead is attached to the electrode pad below the left clavicle, and the LL lead is attached to the electrode pad on the left lower rib cage. You can monitor either limb leads I, II, or III by turning the lead selector on the monitor. Although you can't monitor chest leads ($V_1$ to $V_6$) with a three-lead-

wire system, you can monitor modified chest leads that provide similar information. To monitor any of these leads, reposition the LL lead to the appropriate position for the chest lead you want to monitor, and turn the lead selector on the monitor to lead III. Examples of modified chest lead $V_1$ ($MCL_1$) and modified chest lead $V_6$ ($MCL_6$) are shown in Figure 4-4.

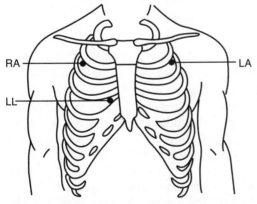

Modified Chest Lead $V_1$ ($MCL_1$)

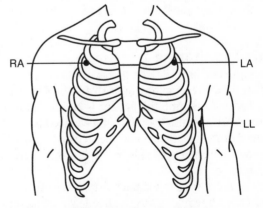

Modified Chest Lead $V_6$ ($MCL_6$)

**Figure 4-4.** Hardwire monitoring—Three-leadwire system: Leads $MCL_1$ and $MCL_6$. Modified chest leads can be monitored with the three-leadwire system by repositioning the left leg (LL) lead to the chest position desired and turning the lead selector on the monitor to lead III.

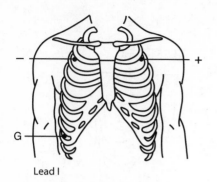

Lead I

Negative lead – 2nd interspace
right midclavicular line

Positive lead – 2nd interspace
left midclavicular line

Ground lead – 8th interspace
right midclavicular line

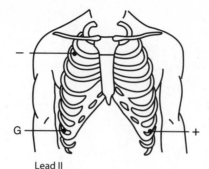

Lead II

Negative lead – 2nd interspace
right midclavicular line

Positive lead – 8th interspace
left midclavicular line

Ground lead – 8th interspace
right midclavicular line

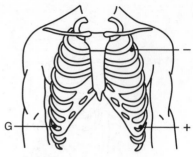

Lead III

Negative lead – 2nd interspace
left midclavicular line

Positive lead – 8th interspace
left midclavicular line

Ground lead – 8th interspace
right midclavicular line

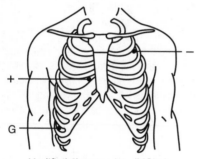

Modified Chest Lead V₁ (MCL₁)

Negative lead – 2nd interspace
left midclavicular line

Positive lead – 4th interspace
right sternal border

Ground lead – 8th interspace
right midclavicular line

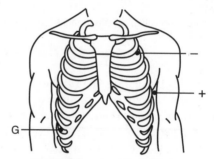

Modified Chest Lead V₆ (MCL₆)

Negative lead – 2nd interspace
left midclavicular line

Positive lead – 5th interspace
left midaxillary line

Ground lead – 8th interspace
right midclavicular line

**Figure 4-6.** Telemetry monitoring: Three-leadwire system.
The three-leadwire system uses three electrode pads and three leadwires. The leadwires are connected to positive, negative, or ground connections on the telemetry transmitter and attached to specific lead positions (lead I, lead II, lead III, lead $MCL_1$, or lead $MCL_6$). Only one lead position can be monitored at a time. A lead selector isn't available.

## Telemetry monitoring

Wireless monitoring, or telemetry, gives your patient more freedom than hardwire monitoring. Instead of being connected to a bedside monitor, the patient is connected to a portable monitor transmitter, which can be placed in a pajama pocket or in a telemetry pouch. Telemetry monitoring systems are available in a five-leadwire system and a three-leadwire system.

The *five-leadwire system* for telemetry (Figure 4-5) is connected in the same manner as the five-leadwire system for hardwire monitoring with the four limb positions (RA, LA, RL, LL) in the conventional locations and the chest leads placed in the desired $V_1$ to $V_6$ location. With this system you can monitor any of the 12 leads using a lead selector on the monitor. Leads placed in the limb positions as shown in Figure 4-5 allow you to view leads I, II, III, $AV_R$, $AV_L$, and $AV_F$. To view chest leads $V_1$ through $V_6$, the chest lead must be placed in the specific chest lead position desired.

The *three-leadwire system* for telemetry (Figure 4-6) uses three electrode pads and three lead wires. The lead wires are connected to positive, negative, and ground connections on the telemetry transmitter and attached to electrode pads placed in specific chest lead positions (leads I, II, III, $MCL_1$, and $MCL_6$). These leads record electrical forces viewed between two electrodes, one designated negative and one des-

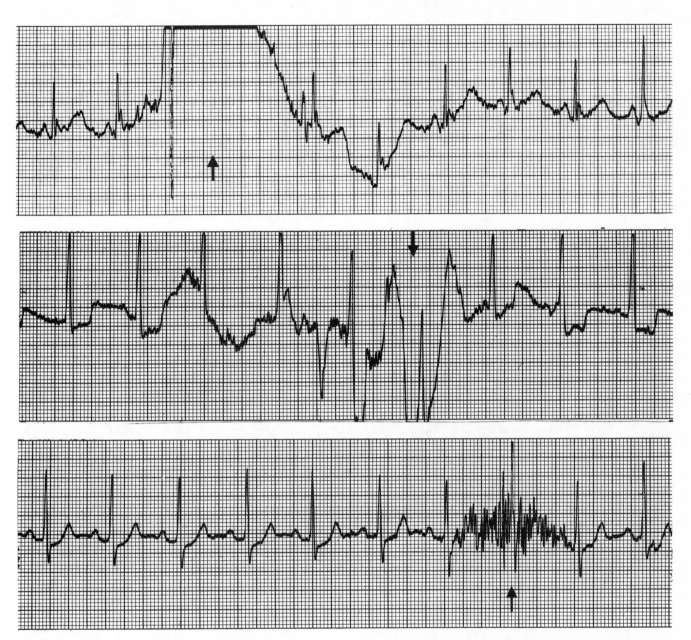

**Figure 4-7.** Patient movement. *Cause:* Strips above show patient turning in bed or extremity movement. *Solution:* Problem is usually intermittent and no correction is necessary. Movement artifact can be reduced by avoiding placement of electrode pads in areas where extremity movement is greatest (bony areas such as the clavicles).

ignated positive. Only one lead position can be monitored at a time, and a lead selector on the monitor isn't available.

## Applying the electrode pads

Proper attachment of the electrode pads to the skin is the most important step in obtaining a good quality ECG tracing. Unless there is good contact between the skin and the electrode pad, distortions of the ECG tracing (artifacts) may appear. An artifact is any abnormal wave, spike, or movement on the ECG tracing that isn't generated by the elec-

trical activity of the heart. The procedure for attaching the electrodes is as follows:

■ **Choose monitor lead position.** It's helpful to assess the 12-lead ECG to ascertain which lead provides the best QRS complex voltage and P wave identification.

■ **Prepare the skin.** Shave the sites, if necessary, using a razor; hair interferes with good contact between the electrode pad and the skin. Wipe sites with an alcohol or acetone pad to remove skin oil, and allow them to dry. Then gently abrade the skin. A dry washcloth may be used, or some companies produce electrode pads with a small amount of abrasive material attached to the pad's peel-off section; these work extremely well. If the patient is perspiring, apply a thin coat of tincture of benzoin, and allow it to dry.

■ **Attach the electrode pads.** Remove pads from packaging, and check them for moist conductive gel; dried gel can cause loss of the ECG signal. Place an electrode pad on each prepared site, pressing firmly around periphery of the pad and avoiding bony areas, such as the clavicles or prominent rib markings.

■ **Connect the leadwires.** Attach appropriate leadwires to the electrode pads according to established electrode-lead positions.

## Troubleshooting monitor problems

Many problems may be encountered during cardiac monitoring. The most common problems are related to patient movement, interference from equipment in or near the patient room, weak ECG signals, poor choice of monitor lead or electrode placement, and poor contact between the skin and electrode-lead attachments. Monitor problems can cause artifacts on the ECG tracing, making identification of the cardiac rhythm difficult or triggering false monitor alarms (high-rate alarms and low-rate alarms). Some problems are potentially serious and require intervention, whereas others are temporary, non-life-threatening occurrences that will correct themselves. The nurse and monitor technician need to be proficient in recognizing monitoring problems, identifying probable causes, and seeking solutions to correct the problems. The most common monitoring problems are discussed below.

### False high-rate alarms

High-voltage artifact potentials are commonly interpreted by the monitor as QRS complexes and activate the high-rate alarm (Figure 4-7). Most high-voltage artifacts are related to muscle movements from turning in bed or moving the extremities. Seizure activity can also produce high-voltage artifact potentials.

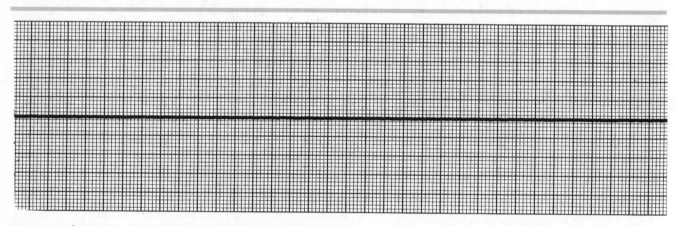

**Figure 4-8.** Continuous straight line. *Cause:* Dried conductive gel, disconnected lead wire, or disconnected electrode pad. *Solution:* Check electrode-lead system; re-prep and re-attach electrodes and leads as necessary. *Note:* A straight line may also indicate the absence of electrical activity in the heart; the patient must be evaluated immediately for the presence of a pulse.

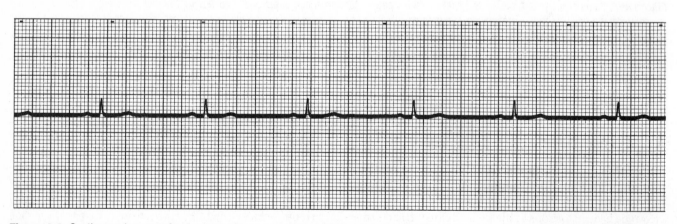

**Figure 4-9.** Continuous low waveform voltage. *Cause:* Low voltage QRS complexes. *Solution:* Turn up amplitude (gain) knob on monitor or change lead positions.

# False low-rate alarms

Any disturbance in the transmission of the electrical signal from the skin electrode to the monitoring system can activate a false low-rate alarm (Figures 4-8, 4-9, and 4-10). This problem is usually caused by ineffective contact between the skin and the electrode-leadwire system resulting from dried conductive gel, a loose electrode, or a disconnected leadwire. Low-voltage QRS complexes can also activate the low-rate alarm. If the ventricular waveforms aren't tall enough,

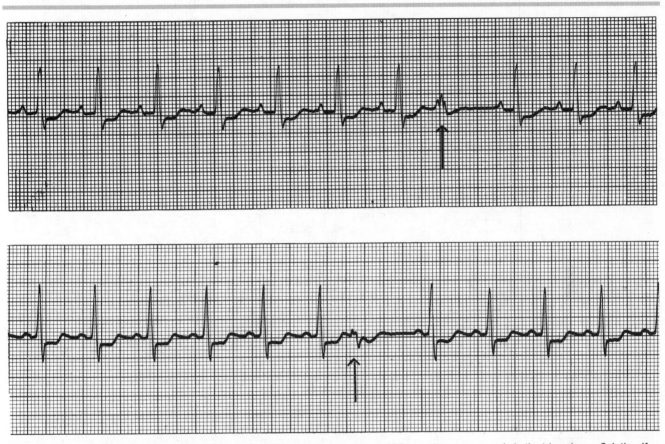

**Figure 4-10.** Intermittent low waveform voltage. *Cause:* Intermittent low voltage QRS complexes are seen in both strips above. *Solution:* If the problem is frequent and activates the low rate alarm, change lead positions.

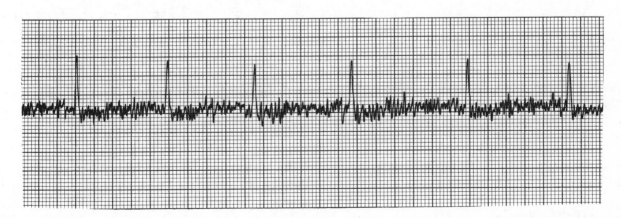

**Figure 4-11.** Continuous muscle tremor. *Cause:* Muscle tremors are usually related to tense or nervous patients or those shivering from cold or a chill. *Solution:* Treat cause.

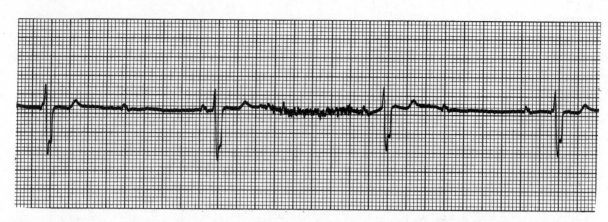

**Figure 4-12.** Intermittent muscle tremor. *Cause:* Muscle tremors that occur intermittently. *Solution:* Correction is usually unnecessary. *Note:* In this strip, the patient has two P waves preceding each QRS complex (second-degree atrioventricular block, Mobitz II). If the muscle tremors were continuous (as in Figure 4-11), you would be unable to identify this serious arrhythmia.

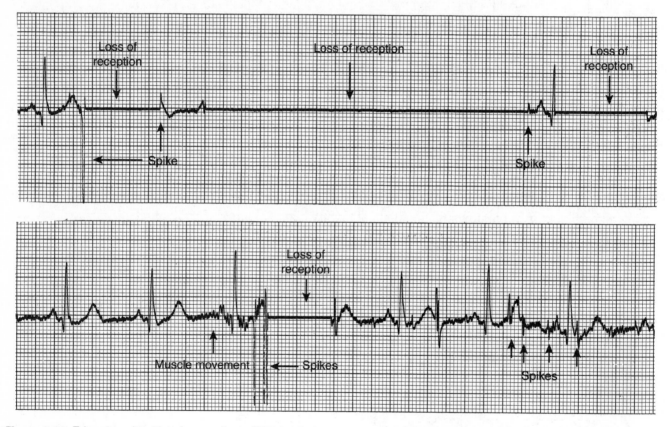

**Figure 4-13.** Telemetry-related interference. *Cause:* ECG signals are poorly received over the telemetry system causing sharp spikes and sometimes loss of signal reception. This problem is usually related to weak batteries or the transmitter being used in the outer fringes of the reception area for the base station receiver. *Solution:* Change batteries; keep patient in reception area of base station receivers.

the monitor detects no electrical activity and will sound the low-rate alarm.

## Muscle tremors

Muscle tremors (Figures 4-11 and 4-12) can occur in tense, nervous patients or those shivering from cold or having a chill. The ECG baseline has an uneven, coarsely jagged appearance, obscuring the waveforms on the ECG tracing. The problem may be continuous or intermittent.

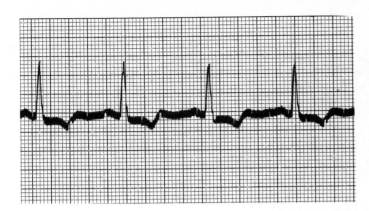

**Figure 4-14.** Electrical interference (AC interference). *Cause:* Patient using electrical equipment (electric razor, hair dryer); multiple electrical equipment in use in room; improperly grounded equipment; loose electrical connections or exposed wiring. *Solution:* If patient is using electrical equipment, problem is transient and will correct itself. If patient is not using electrical equipment, unplug all equipment not in continuous use, remove from service and report any equipment with breaks or wires showing, and ask the electrical engineer to check the wiring.

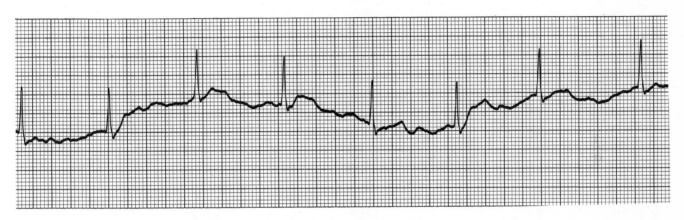

**Figure 4-15.** Wandering baseline. *Cause:* Exaggerated respiratory movements usually seen in patients in respiratory distress (patients with chronic obstructive pulmonary disease). *Solution:* Avoid placing electrode pads in areas where movements of the accessory muscles are most exaggerated (which can be anywhere on the anterior chest wall). Place the pads on the upper back or top of the shoulders if necessary.

## Telemetry-related interference

Telemetry-related artifacts occur when the ECG signals are poorly received over a telemetry monitoring system (Figure 4-13). Weak ECG signals are caused by weak batteries or by the transmitter being used in the outer fringes of the reception area of the base station receiver, resulting in sharp spikes or straight lines on the ECG tracing.

## Electrical interference (AC interference)

Electrical interference (Figure 4-14) can occur when multiple pieces of electrical equipment are in use in the patient's room; when the patient is using an electrical appliance, such as an electric razor or hair dryer; when improperly grounded equipment is in use; or when loose or exposed wiring is present. This type of interference results in an artifact with a wide baseline consisting of a continuous series of fine, even, rapid spikes, which can obscure the components of the ECG tracing.

## Wandering baseline

A wandering baseline (Figure 4-15) is a monitor pattern that wanders up and down on the monitor screen or ECG trac-

ing and is caused by exaggerated respiratory movements commonly seen in patients with respiratory distress. This type of artifact makes it difficult to identify the cardiac rhythm as well as changes in the ST segment and T wave.

# 5

# Analyzing a rhythm strip

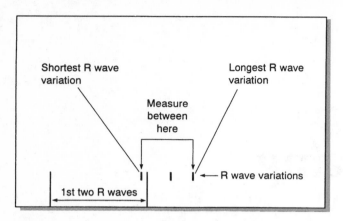

**Figure 5-1.** Index card.

There are five basic steps to be followed in analyzing a rhythm strip. Each step should be followed in sequence. Eventually, this will become a habit and will enable you to identify a strip quickly and accurately.

## Step 1: Determine the regularity (rhythm) of the R waves

Starting at the left side of the rhythm strip, place an index card above the first two R waves (Figure 5-1). Using a sharp pencil, mark on the index card above the two R waves. Measure from R wave to R wave across the rhythm strip, marking on the index card any variation in R-wave regularity. If the rhythm varies by 0.12 second (3 squares) or more between the shortest and longest R-wave variation marked on the index card, the rhythm is irregular. If the rhythm doesn't vary or varies by less than 0.12 second, the rhythm is considered regular.

Calipers may also be used, instead of an index card, to determine regularity of the rhythm strip. R-wave regularity is assessed in the same manner as with the index card, by placing the two caliper points on top of two consecutive R waves and proceeding left to right across the rhythm strip, noting any variation in the R-R regularity.

The author prefers the index card method, because each R-wave variation (however slight) can be marked and measured to determine if a 0.12 second or greater variance exists between the shorter and longer R-wave variations. With calipers, a variation in the R-wave regularity may be noted, but without marking and measuring between the shortest and longest R-wave variations, there is no way to determine how irregular the rhythm is. Examples of rhythm measurements are shown in Figures 5-2, 5-3, and 5-4.

## Step 2: Calculate the heart rate

This measurement will always refer to the ventricular rate unless the atrial and ventricular rates differ, in which case both will be given. The ventricular rate is usually determined by looking at a 6-second rhythm strip. The top of the electrocardiogram paper is marked at 3-second intervals; two intervals equal 6 seconds (Figure 5-5). Several methods can be used to calculate heart rate. These methods differ according to the regularity or irregularity of the rhythm.

### Regular rhythms
Two methods can be used to calculate heart rate in regular rhythms:
- Rapid rate calculation – Count the number of R waves in a 6-second strip and multiply by 10 (6 seconds × 10 = 60 seconds, or the heart rate per minute). This method provides an approximate heart rate in beats per minute, is fast and simple, and can be used with both regular and irregular rhythms.
- Precise rate calculation – Count the number of small squares between two consecutive R waves (Figure 5-6) and refer to the conversion table printed on page 370 of the book. Although this method is accurate, it can be used only for regular rhythms. If a conversion table isn't available, divide the number of small squares between the two consecutive R waves into 1,500 (the number of small squares in a 1-minute rhythm strip). The heart rates for regular rhythms in the answer keys were determined by the precise rate calculation method.

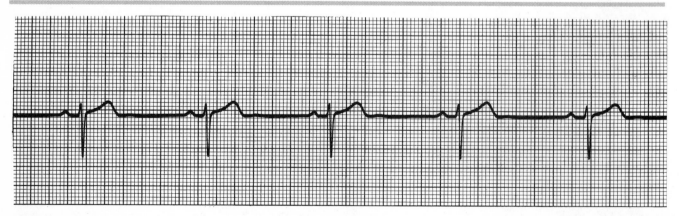

**Figure 5-2.** Regular rhythm; R-R intervals do not vary.

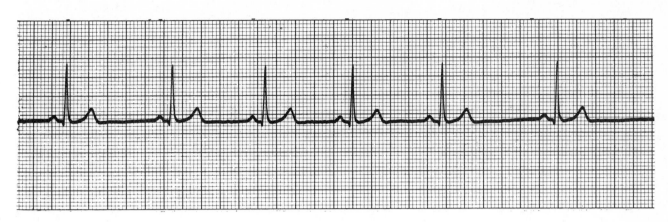

**Figure 5-3.** Irregular rhythm; R-R intervals vary by 0.32 second.

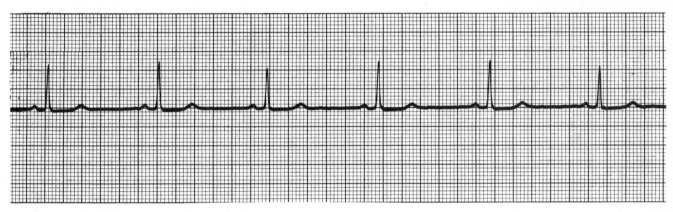

**Figure 5-4.** Regular rhythm; R-R intervals vary by 0.04 second.

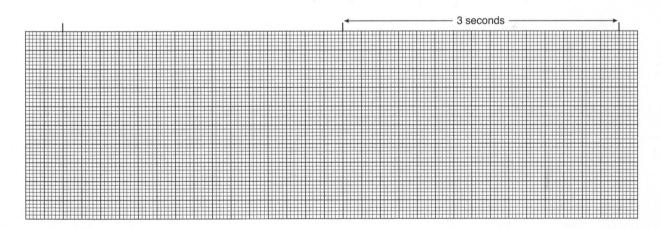

**Figure 5-5.** ECG graph paper.

## Irregular rhythms

Only **rapid rate calculation** is used to calculate heart rate in irregular rhythms. Count the number of R waves in a 6-second strip and multiple by 10 (Figure 5-7), or count the number of R waves in a 3-second strip and multiply by 20 (3 seconds × 20 = 60 seconds, or the heart rate per minute).

## Other hints

When interpreting the rhythm strip, describe the basic underlying rhythm first, then add additional information, such as normal sinus rhythm (the underlying rhythm) with frequent premature ventricular complexes.

When rhythm strips have premature beats (Figure 5-8), the premature beats aren't included in the calculation of the

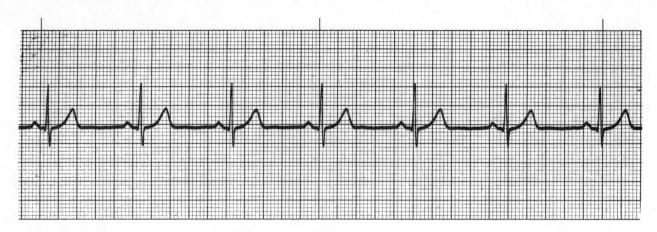

**Figure 5-6.** Regular rhythm; 25 small squares between R waves = 60 heart rate.

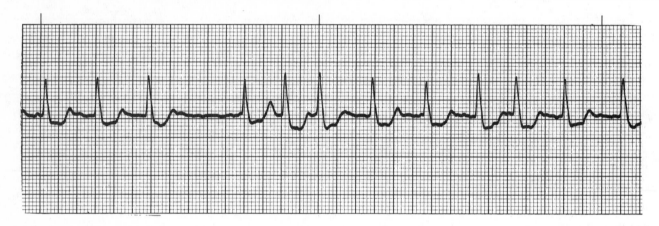

**Figure 5-7.** Irregular rhythm; 11 R waves × 10 = 110 heart rate.

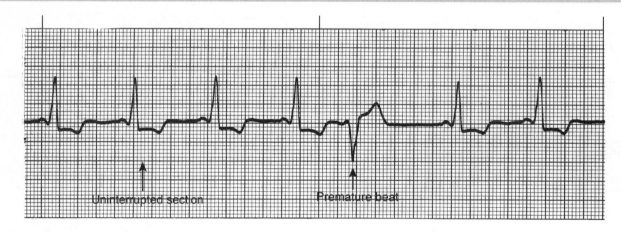

**Figure 5-8.** Rhythm with premature beat.

rate. Count the rate in the uninterrupted section; this is the underlying rhythm. In this example, the uninterrupted section is regular and the heart rate is 68 beats/minute (22 squares between R waves = 68).

When rhythm strips have more than one rhythm on a 6-second strip (Figure 5-9), rates must be calculated for each rhythm. This will aid in the identification of each rhythm.

In the example, the first rhythm is irregular and the heart rate is 140 beats/minute (7 R waves in 3 seconds × 20 = 140). The second rhythm is regular and the heart rate is 250 beats/minute (6 squares between R waves = 250).

When a rhythm covers less than 3 seconds on a rhythm strip (Figure 5-10), rate calculation is difficult but not impossible. In the example, the first rhythm takes up half of a

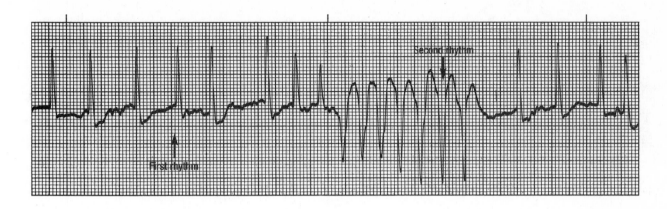

**Figure 5-9.** Rhythm strip with two different rhythms.

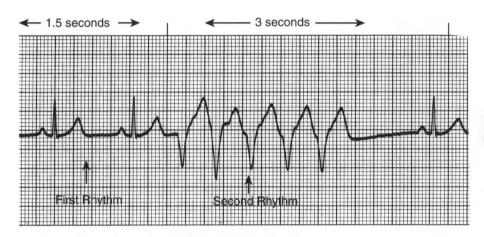

**Figure 5-10.** Calculating rate when a rhythm covers less than 3 seconds.

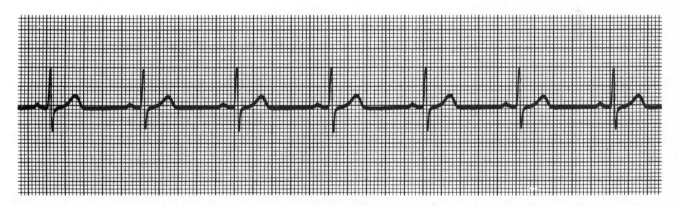

**Figure 5-11.** Normal P waves.

3-second interval. There are only two R waves; therefore, you can't determine if the rhythm is regular or irregular. In this situation, multiply the two R waves by 40 (1½ seconds × 40 = 60 seconds, or the heart rate per minute) to obtain an approximate heart rate of 80 beats/minute. The second rhythm is regular, with a heart rate of 167 beats/minute (9 small squares between R waves = 167).

## Step 3: Identify and examine P waves

Analyze the P waves—one P wave should precede each QRS complex. All P waves should be identical (or near identical) in size, shape, and position. In Figure 5-11 there is one P wave to each QRS complex, and all P waves are identical in size, shape, and position. In Figure 5-12 there is one P wave

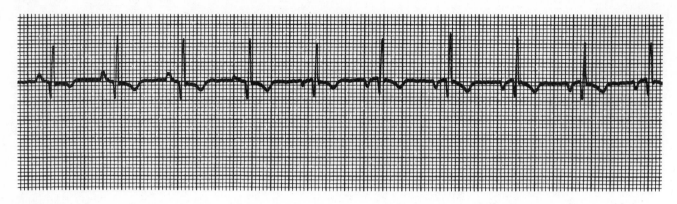

**Figure 5-12.** Abnormal P waves.

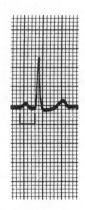

**Figure 5-13.** PR interval 0.16 second.

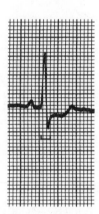

**Figure 5-15.** QRS complex 0.10 second.

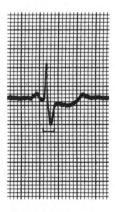

**Figure 5-14.** QRS complex 0.12 second.

**Box 5-1.**
### Rhythm strip analysis

1. Determine regularity (rhythm).
2. Calculate rate.
3. Examine P waves.
4. Measure PR interval.
5. Measure QRS complex.

to each QRS complex, but the P waves vary in size, shape, and position.

## Step 4: Measure the PR interval

Measure from the beginning of the P wave as it leaves baseline to the beginning of the QRS complex. Count the number of squares contained in this interval and multiply by 0.04 second. In Figure 5-13 the PR interval is 0.16 second (4 squares × 0.04 second = 0.16 second).

## Step 5: Measure the QRS complex

Measure from the beginning of the QRS complex as it leaves baseline until the end of the QRS complex when the ST segment begins. Count the number of squares in this measurement and multiply by 0.04 second. In Figure 5-14 the QRS complex takes up 3 squares and represents 0.12 second (3 squares × 0.04 second = 0.12 second). In Figure 5-15 the QRS complex takes up 2½ squares and represents 0.10 second (2½ square × 0.04 second = 0.10 second).

If rhythm strips are analyzed using a systematic step-by-step approach (Box 5-1), accurate interpretation will be achieved most of the time.

# Rhythm strip practice: Analyzing rhythm strips

Analyze the following rhythm strips using the five-step process discussed in this chapter. Check your answers with the answer key in the appendix.

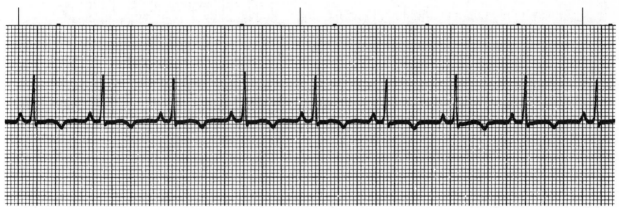

**Strip 5-1.** Rhythm: _____ Rate: _____ P wave: _____
PR interval: _____ QRS complex: _____

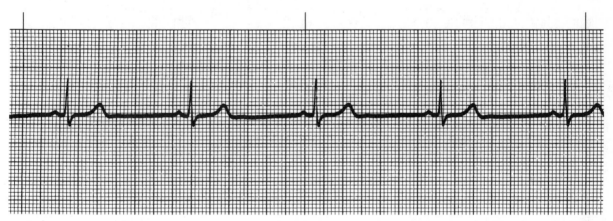

**Strip 5-2.** Rhythm: _____ Rate: _____ P wave: _____
PR interval: _____ QRS complex: _____

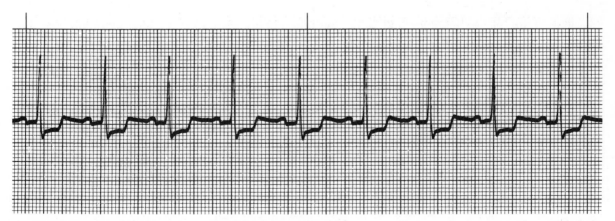

**Strip 5-3.** Rhythm: _____ Rate: _____ P wave: _____
PR interval: _____ QRS complex: _____

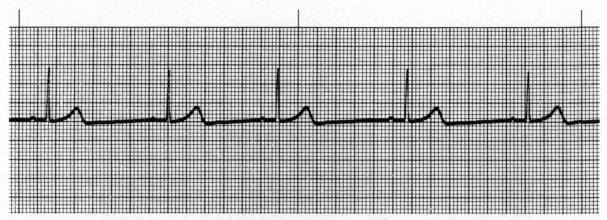

**Strip 5-4.** Rhythm: _____ Rate: _____ P wave: _____

PR interval: _____ QRS complex: _____

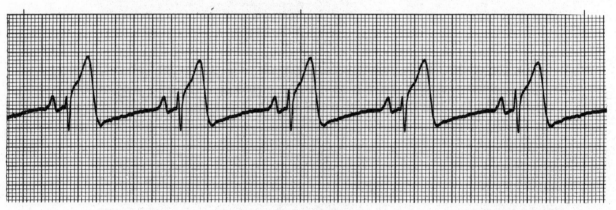

**Strip 5-5.** Rhythm: _____ Rate: _____ P wave: _____

PR interval: _____ QRS complex: _____

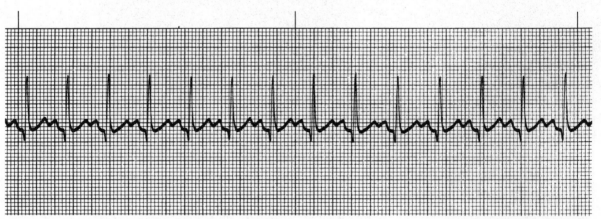

**Strip 5-6.** Rhythm: _____ Rate: _____ P wave: _____

PR interval: _____ QRS complex: _____

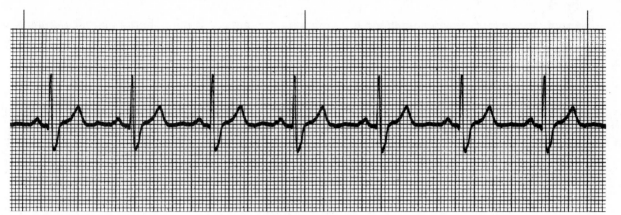

**Strip 5-7.** Rhythm: _____ Rate: _____ P wave: _____

           PR interval: _____ QRS complex: _____

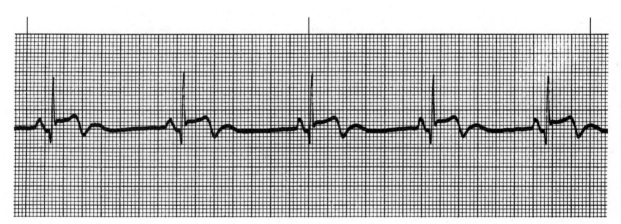

**Strip 5-8.** Rhythm: _____ Rate: _____ P wave: _____

           PR interval: _____ QRS complex: _____

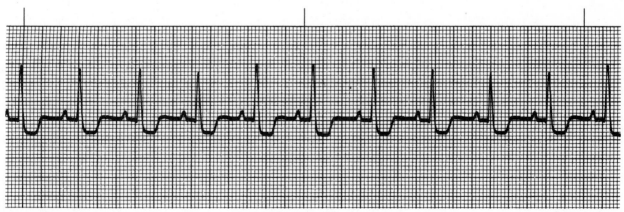

**Strip 5-9.** Rhythm: _____ Rate: _____ P wave: _____

           PR interval: _____ QRS complex: _____

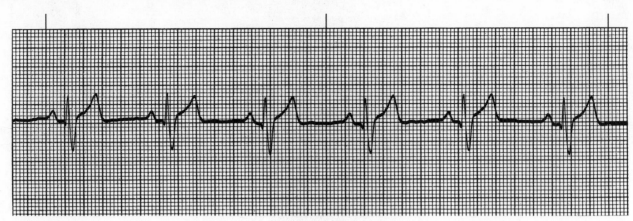

**Strip 5-10.** Rhythm: _____ Rate: _____ P wave: _____

PR interval: _____ QRS complex: _____

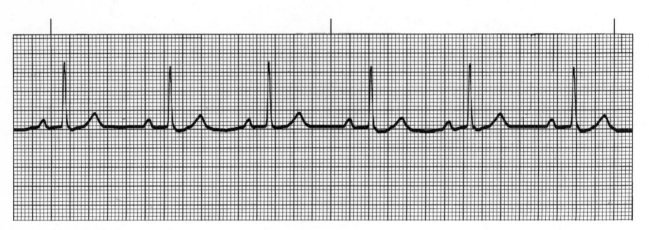

**Strip 5-11.** Rhythm: _____ Rate: _____ P wave: _____

PR interval: _____ QRS complex: _____

# 6 Sinus arrhythmias

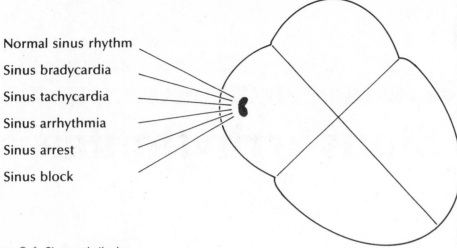

Normal sinus rhythm

Sinus bradycardia

Sinus tachycardia

Sinus arrhythmia

Sinus arrest

Sinus block

**Figure 6-1.** Sinus arrhythmias

## Overview

The term *arrhythmia* (also called *dysrhythmia*) is very general, referring to all rhythms other than the normal rhythm of the heart (normal sinus rhythm). Sinus arrhythmias (Figure 6-1) result from disturbances in impulse discharge or impulse conduction from the sinus node. The sinus node retains its role as pacemaker of the heart but discharges impulses too fast (sinus tachycardia) or too slow (sinus bradycardia); discharges impulses irregularly (sinus arrhythmia); or fails to initiate an impulse (sinus arrest); or the impulses initiated are blocked as they exit the sinoatrial (SA) node (sinus exit block). Sinus bradycardia, sinus tachycardia, sinus arrhythmia, sinus arrest, and sinus block are all considered arrhythmias. However, sinus bradycardia at rest, sinus tachycardia with exercise, and respiratory sinus arrhythmia are all normal findings.

The regulation of the heart rate is controlled by the autonomic nervous system. The autonomic nerve supply to the heart consists of two opposing groups of fibers: the *sympathetic nerves* and the *parasympathetic nerves*. Sympathetic stimulation produces an increase in heart rate, an increase in conduction through the atrioventricular (AV) node, and an increase in the strength of myocardial contraction. Parasympathetic stimulation (from the vagus nerve) produces a slowing of the heart rate, a decrease in conduction through the AV node, and a slight decrease in the strength of myocardial contraction. Thus, the sympathetic nervous system acts as a cardiac accelerator, and the parasympathetic system acts as a cardiac inhibitor. Normally, these systems

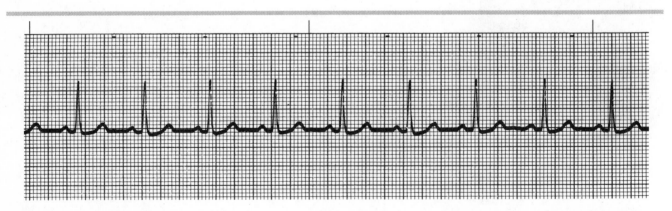

| **Figure 6-2.** | **Normal sinus rhythm** |
|---|---|
| Rhythm: | Regular |
| Rate: | 84 beats/minute |
| P waves: | Normal and precede each QRS |
| PR interval: | 0.14 to 0.16 second |
| QRS complex: | 0.06 to 0.08 second |

are balanced, maintaining a heart rate between 60 and 100 beats/minute.

# Normal sinus rhythm

Normal sinus rhythm (Figure 6-2 and Box 6-1) reflects the heart's normal electrical activity. Normally, the impulse originates in the SA node, travels through the atria, and reaches the AV node where there is a brief pause. Leaving the AV node, the electrical impulse travels down the right and left bundle branches through the Purkinje fibers to the ventricular myocardium. In normal sinus rhythm the atria contract first, then the ventricles, a sequence that produces efficient heartbeats. Normal sinus rhythm is regular with a heart rate between 60 and 100 beats/minute. The P waves are normal in size, shape, and direction; positive in lead II, with one P wave preceding each QRS complex. The duration of the PR interval and the QRS complex is each within normal limits. Normal sinus rhythm is the normal rhythm of the heart. No treatment is indicated.

**Box 6-1.**
## Normal sinus rhythm: Identifying ECG features

| | |
|---|---|
| **Rhythm**: | Regular |
| **Rate**: | 60 to 100 beats/minute |
| **P waves**: | Normal in size, shape, and direction; positive in lead II; one P wave precedes each QRS complex |
| **PR interval**: | Normal (0.12 to 0.20 second) |
| **QRS complex**: | Normal (0.10 second or less) |

# Sinus tachycardia

Sinus tachycardia (Figure 6-3 and Box 6-2) is a rhythm that originates in the SA node and discharges impulses regularly at a rate between 100 and 180 beats/minute. The P waves are normal in size, shape, and direction; and positive in lead II, with one P wave preceding each QRS complex. The duration of the PR interval and the QRS complex is each within normal limits. The distinguishing feature of this rhythm is the sinus origin and the rate between 100 and 180 beats/minute.

**Box 6-2.**
## Sinus tachycardia: Identifying ECG features

| | |
|---|---|
| **Rhythm**: | Regular |
| **Rate**: | 100 to 180 beats/minute |
| **P waves**: | Normal in size, shape, and direction; positive in lead II; one P wave precedes each QRS complex |
| **PR interval**: | Normal (0.12 to 0.20 second) |
| **QRS complex**: | Normal (0.10 second or less) |

Sinus tachycardia is the normal response of the heart to the body's demand for an increase in blood flow (such as exercise and excitement). The sinus node gradually increases its rate in response to the needs of the body. When these needs no longer exist, the heart rate gradually slows down. Sinus tachycardia begins and ends gradually in contrast to other tachycardias, which begin and end suddenly.

Sinus tachycardia can be caused by anything that stimulates the sympathetic nervous system or anything that inhibits the parasympathetic nervous system. Factors commonly associated with sinus tachycardia are:
- excitement, exertion, exercise
- fever, infections, septic shock

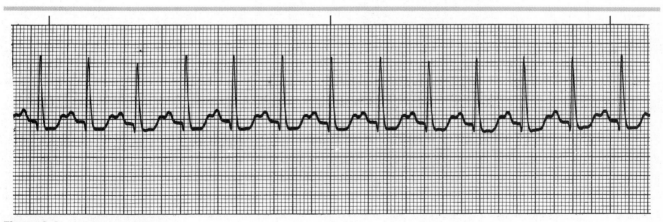

**Figure 6-3.  Sinus tachycardia**

| | |
|---|---|
| **Rhythm**: | Regular |
| **Rate**: | 115 beats/minute |
| **P waves**: | Sinus |
| **PR interval**: | 0.16 to 0.18 second |
| **QRS complex**: | 0.08 to 0.10 second |

- hypoxia, hypovolemia, hypotension, heart failure, hyperthyroidism
- pain, pulmonary embolism (Sinus tachycardia is the most common arrhythmia seen with pulmonary embolism.)
- anxiety, anemia
- myocardial ischemia, myocardial infarction (Sinus tachycardia persisting after an acute infarct implies extensive heart damage and is generally a bad prognostic sign.)
- drugs that increase sympathetic tone (such as epinephrine, norepinephrine, dopamine, dobutamine, tricyclic antidepressants, isuprel, cocaine, and nitroprusside)
- drugs that decrease parasympathetic tone (such as atropine)
- smoking, consumption of alcohol, and ingestion of beverages containing caffeine.

Sinus tachycardia in healthy individuals is usually a benign arrhythmia and doesn't require aggressive treatment. When its cause (such as fever or anxiety) is removed or treated, sinus tachycardia resolves gradually on its own. However, sinus tachycardia is a warning sign and should never be ignored, especially in a cardiac patient. Sinus tachycardia may be one of the first signs of left-sided heart failure. A rapid heart rate increases the workload of the heart and its oxygen requirements. Persistent tachycardia can cause decreased stroke volume, decreased cardiac output, and decreased coronary perfusion secondary to a decrease in the diastolic filling time that occurs with rapid heart rates. Treatment of sinus tachycardia should be directed, not at the rapid heart rate itself, but to correcting the underlying cause of the arrhythmia.

## Sinus bradycardia

Sinus bradycardia (Figure 6-4 and Box 6-3) is a rhythm that originates in the SA node and discharges impulses regularly at a rate between 40 and 60 beats/minute. The P waves are normal in size, shape, and direction; positive in lead II, with one P wave preceding each QRS complex. The duration of the PR interval and the QRS complex is each within normal limits. The distinguishing feature of this rhythm is the sinus origin and a heart rate between 40 and 60 beats/minute.

### Box 6-3.
### Sinus bradycardia: Identifying ECG features

| | |
|---|---|
| Rhythm: | Regular |
| Rate: | 40 to 60 beats/minute |
| P waves: | Normal in size, shape, and direction; positive in lead II; one P wave precedes each QRS complex |
| PR interval: | Normal (0.12 to 0.20 second) |
| QRS complex: | Normal (0.10 second or less) |

Sinus bradycardia is the normal response of the heart to relaxation or sleeping when the parasympathetic effect on cardiac automaticity dominates over the sympathetic effect. It's common among trained athletes who may have a resting or sleeping pulse rate as low as 35 beats/minute. Mild sinus bradycardia may actually be beneficial in some patients (for example, in those with an acute MI) because of the decrease in workload on the heart.

Sinus bradycardia can be caused by anything that increases parasympathetic tone or decreases sympathetic tone. It commonly occurs with the following:

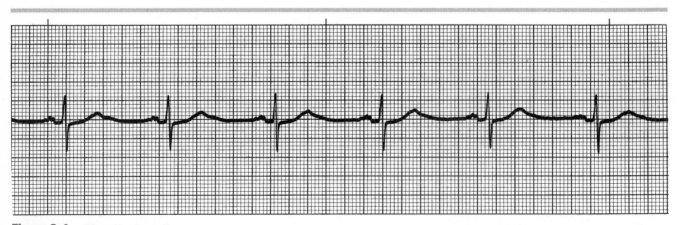

| Figure 6-4. | Sinus bradycardia |
|---|---|
| Rhythm: | Regular |
| Rate: | 54 beats/minute |
| P waves: | Sinus |
| PR interval: | 0.20 second |
| QRS complex: | 0.06 to 0.08 second |
| Note: | A notched P wave is usually indicative of left atrial hypertrophy. |

■ as a normal variant (Many people have a resting heart rate that is less than 60 beats/minute.)

■ in acute inferior wall myocardial infarction involving the right coronary artery, which usually supplies blood to the SA node

■ as a "reperfusion rhythm" after coronary angioplasty or after treatment with thrombolytics

■ vagal stimulation from vomiting, " bearing down" (Valsalva's maneuver), or carotid sinus massage

■ vasovagal reactions (These reactions—a sudden increase in vagal tone accompanied by vascular dilation—are seen with pain, nausea, vomiting, fright, or sudden stressful situations. They may result in marked bradycardia [a heart rate less than 30 beats/minute] and hypotension. The combination of these two components results in a decrease in cardiac output so severe that it may cause fainting [vasovagal syncope]. The situation is usually reversed when the individual is placed into a recumbent position, thereby increasing venous return to the heart. If fainting occurs with the individual in the recumbent position, it can usually be reversed with leg elevation.)

■ carotid sinus hypersensitivity syndrome, sleep apnea syndrome

■ decreased metabolic rate (hypothyroidism, hypothermia, sleep); hyperkalemia

■ sudden movement from recumbent to an upright position (common in the elderly)

■ increased intracranial pressure (Sudden appearance of sinus bradycardia in a patient with cerebral edema or subdural hematoma is an important clinical observation.)

■ drugs such as digitalis, calcium channel blockers, and beta blockers

■ degenerative disease of the sinus node (sick sinus syndrome). Persistent sinus bradycardia is the most common and often the earliest manifestation of sick sinus syndrome.

Sick sinus syndrome is a dysfunctioning sinus node, which is manifested on the ECG by marked bradyarrhythmias alternating with episodes of tachyarrhythmias and is commonly accompanied by symptoms of hemodynamic compromise (such as dizziness, syncope, chest pain, and heart failure). This syndrome has also been called *tachy-brady syndrome*. Permanent pacemaker implantation is recommended once patients become symptomatic.

Sinus bradycardia doesn't require treatment unless the patient becomes symptomatic. If the arrhythmia is accompanied by hypotension, diaphoresis, chest pain, dyspnea, decreased level of consciousness, a decrease in urine output, or other signs or symptoms of hemodynamic compromise, treatment is necessary. A simple maneuver such as asking the patient to cough, which decreases vagal tone, might be tried initially in an attempt to increase the heart rate. If sinus bradycardia persists, the treatment of choice is atropine, a parasympatholytic drug that inhibits parasympathetic tone, increasing the heart rate. The usual dose is 0.5 mg I.V. push every 5 minutes until the bradycardia is resolved or a maximum dose of 3 mg is given. Atropine must be administered correctly—atropine administered too slowly or in doses less than 0.5 mg exert a sympatholytic effect (inhibits sympathetic tone) and can further decrease the heart rate. If the arrhythmia still doesn't resolve after the atropine is administered, a transcutaneous (external) or transvenous pacemaker may be needed. All medications that cause a decrease in heart rate should be reviewed and discontinued if indicated. For chronic bradycardia, permanent pacing may be indicated.

## Sinus arrhythmia

Sinus arrhythmia (Figure 6-5 and Box 6-4) is a rhythm that originates in the sinus node and discharges impulses irreg-

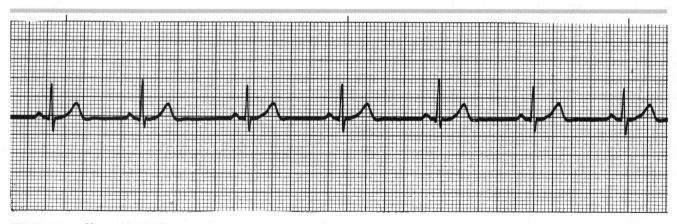

**Figure 6-5.    Sinus arrhythmia**
**Rhythm:**         Irregular
**Rate:**           60 beats/minute
**P waves:**        Normal in configuration; precede each QRS
**PR interval:**    0.12 to 0.14 second
**QRS complex:** 0.06 to 0.08 second

ularly. The heart rate may be normal (60 to 100 beats/minute), but is commonly associated with sinus bradycardia. The P waves are normal in size, shape, and direction; and positive in lead II, with one P wave preceding each QRS complex. The duration of the PR interval and the QRS complex is each within normal limits. The distinguishing feature of this rhythm is the sinus origin and the rhythm irregularity.

## Box 6-4.
### Sinus arrhythmia: Identifying ECG features

| | |
|---|---|
| **Rhythm:** | Irregular |
| **Rate:** | Normal (60 to 100 beats/minute) or slow (less than 60 beats/minute) |
| **P waves:** | Normal in size, shape, and direction; positive in lead II; one P wave precedes each QRS complex |
| **PR interval:** | Normal (0.12 to 0.20 second) |
| **QRS complex:** | Normal (0.10 second or less) |

Sinus arrhythmia is a normal phenomenon thought to be caused by variations in autonomic tone and is commonly associated with the phases of respiration. Heart rate tends to increase gradually with inspiration and decrease gradually with expiration. Sinus arrhythmia is an extremely common finding among children and young adults. Although sinus arrhythmia may also occur in the elderly, it's usually unrelated to the phases of respiration in this age-group and sometimes the precursor of sick sinus syndrome. Sinus arrhythmia doesn't usually require treatment unless it's accompanied by a bradycardia that causes hemodynamic compromise.

## Sinus pause (sinus arrest and sinus exit block)

*Sinus pause* is a broad term used to describe rhythms in which there is a sudden failure of the SA node to initiate or conduct an impulse. Two rhythms fall under this category: *sinus arrest* and *sinus exit block*. Sinus arrest and sinus exit block, two separate arrhythmias with different pathophysiologies (Figures 6-6, 6-7, and 6-8 and Box 6-5), are discussed together here because distinguishing between them is at times difficult, and because their treatment and clinical significance are the same.

Both sinus arrest and sinus exit block originate in the sinus node and are characterized by a sudden pause in the sinus rhythm in which one or more beats (cardiac cycles) is missing. The P waves in the underlying rhythm will be normal in size, shape, and direction and positive in lead II, with one P wave preceding each QRS complex. The duration of the PR interval and the QRS complex in the underlying rhythm is each within normal limits. The distinguishing feature of both rhythms is the abrupt pause in the underlying sinus rhythm in which one or more PQRST sequences are missing, followed by a resumption of the basic rhythm after the pause.

## Box 6-5.
### Sinus arrest and sinus exit block: Identifying ECG features

| | |
|---|---|
| **Rhythm:** | Basic rhythm usually regular; there is a sudden pause in the basic rhythm (causing irregularity) with one or more missing beats; heart rate may slow down for several beats after pause (temporary rate suppression) but returns to basic rate |
| **Rate:** | Basic rhythm normal (60 to 100 beats/minute) or slow (less than 60 beats/minute) |
| **P waves:** | Sinus P waves with basic rhythm; absent during pause |
| **PR interval:** | Normal (0.12 to 0.20 second) with basic rhythm; absent during pause |
| **QRS complex:** | Normal (0.10 second or less) with basic rhythm; absent during pause |

#### *Differentiating features*
| | |
|---|---|
| **Sinus block:** | Basic rhythm (R-R regularity) resumes on time after pause |
| **Sinus arrest:** | Basic rhythm (R-R regularity) doesn't resume on time after pause |

Sinus arrest is caused by a failure of the SA node to initiate an impulse and is therefore a disorder of automaticity. This failure in the automaticity of the SA node upsets the timing of the sinus node discharge, and the underlying rhythm won't resume on time after the pause.

With sinus exit block, an electrical impulse is initiated by the SA node, but is blocked as it exits the sinus node, preventing conduction of the impulse to the atria. Thus, SA exit block is a disorder of conductivity. Because the regularity of the sinus node discharge isn't interrupted (just blocked), the underlying rhythm will resume on time after the pause. Once the rhythm resumes after the pause (in both sinus arrest and sinus exit block) it's common for the rate to be slower for several cycles (temporary rate suppression). This will cause a brief irregularity in rhythm, but after several cycles the basic rate and rhythm will return. An example of rate suppression is shown in Figure 6-8.

Differentiating between the two rhythms involves comparing the length of the pause with the underlying P-P or R-R interval to determine if the underlying rhythm resumes on time after the pause. This is useful only if the underlying rhythm is regular. If the underlying rhythm is irregular, as in sinus arrhythmia (Figure 6-9), it's impossible to distinguish sinus arrest from sinus exit block on the surface electrocardiogram. In this case the rhythm would best be interpreted using the broad term *sinus pause,* indicating

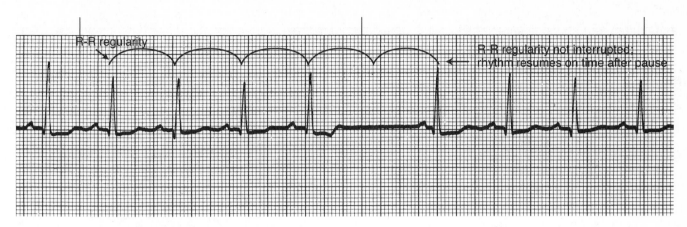

**Figure 6-6.    Normal sinus rhythm with sinus block**

| | |
|---|---|
| **Rhythm:** | Basic rhythm regular; irregular during pause |
| **Rate:** | Basic rhythm 84 beats/minute |
| **P waves:** | Normal in basic rhythm; absent during pause |
| **PR interval:** | 0.16 to 0.18 second in basic rhythm; absent during pause |
| **QRS complex:** | 0.08 to 0.10 second in basic rhythm; absent during pause |
| **Comment:** | ST segment depression is present. |

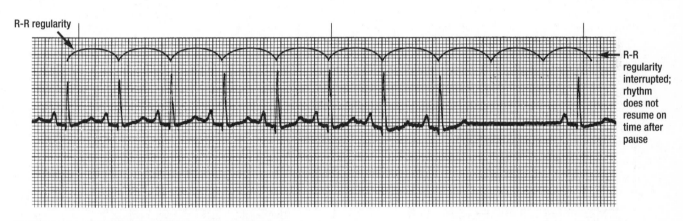

**Figure 6-7.    Normal sinus rhythm with sinus arrest**

| | |
|---|---|
| **Rhythm:** | Basic rhythm regular, irregular during pause |
| **Rate:** | Basic rhythm 94 beats/minute |
| **P waves:** | Normal in basic rhythm; absent during pause |
| **PR interval:** | 0.16 to 0.18 second in basic rhythm; absent during pause |
| **QRS complex:** | 0.06 to 0.08 second in basic rhythm; absent during pause |

that either rhythm could be present. From a clinical viewpoint, distinguishing between sinus arrest and sinus block usually isn't essential.

Sinus arrest or sinus exit block can be caused by numerous factors, including:

- increase in vagal (parasympathetic) tone on the SA node
- myocardial ischemia or infarction
- use of certain drugs (such as digitalis, beta blockers, or calcium channel blockers).

The pauses associated with sinus arrest or sinus block may be short and produce no symptoms or long and produce symptoms of hypotension, dizziness, or syncope. An-

other danger to long pauses is that the SA node may lose pacemaker control. When the sinus node slows down below its minimum firing rate of 60 beats/minute because of bradycardia or a pause in the underlying rhythm, an opportunity is provided for pacemaker cells in other areas of the conduction system to usurp control from the sinus node and become the dominant pacemaker of the heart. The term *ectopic* is commonly applied to rhythms that originate from any site other than the SA node. Ectopic sites in the atria, AV node, or ventricles may assume pacemaker control for one beat, several beats, or continuously. As in sinus bradycardia, asking the patient to cough might cause a decrease

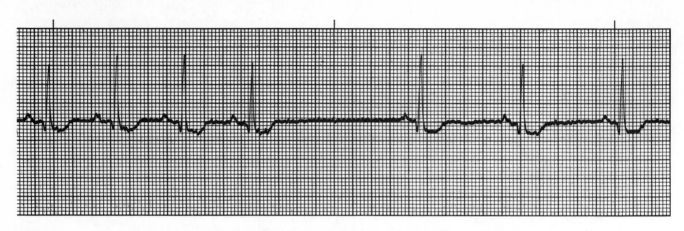

**Figure 6-8.    Normal sinus rhythm with sinus arrest; rate suppression is present following pause**
**Rhythm:**      Basic rhythm regular; irregular during pause
**Rate:**        Basic rhythm rate 84 beats/minute; rate slows to 56 beats/minute following pause (temporary rate suppression may occur
                 following a pause in the basic rhythm)
**P waves:**     Sinus in basic rhythm; absent during pause
**PR interval:** 0.16 to 0.18 second in basic rhythm; absent during pause
**QRS complex:** 0.08 to 0.10 second in basic rhythm; absent during pause

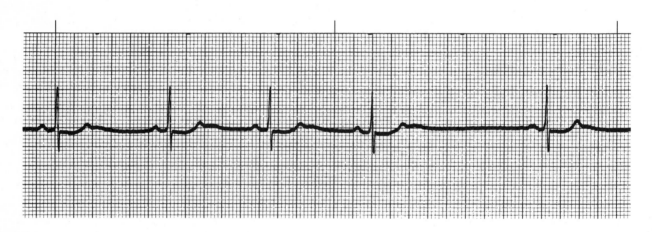

**Figure 6-9.    Sinus arrhythmia with sinus pause**
**Rhythm:**      Basic rhythm irregular
**Rate:**        Basic rhythm 60 beats/minute
**P waves:**     Normal in basic rhythm; absent during pause
**PR interval:** 0.16 to 0.18 second in basic rhythm; absent during pause
**QRS complex:** 0.06 second in basic rhythm; absent during pause
**Comment:**     Because of the irregularity of the basic rhythm, sinus arrest can't be differentiated from sinus block, and the rhythm is
                 interpreted using the broad term sinus pause, indicating that either rhythm could be present.
**Comment:**     ST segment depression and a U wave are present

in vagal tone and result in sinus node recovery. If sinus arrest or sinus exit block produces symptoms, the arrhythmias are treated the same as in symptomatic sinus bradycardia. In addition, all medications that depress sinus node discharge or conduction should be stopped.

A summary of the identifying ECG features of sinus arrhythmias can be found in Table 6-1.

Table 6-1.

## Sinus arrhythmias: Summary of identifying ECG features

| | Rhythm | Rate (beats/minute) | P waves (lead II) | PR interval | QRS complex |
|---|---|---|---|---|---|
| **Normal sinus rhythm** | Regular | 60 to 100 | Positive in lead II; normal in size, shape, and direction; one P wave precedes each QRS complex | Normal (0.12 to 0.20 second) | Normal (0.10 second or less) |
| **Sinus bradycardia** | Regular | 40 to 60 | Positive in lead II; normal in size, shape, and direction; one P wave precedes each QRS complex | Normal (0.12 to 0.20 second) | Normal (0.10 second or less) |
| **Sinus tachycardia** | Regular | 100 to 180 | Positive in lead II; normal in size, shape, and direction; one P wave precedes each QRS complex | Normal (0.12 to 0.20 second) | Normal (0.10 second or less) |
| **Sinus arrhythmia** | Irregular | 60 to 100 (normal) or < 60 (slow) | Positive in lead II; normal in size, shape, and direction; one P wave precedes each QRS complex | Normal (0.12 to 0.20 second) | Normal (0.10 second or less) |
| **Sinus block and sinus arrest** | Basic rhythm usually regular; there is a sudden pause in the basic rhythm (causing irregularity) with one or more missing beats; temporary rate suppression common following pause | 60 to 100 (normal) or < 60 (slow) | Sinus P waves with basic rhythm; absent during pause | Normal (0.12 to 0.20 second) with basic rhythm; absent during pause | Normal (0.10 second or less) with basic rhythm; absent during pause |

| *Differentiating features* | |
|---|---|
| Sinus block: | Basic rhythm resumes on time after pause |
| Sinus arrest: | Basic rhythm does not resume on time after pause |

*Note:* If the basic rhythm is irregular (sinus arrhythmia), sinus arrest can't be differentiated from sinus block, and the rhythm is interpreted as sinus arrhythmia with sinus pause.

# Rhythm strip practice: Sinus arrhythmias

For each of the following rhythm strips:
- determine the rhythm regularity, ventricular rate and, if it differs from the ventricular rate, the atrial rate
- identify and examine P waves
- measure the duration of the PR interval and QRS complex
- interpret the rhythm.

All rhythm strips are lead II unless otherwise noted. Check your answers with the answer key in the appendix.

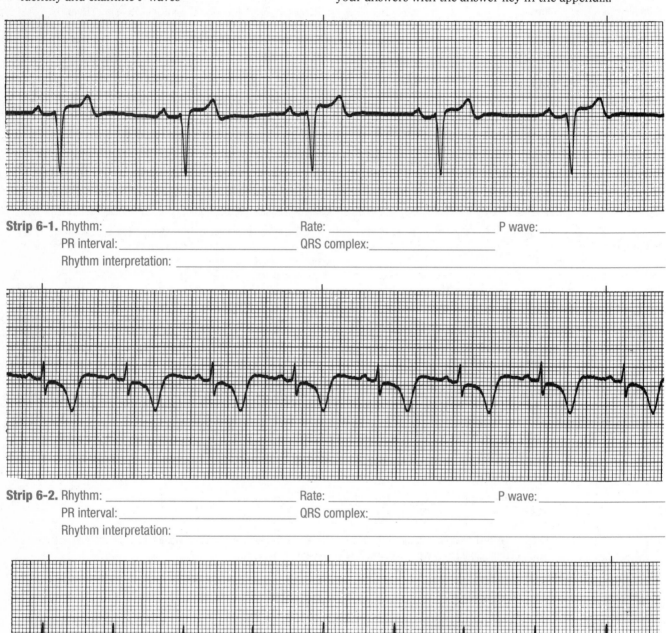

**Strip 6-1.** Rhythm: _____ Rate: _____ P wave: _____

PR interval: _____ QRS complex: _____

Rhythm interpretation: _____

**Strip 6-2.** Rhythm: _____ Rate: _____ P wave: _____

PR interval: _____ QRS complex: _____

Rhythm interpretation: _____

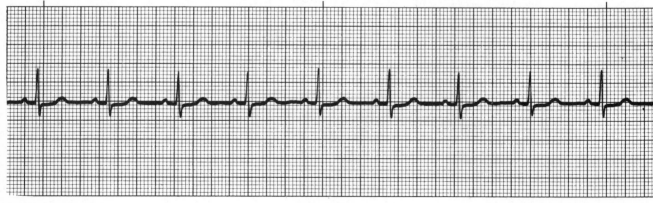

**Strip 6-3.** Rhythm: _____ Rate: _____ P wave: _____

PR interval: _____ QRS complex: _____

Rhythm interpretation: _____

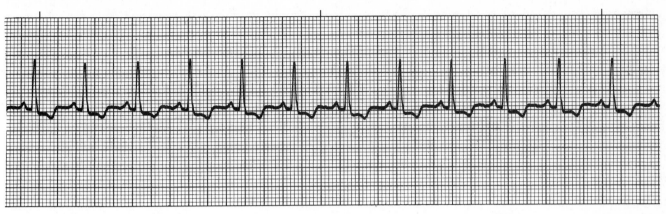

**Strip 6-4.** Rhythm: _____ Rate: _____ P wave: _____
PR interval: _____ QRS complex: _____
Rhythm interpretation: _____

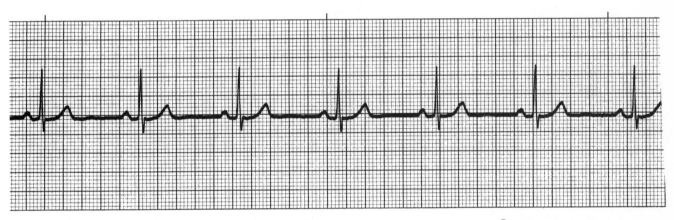

**Strip 6-5.** Rhythm: _____ Rate: _____ P wave: _____
PR interval: _____ QRS complex: _____
Rhythm interpretation: _____

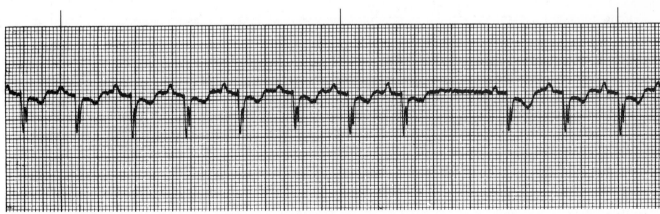

**Strip 6-6.** Rhythm: _____ Rate: _____ P wave: _____
PR interval: _____ QRS complex: _____
Rhythm interpretation: _____

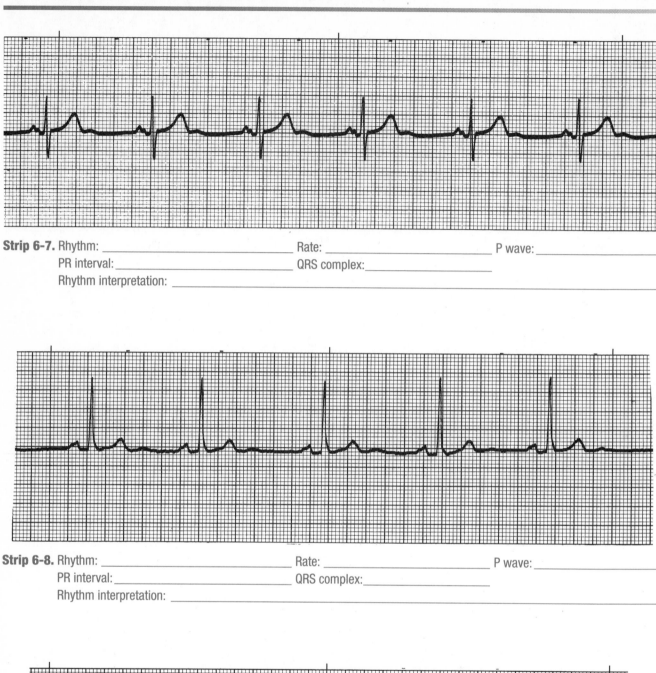

**Strip 6-7.** Rhythm: _____ Rate: _____ P wave: _____

PR interval: _____ QRS complex: _____

Rhythm interpretation: _____

**Strip 6-8.** Rhythm: _____ Rate: _____ P wave: _____

PR interval: _____ QRS complex: _____

Rhythm interpretation: _____

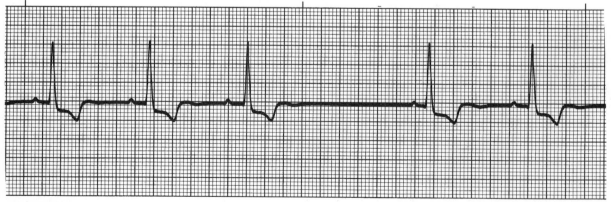

**Strip 6-9.** Rhythm: _____ Rate: _____ P wave: _____

PR interval: _____ QRS complex: _____

Rhythm interpretation: _____

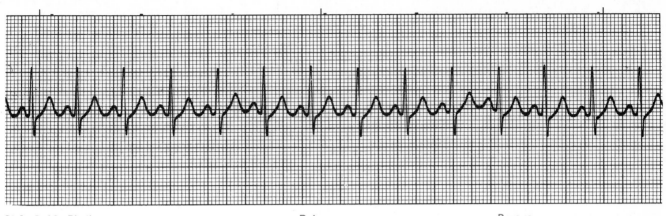

**Strip 6-10.** Rhythm:_____ Rate:_____ P wave:_____

PR interval: _____ QRS complex:_____

Rhythm interpretation: _____

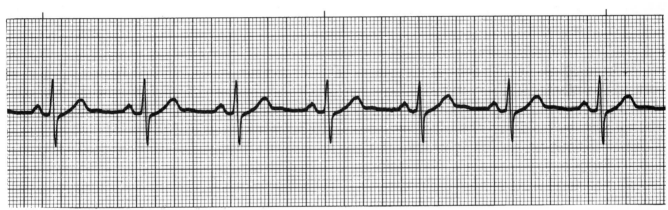

**Strip 6-11.** Rhythm:_____ Rate:_____ P wave:_____

PR interval: _____ QRS complex:_____

Rhythm interpretation: _____

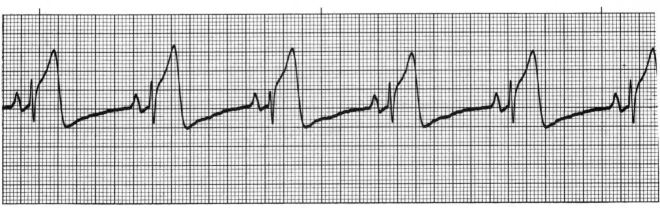

**Strip 6-12.** Rhythm:_____ Rate:_____ P wave:_____

PR interval: _____ QRS complex:_____

Rhythm interpretation: _____

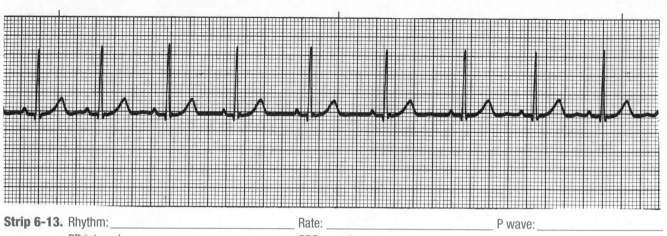

**Strip 6-13.** Rhythm: _____ Rate: _____ P wave: _____

PR interval: _____ QRS complex: _____

Rhythm interpretation: _____

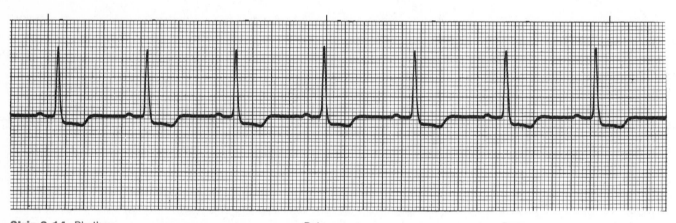

**Strip 6-14.** Rhythm: _____ Rate: _____ P wave: _____

PR interval: _____ QRS complex: _____

Rhythm interpretation: _____

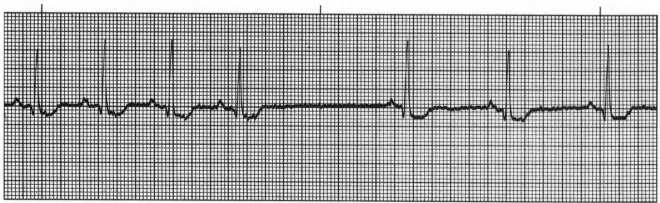

**Strip 6-15.** Rhythm: _____ Rate: _____ P wave: _____

PR interval: _____ QRS complex: _____

Rhythm interpretation: _____

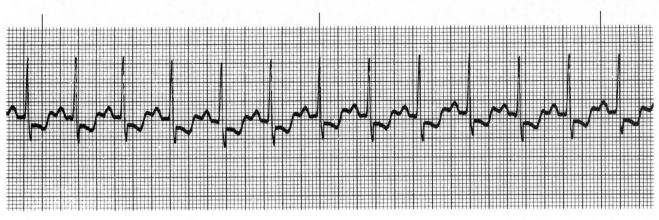

**Strip 6-16.** Rhythm:_____ Rate:_____ P wave:_____

PR interval:_____ QRS complex:_____

Rhythm interpretation:_____

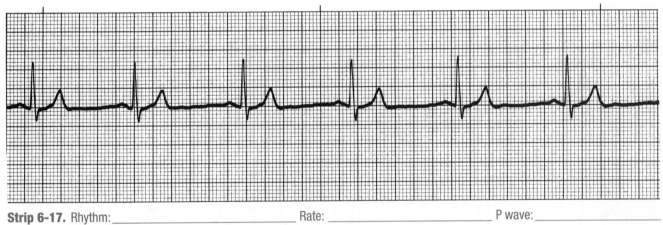

**Strip 6-17.** Rhythm:_____ Rate:_____ P wave:_____

PR interval:_____ QRS complex:_____

Rhythm interpretation:_____

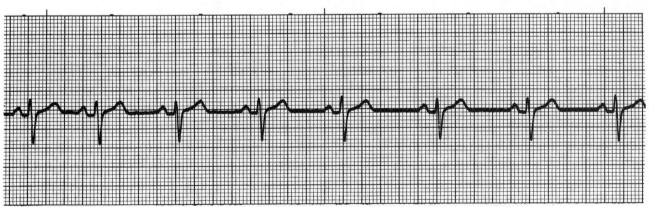

**Strip 6-18.** Rhythm:_____ Rate:_____ P wave:_____

PR interval:_____ QRS complex:_____

Rhythm interpretation:_____

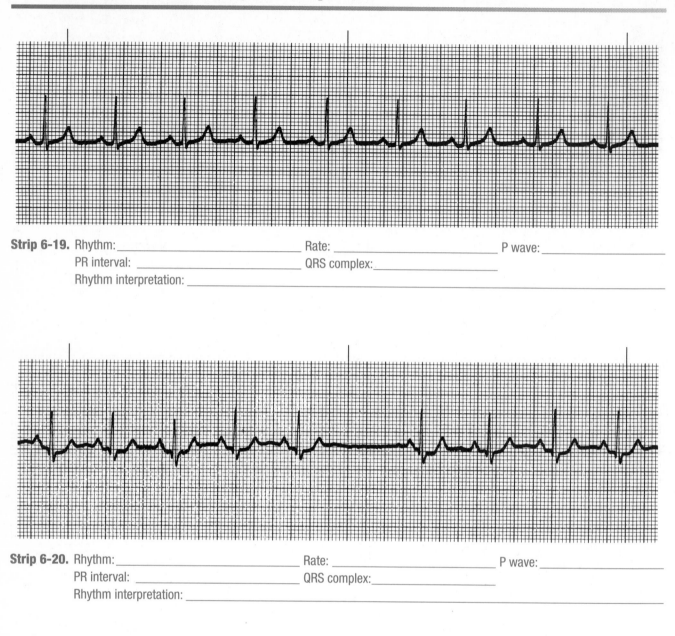

**Strip 6-19.** Rhythm:_____ Rate:_____ P wave:_____

PR interval:_____ QRS complex:_____

Rhythm interpretation:_____

**Strip 6-20.** Rhythm:_____ Rate:_____ P wave:_____

PR interval:_____ QRS complex:_____

Rhythm interpretation:_____

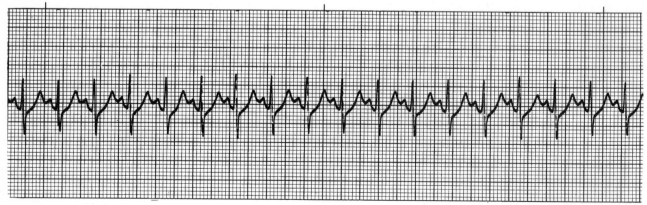

**Strip 6-21.** Rhythm:_____ Rate:_____ P wave:_____

PR interval:_____ QRS complex:_____

Rhythm interpretation:_____

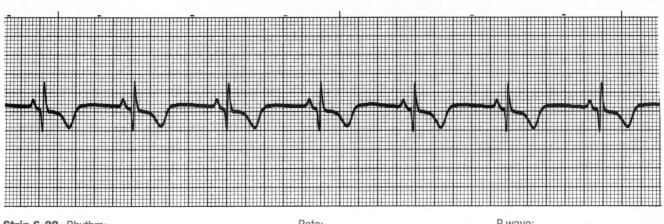

**Strip 6-22.** Rhythm:_____ Rate:_____ P wave:_____

PR interval:_____ QRS complex:_____

Rhythm interpretation:_____

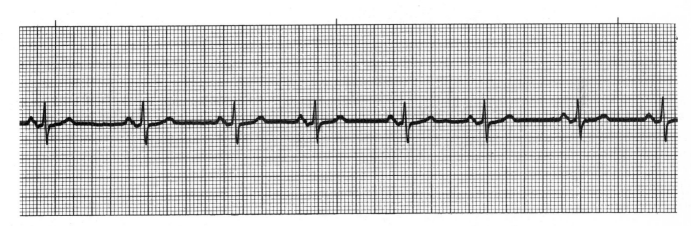

**Strip 6-23.** Rhythm:_____ Rate:_____ P wave:_____

PR interval:_____ QRS complex:_____

Rhythm interpretation:_____

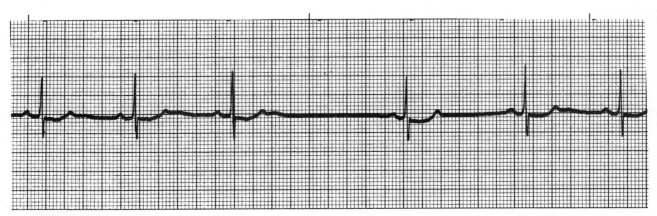

**Strip 6-24.** Rhythm:_____ Rate:_____ P wave:_____

PR interval:_____ QRS complex:_____

Rhythm interpretation:_____

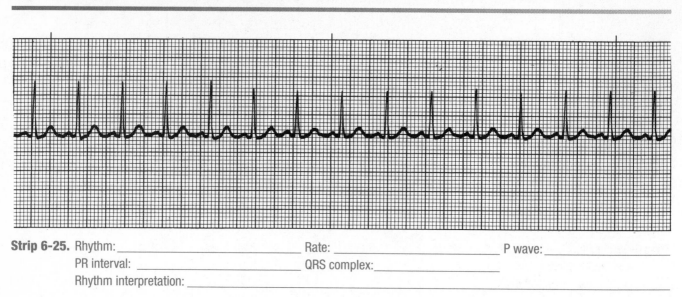

**Strip 6-25.** Rhythm:_____ Rate:_____ P wave:_____

PR interval:_____ QRS complex:_____

Rhythm interpretation:_____

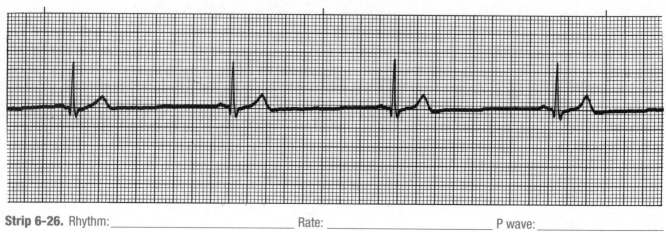

**Strip 6-26.** Rhythm:_____ Rate:_____ P wave:_____

PR interval:_____ QRS complex:_____

Rhythm interpretation:_____

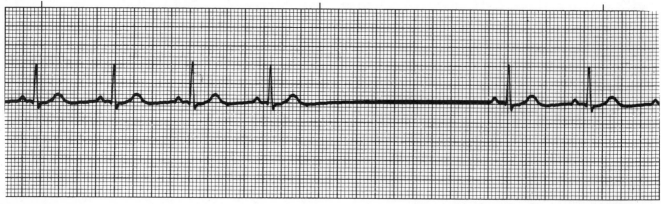

**Strip 6-27.** Rhythm:_____ Rate:_____ P wave:_____

PR interval:_____ QRS complex:_____

Rhythm interpretation:_____

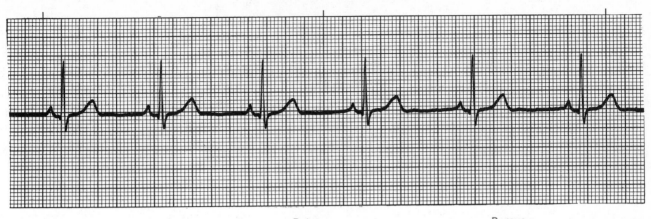

**Strip 6-28.** Rhythm: _____ Rate: _____ P wave: _____
PR interval: _____ QRS complex: _____
Rhythm interpretation: _____

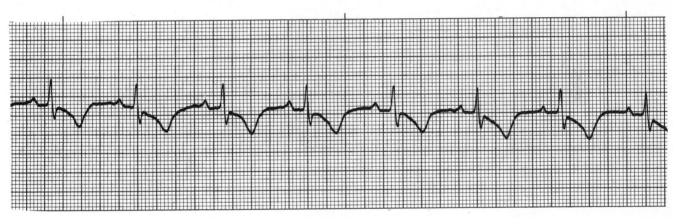

**Strip 6-29.** Rhythm: _____ Rate: _____ P wave: _____
PR interval: _____ QRS complex: _____
Rhythm interpretation: _____

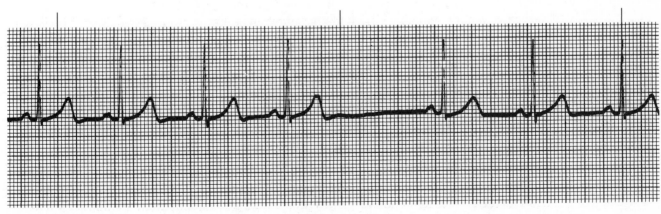

**Strip 6-30.** Rhythm: _____ Rate: _____ P wave: _____
PR interval: _____ QRS complex: _____
Rhythm interpretation: _____

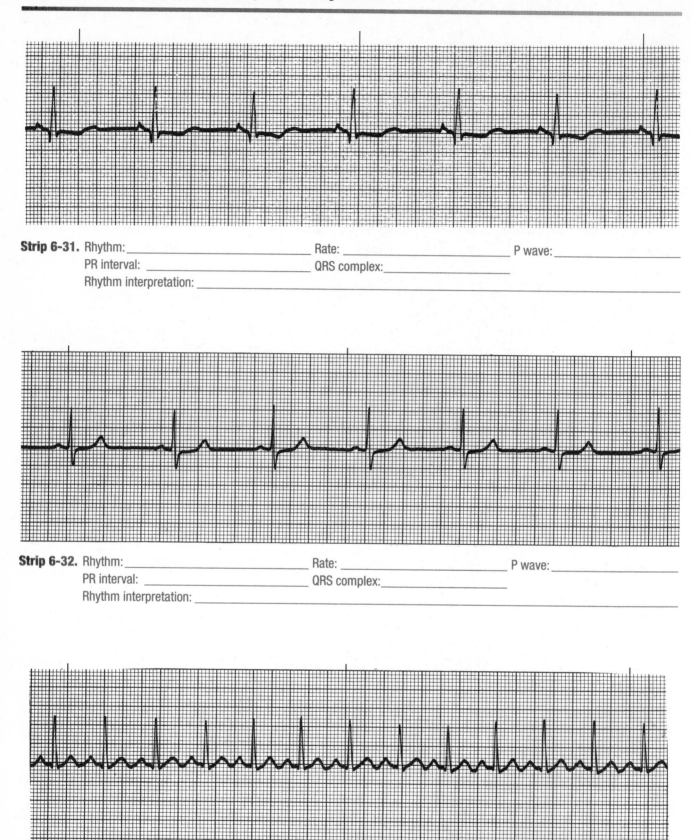

**Strip 6-31.** Rhythm:_____ Rate: _____ P wave:_____
PR interval: _____ QRS complex:_____
Rhythm interpretation: _____

**Strip 6-32.** Rhythm:_____ Rate: _____ P wave:_____
PR interval: _____ QRS complex:_____
Rhythm interpretation: _____

**Strip 6-33.** Rhythm:_____ Rate: _____ P wave:_____
PR interval: _____ QRS complex:_____
Rhythm interpretation: _____

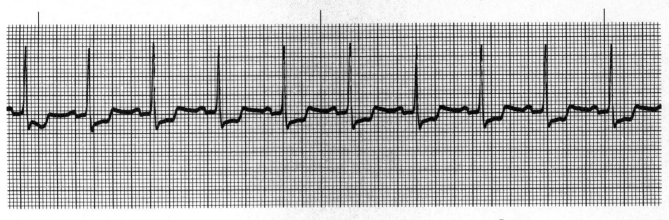

**Strip 6-34.** Rhythm:_____ Rate:_____ P wave:_____

PR interval: _____ QRS complex:_____

Rhythm interpretation: _____

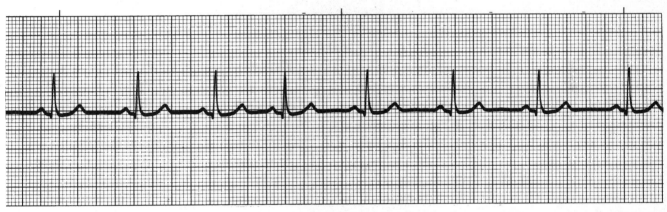

**Strip 6-35.** Rhythm:_____ Rate:_____ P wave:_____

PR interval: _____ QRS complex:_____

Rhythm interpretation: _____

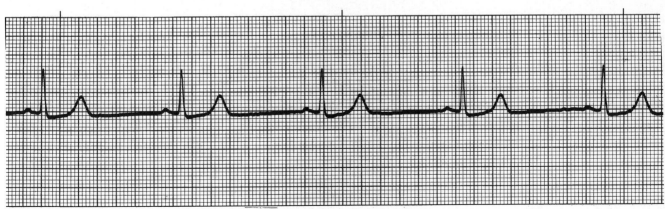

**Strip 6-36.** Rhythm:_____ Rate:_____ P wave:_____

PR interval: _____ QRS complex:_____

Rhythm interpretation: _____

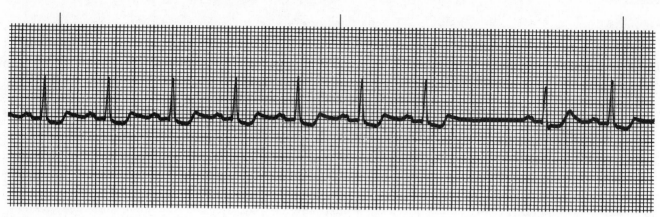

**Strip 6-37.** Rhythm: _____ Rate: _____ P wave: _____
PR interval: _____ QRS complex: _____
Rhythm interpretation: _____

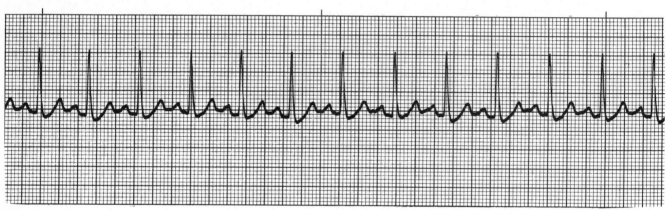

**Strip 6-38.** Rhythm: _____ Rate: _____ P wave: _____
PR interval: _____ QRS complex: _____
Rhythm interpretation: _____

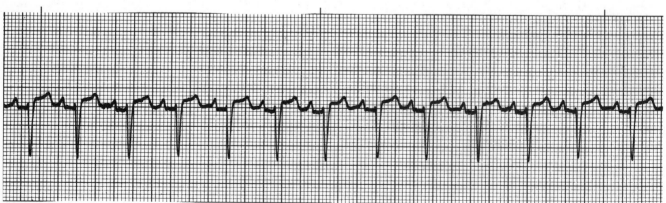

**Strip 6-39.** Rhythm: _____ Rate: _____ P wave: _____
PR interval: _____ QRS complex: _____
Rhythm interpretation: _____

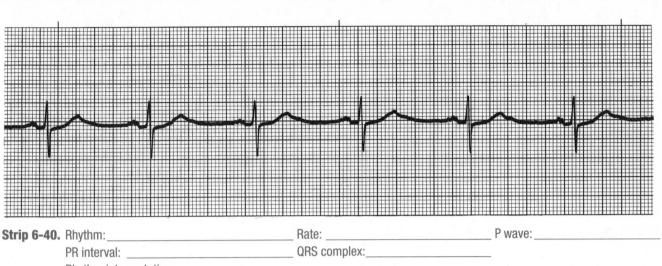

**Strip 6-40.** Rhythm:_____ Rate:_____ P wave:_____

PR interval: _____ QRS complex:_____

Rhythm interpretation: _____

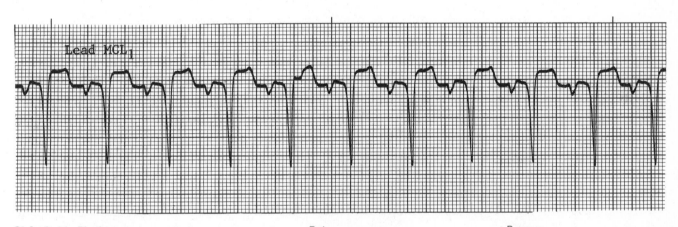

**Strip 6-41.** Rhythm:_____ Rate:_____ P wave:_____

PR interval: _____ QRS complex:_____

Rhythm interpretation: _____

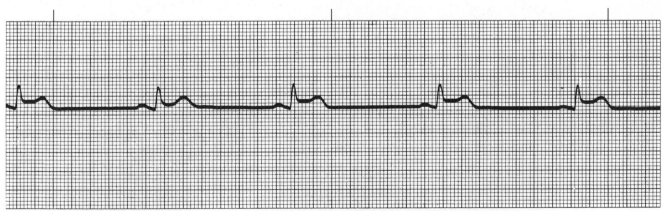

**Strip 6-42.** Rhythm:_____ Rate:_____ P wave:_____

PR interval: _____ QRS complex:_____

Rhythm interpretation: _____

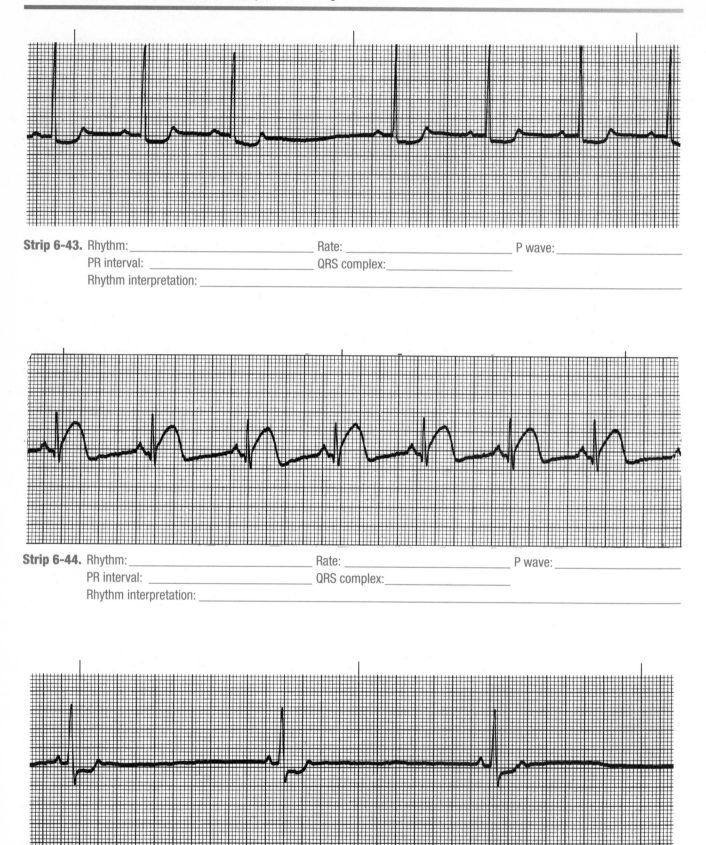

**Strip 6-43.** Rhythm:_____ Rate:_____ P wave:_____

PR interval:_____ QRS complex:_____

Rhythm interpretation:_____

**Strip 6-44.** Rhythm:_____ Rate:_____ P wave:_____

PR interval:_____ QRS complex:_____

Rhythm interpretation:_____

**Strip 6-45.** Rhythm:_____ Rate:_____ P wave:_____

PR interval:_____ QRS complex:_____

Rhythm interpretation:_____

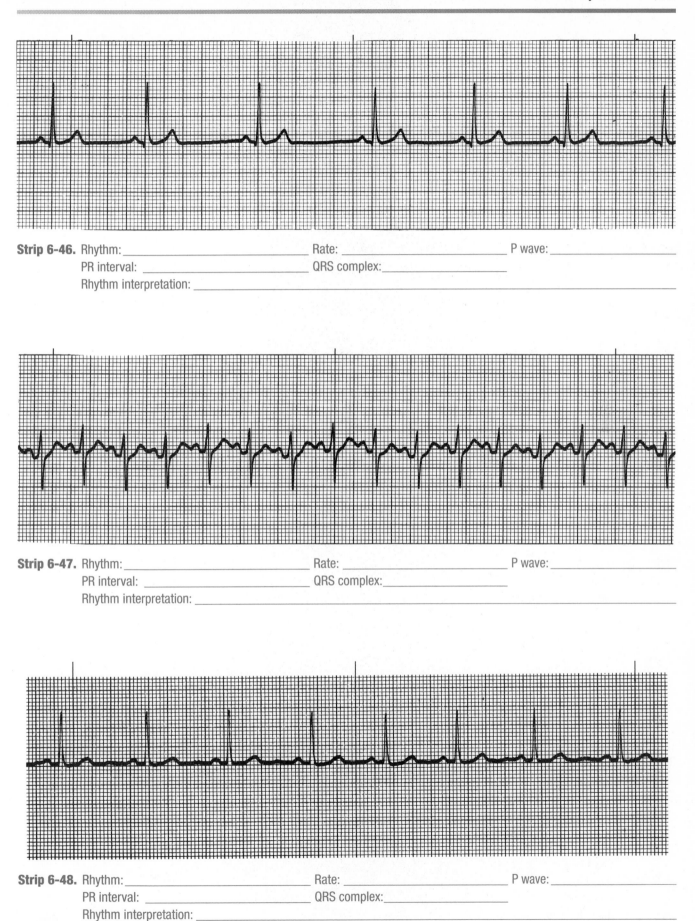

**Strip 6-46.** Rhythm:_____ Rate:_____ P wave:_____
PR interval: _____ QRS complex:_____
Rhythm interpretation: _____

**Strip 6-47.** Rhythm:_____ Rate:_____ P wave:_____
PR interval: _____ QRS complex:_____
Rhythm interpretation: _____

**Strip 6-48.** Rhythm:_____ Rate:_____ P wave:_____
PR interval: _____ QRS complex:_____
Rhythm interpretation: _____

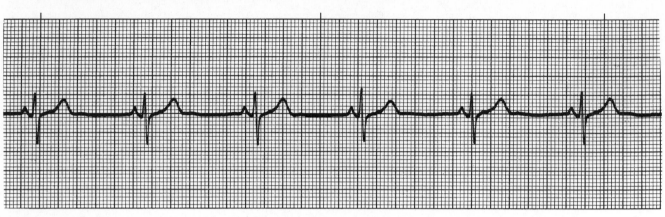

**Strip 6-49.** Rhythm: _____ Rate: _____ P wave: _____

PR interval: _____ QRS complex: _____

Rhythm interpretation: _____

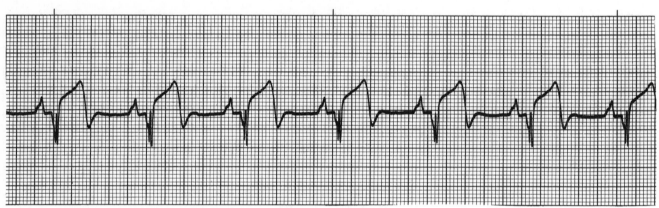

**Strip 6-50.** Rhythm: _____ Rate: _____ P wave: _____

PR interval: _____ QRS complex: _____

Rhythm interpretation: _____

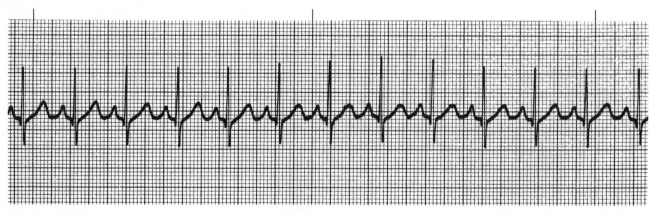

**Strip 6-51.** Rhythm: _____ Rate: _____ P wave: _____

PR interval: _____ QRS complex: _____

Rhythm interpretation: _____

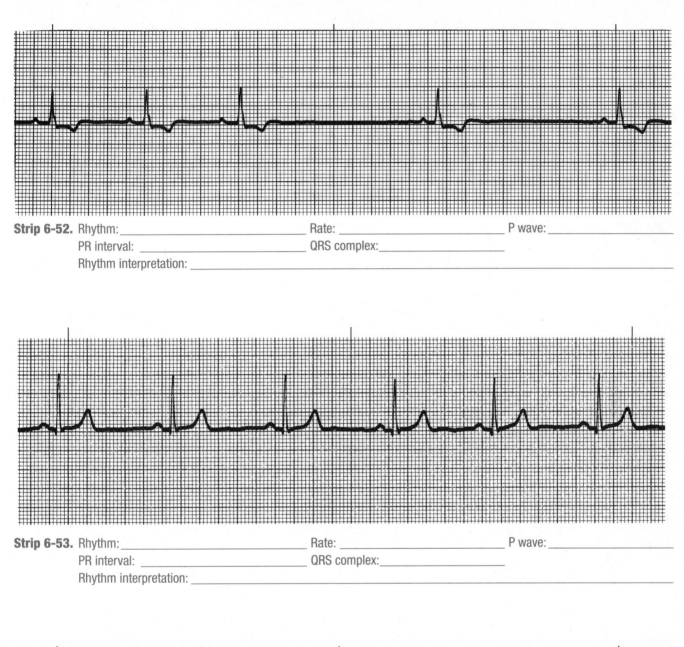

**Strip 6-52.** Rhythm:_____ Rate:_____ P wave:_____

PR interval:_____ QRS complex:_____

Rhythm interpretation:_____

**Strip 6-53.** Rhythm:_____ Rate:_____ P wave:_____

PR interval:_____ QRS complex:_____

Rhythm interpretation:_____

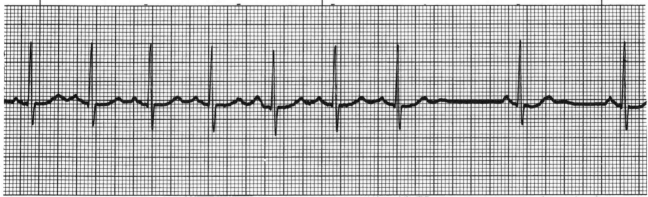

**Strip 6-54.** Rhythm:_____ Rate:_____ P wave:_____

PR interval:_____ QRS complex:_____

Rhythm interpretation:_____

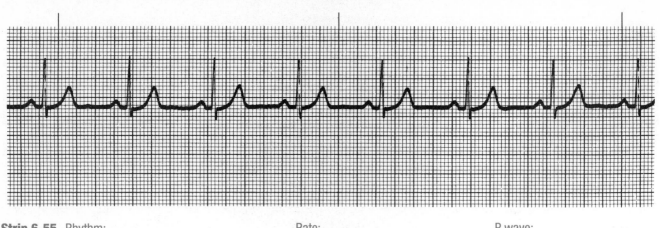

**Strip 6-55.** Rhythm: _____ Rate: _____ P wave: _____

PR interval: _____ QRS complex: _____

Rhythm interpretation: _____

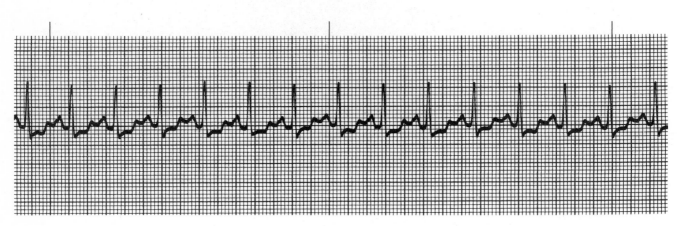

**Strip 6-56.** Rhythm: _____ Rate: _____ P wave: _____

PR interval: _____ QRS complex: _____

Rhythm interpretation: _____

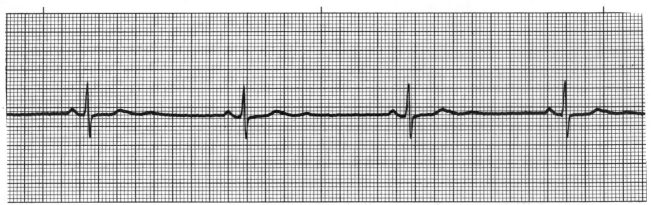

**Strip 6-57.** Rhythm: _____ Rate: _____ P wave: _____

PR interval: _____ QRS complex: _____

Rhythm interpretation: _____

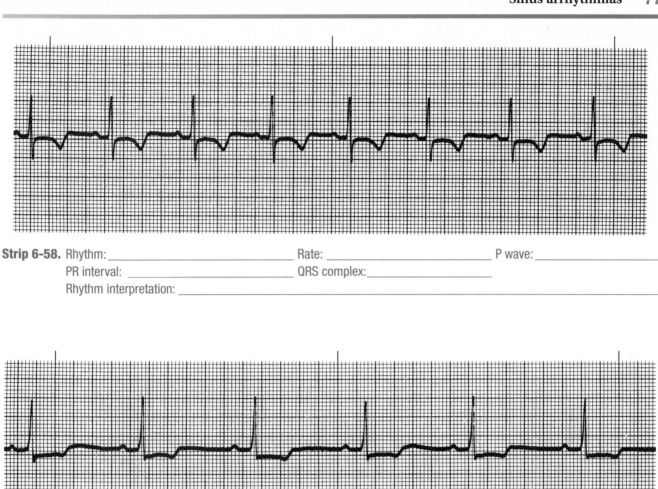

**Strip 6-58.** Rhythm: _____ Rate: _____ P wave: _____
PR interval: _____ QRS complex: _____
Rhythm interpretation: _____

**Strip 6-59.** Rhythm: _____ Rate: _____ P wave: _____
PR interval: _____ QRS complex: _____
Rhythm interpretation: _____

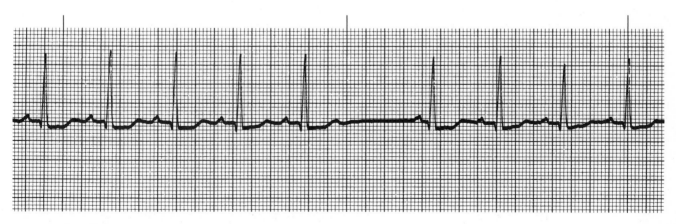

**Strip 6-60.** Rhythm: _____ Rate: _____ P wave: _____
PR interval: _____ QRS complex: _____
Rhythm interpretation: _____

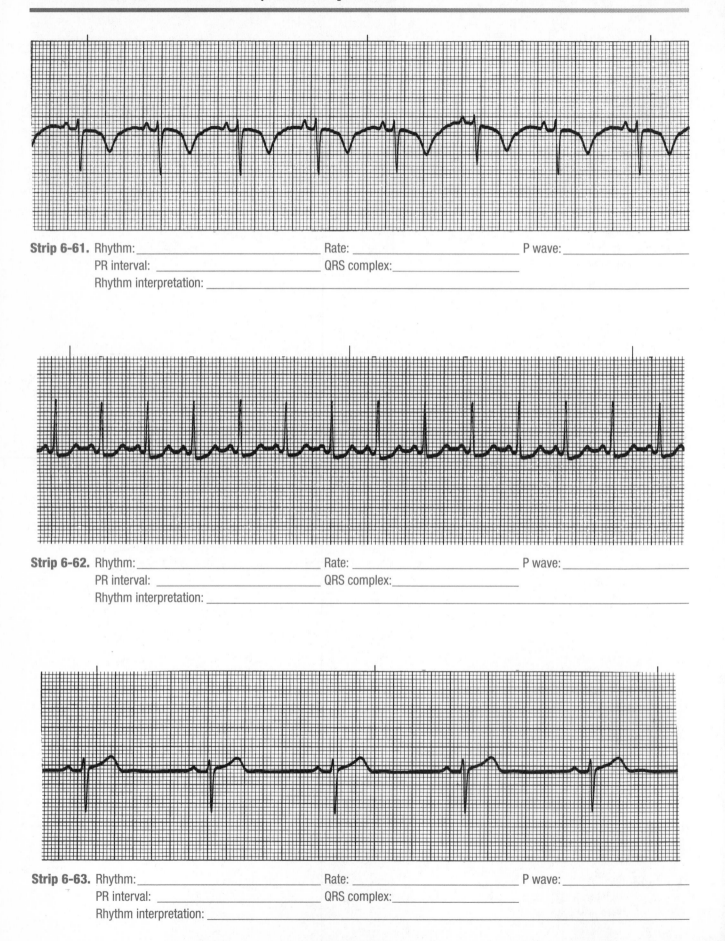

**Strip 6-61.** Rhythm:_____ Rate:_____ P wave:_____
PR interval:_____ QRS complex:_____
Rhythm interpretation:_____

**Strip 6-62.** Rhythm:_____ Rate:_____ P wave:_____
PR interval:_____ QRS complex:_____
Rhythm interpretation:_____

**Strip 6-63.** Rhythm:_____ Rate:_____ P wave:_____
PR interval:_____ QRS complex:_____
Rhythm interpretation:_____

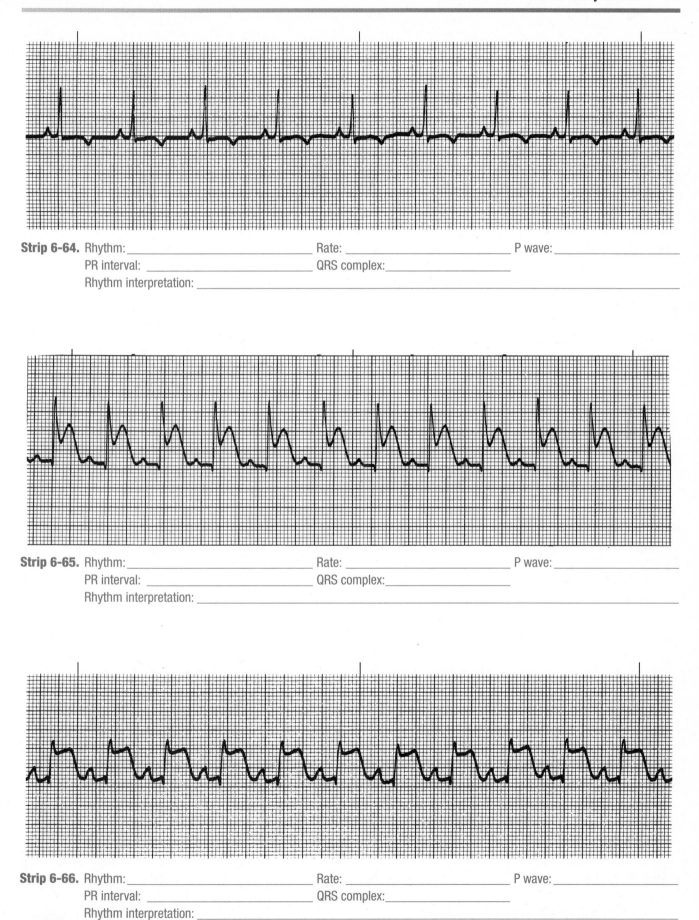

**Strip 6-64.** Rhythm: _____ Rate: _____ P wave: _____

PR interval: _____ QRS complex: _____

Rhythm interpretation: _____

**Strip 6-65.** Rhythm: _____ Rate: _____ P wave: _____

PR interval: _____ QRS complex: _____

Rhythm interpretation: _____

**Strip 6-66.** Rhythm: _____ Rate: _____ P wave: _____

PR interval: _____ QRS complex: _____

Rhythm interpretation: _____

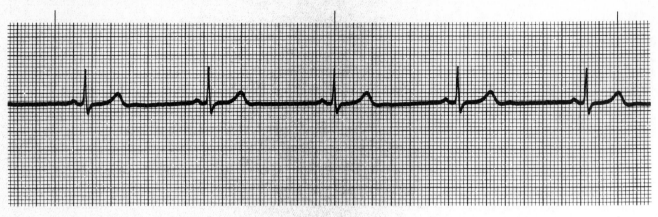

**Strip 6-67.** Rhythm: _____  Rate: _____  P wave: _____
PR interval: _____  QRS complex: _____
Rhythm interpretation: _____

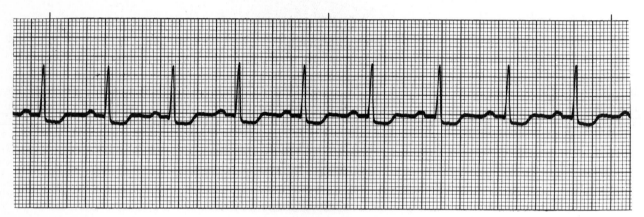

**Strip 6-68.** Rhythm: _____  Rate: _____  P wave: _____
PR interval: _____  QRS complex: _____
Rhythm interpretation: _____

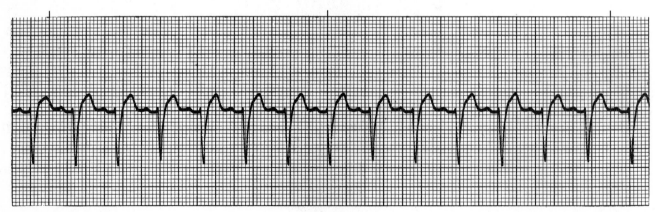

**Strip 6-69.** Rhythm: _____  Rate: _____  P wave: _____
PR interval: _____  QRS complex: _____
Rhythm interpretation: _____

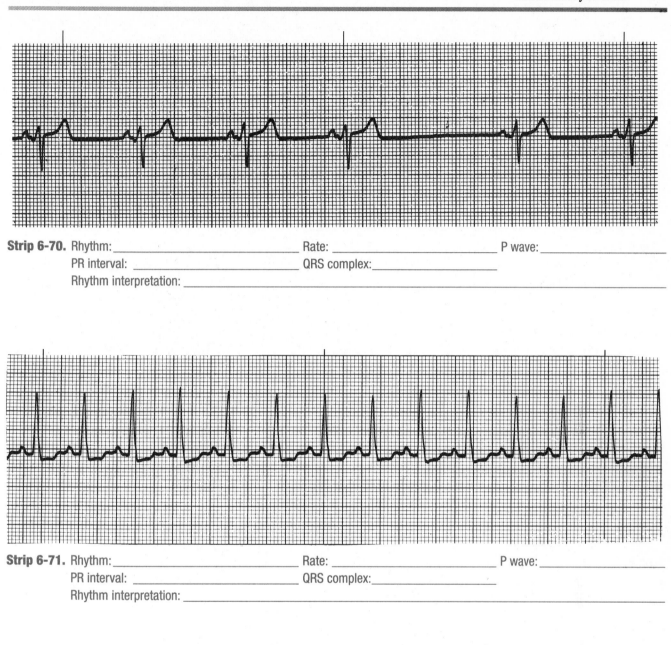

**Strip 6-70.** Rhythm:_____ Rate:_____ P wave:_____

PR interval: _____ QRS complex:_____

Rhythm interpretation: _____

**Strip 6-71.** Rhythm:_____ Rate:_____ P wave:_____

PR interval: _____ QRS complex:_____

Rhythm interpretation: _____

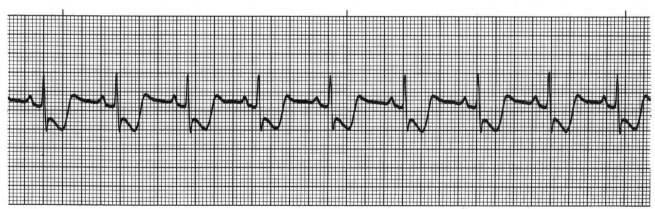

**Strip 6-72.** Rhythm:_____ Rate:_____ P wave:_____

PR interval: _____ QRS complex:_____

Rhythm interpretation: _____

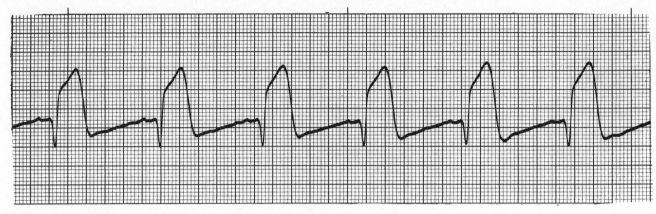

**Strip 6-73.** Rhythm:_____ Rate:_____ P wave:_____

PR interval: _____ QRS complex:_____

Rhythm interpretation: _____

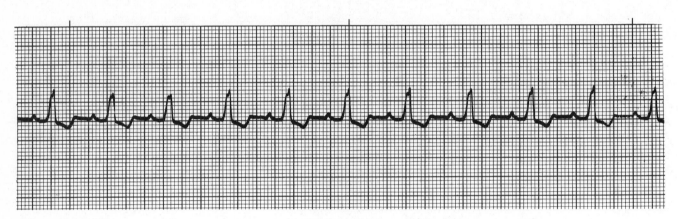

**Strip 6-74.** Rhythm:_____ Rate:_____ P wave:_____

PR interval: _____ QRS complex:_____

Rhythm interpretation: _____

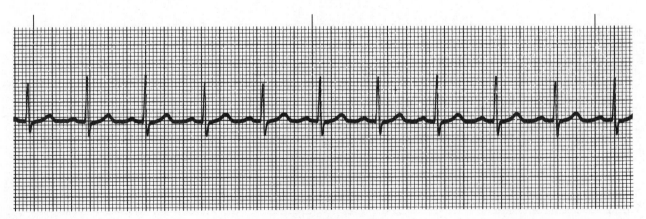

**Strip 6-75.** Rhythm:_____ Rate:_____ P wave:_____

PR interval: _____ QRS complex:_____

Rhythm interpretation: _____

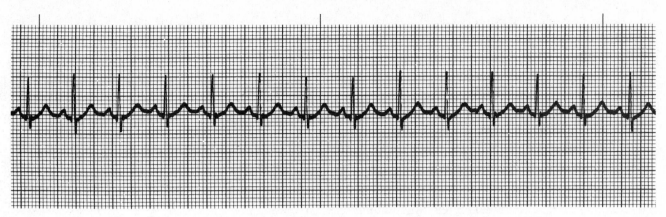

**Strip 6-76.** Rhythm:_____ Rate:_____ P wave:_____

PR interval:_____ QRS complex:_____

Rhythm interpretation:_____

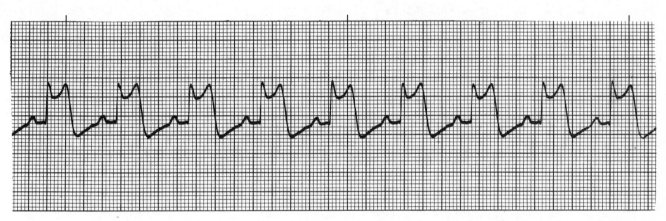

**Strip 6-77.** Rhythm:_____ Rate:_____ P wave:_____

PR interval:_____ QRS complex:_____

Rhythm interpretation:_____

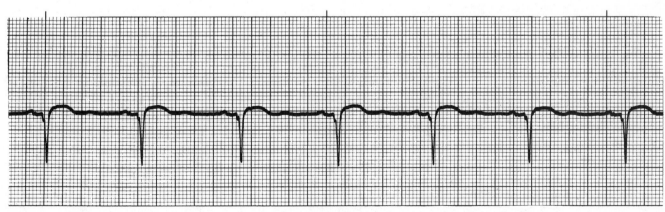

**Strip 6-78.** Rhythm:_____ Rate:_____ P wave:_____

PR interval:_____ QRS complex:_____

Rhythm interpretation:_____

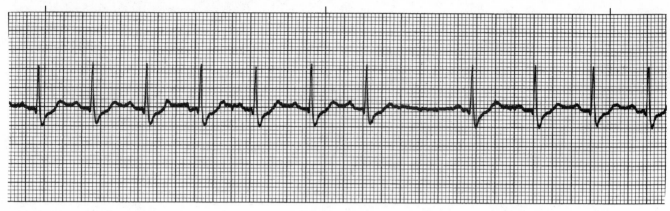

**Strip 6-79.** Rhythm: _____ Rate: _____ P wave: _____

PR interval: _____ QRS complex:_____

Rhythm interpretation: _____

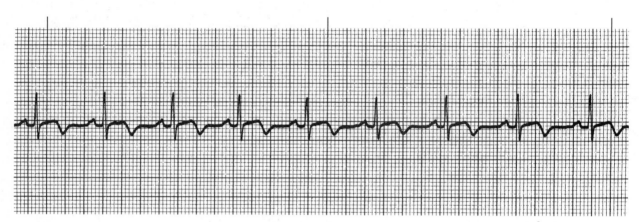

**Strip 6-80.** Rhythm:_____ Rate: _____ P wave: _____

PR interval: _____ QRS complex:_____

Rhythm interpretation: _____

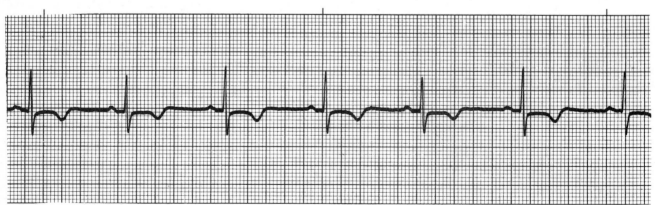

**Strip 6-81.** Rhythm:_____ Rate: _____ P wave: _____

PR interval: _____ QRS complex:_____

Rhythm interpretation: _____

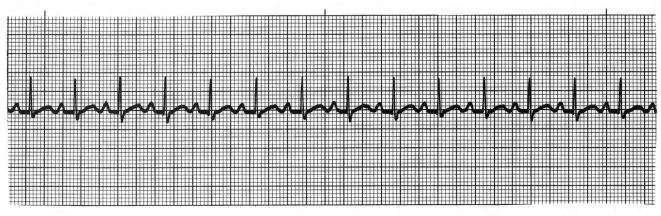

**Strip 6-82.** Rhythm:_____ Rate:_____ P wave:_____
PR interval:_____ QRS complex:_____
Rhythm interpretation:_____

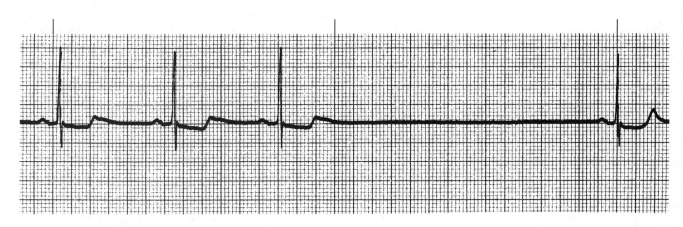

**Strip 6-83.** Rhythm:_____ Rate:_____ P wave:_____
PR interval:_____ QRS complex:_____
Rhythm interpretation:_____

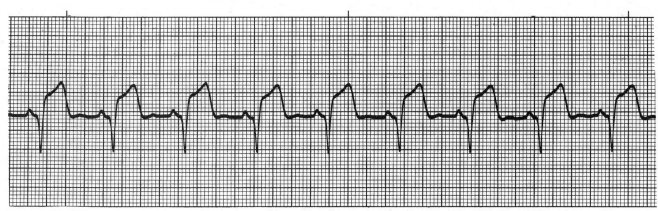

**Strip 6-84.** Rhythm:_____ Rate:_____ P wave:_____
PR interval:_____ QRS complex:_____
Rhythm interpretation:_____

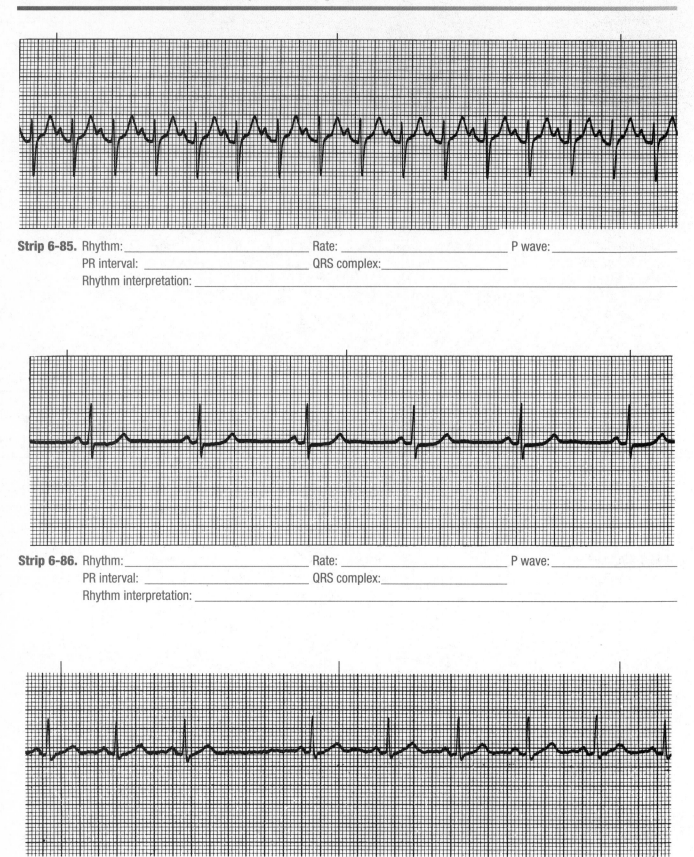

**Strip 6-85.** Rhythm:_____ Rate:_____ P wave:_____
PR interval: _____ QRS complex:_____
Rhythm interpretation: _____

**Strip 6-86.** Rhythm:_____ Rate:_____ P wave:_____
PR interval: _____ QRS complex:_____
Rhythm interpretation: _____

**Strip 6-87.** Rhythm:_____ Rate:_____ P wave:_____
PR interval: _____ QRS complex:_____
Rhythm interpretation: _____

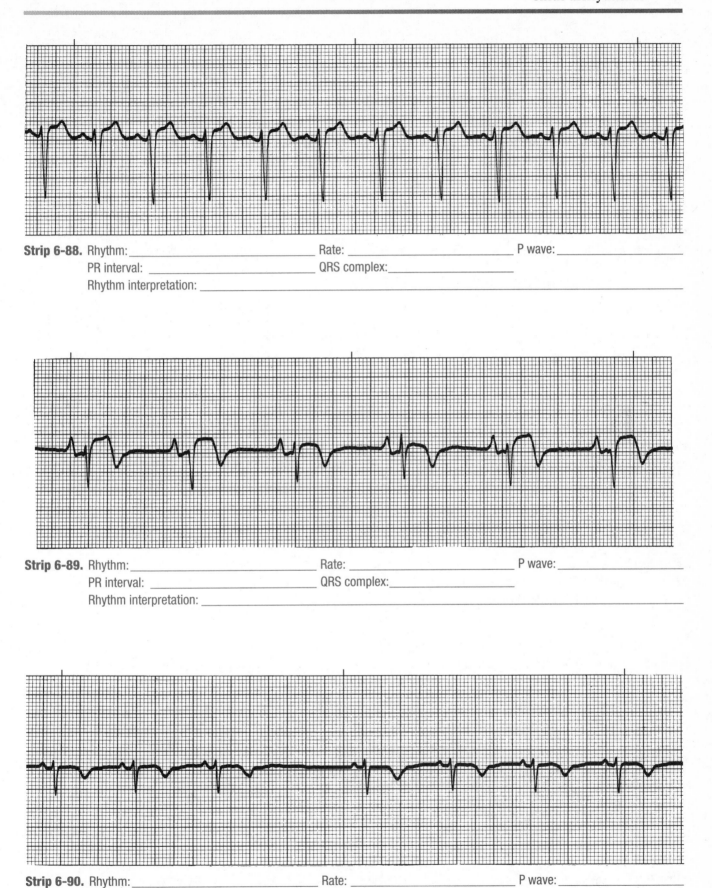

**Strip 6-88.** Rhythm: _____ Rate: _____ P wave: _____

PR interval: _____ QRS complex: _____

Rhythm interpretation: _____

**Strip 6-89.** Rhythm: _____ Rate: _____ P wave: _____

PR interval: _____ QRS complex: _____

Rhythm interpretation: _____

**Strip 6-90.** Rhythm: _____ Rate: _____ P wave: _____

PR interval: _____ QRS complex: _____

Rhythm interpretation: _____

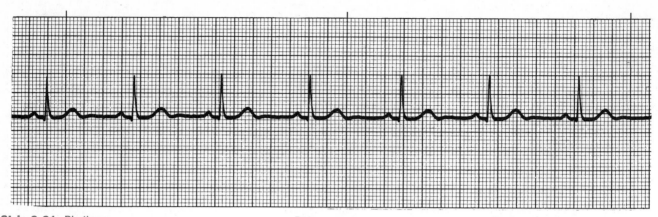

**Strip 6-91.** Rhythm: _____ Rate: _____ P wave: _____

PR interval: _____ QRS complex: _____

Rhythm interpretation: _____

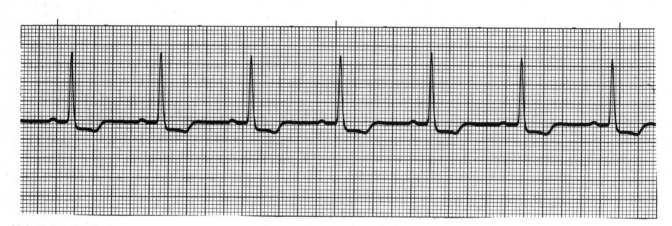

**Strip 6-92.** Rhythm: _____ Rate: _____ P wave: _____

PR interval: _____ QRS complex: _____

Rhythm interpretation: _____

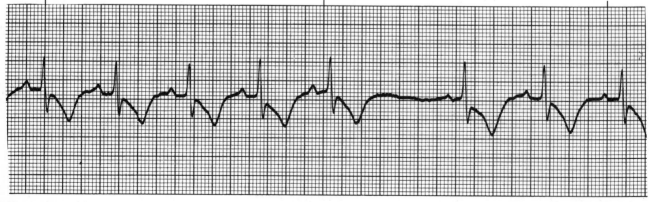

**Strip 6-93.** Rhythm: _____ Rate: _____ P wave: _____

PR interval: _____ QRS complex: _____

Rhythm interpretation: _____

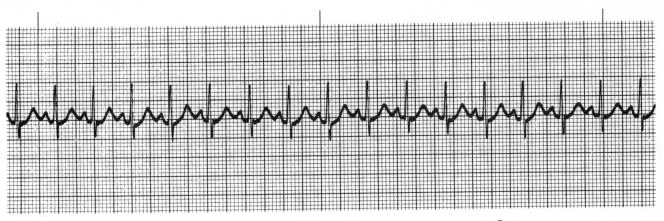

**Strip 6-94.** Rhythm:_____ Rate:_____ P wave:_____

PR interval:_____ QRS complex:_____

Rhythm interpretation:_____

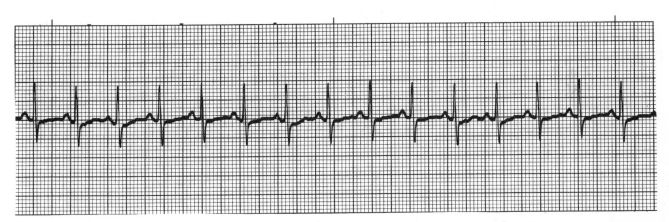

**Strip 6-95.** Rhythm:_____ Rate:_____ P wave:_____

PR interval:_____ QRS complex:_____

Rhythm interpretation:_____

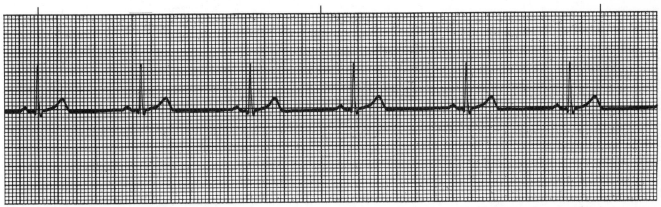

**Strip 6-96.** Rhythm:_____ Rate:_____ P wave:_____

PR interval:_____ QRS complex:_____

Rhythm interpretation:_____

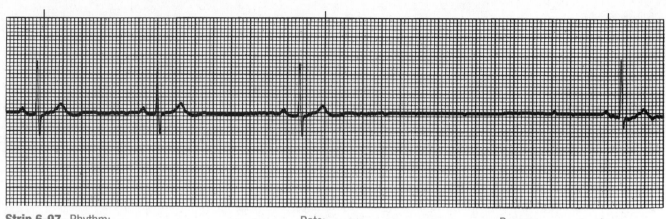

**Strip 6-97.** Rhythm: _____ Rate: _____ P wave: _____

PR interval: _____ QRS complex: _____

Rhythm interpretation: _____

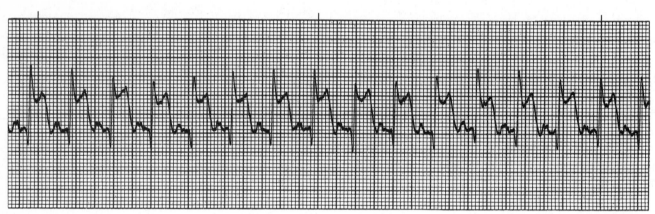

**Strip 6-98.** Rhythm: _____ Rate: _____ P wave: _____

PR interval: _____ QRS complex: _____

Rhythm interpretation: _____

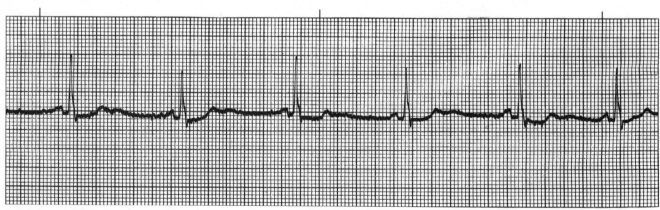

**Strip 6-99.** Rhythm: _____ Rate: _____ P wave: _____

PR interval: _____ QRS complex: _____

Rhythm interpretation: _____

# 7 Atrial arrhythmias

# Overview

Under certain circumstances cardiac cells in any part of the heart may take on the role of pacemaker of the heart. Such a pacemaker is called an *ectopic pacemaker* (a pacemaker other than the sinus node). The result can be abnormal ectopic beats or rhythms. These arrhythmias are identified according to the location of the ectopic pacemaker (for example, atrial, junctional, or ventricular). The three basic mechanisms that are responsible for ectopic beats and rhythms are *altered automaticity, triggered activity,* and *reentry:*

■ **Altered automaticity**—Normally the automaticity of the sinus node exceeds that of all other parts of the conduction system, allowing it to control the heart rate and rhythm. Pacemaker cells in other areas of the heart also have the property of automaticity, including cells in the atria, atrioventricular (AV) junction, and the ventricles. The rates of these other pacemaker sites are slower. Therefore, they're suppressed by the sinus node under normal circumstances. Because the sinus node possesses the faster impulse initiation, it's referred to as the dominant pacemaker. An ectopic pacemaker site, such as the atria, can initiate the cardiac rhythm either because it usurps control from the sinus node by accelerating its own automaticity (enhanced automaticity) or because the sinus node relinquishes its role by decreasing its automaticity.

■ **Triggered activity**—Triggered activity (also called *afterdepolarization*) is an abnormal condition in which myocardial cells may depolarize more than once after stimulation by a single electrical impulse. This can result in atrial, junctional, or ventricular ectopic beats occurring in groups of two (paired or coupled beats), or in bursts of three or more

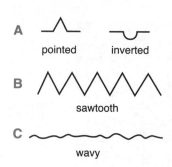

**Figure 7-2.** Atrial P waves.

beats (paroxysms of beats or tachycardia). Triggered activity commonly occurs during repolarization when cells are normally quiet or right after repolarization is complete. Some of the conditions favoring triggered activity include myocardial ischemia, hypoxia, hypomagnesemia, long QT syndrome, slow heart rates, and medications that prolong repolarization.

■ **Reentry**—Normally an impulse spreads through the heart only once. With reentry an impulse can travel through an area of myocardium, depolarize it, and then reenter that same area to depolarize it again. Reentry produces a circular movement of the impulse, which continues as long as it encounters receptive cells. This type of impulse conduction commonly results in rapid heart rates. Myocardial ischemia and hyperkalemia are the two most common causes of reentry. Another cause is the presence of an accessory conduction pathway.

Atrial arrhythmias (Figure 7-1) originate from ectopic sites in the atria. The P waves will be different in configer-

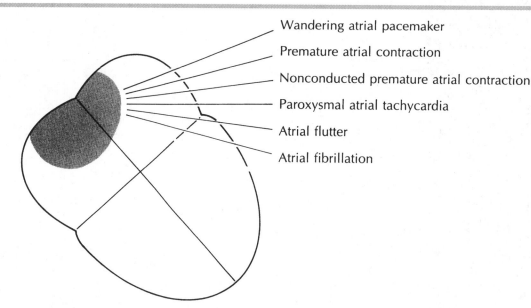

Wandering atrial pacemaker

Premature atrial contraction

Nonconducted premature atrial contraction

Paroxysmal atrial tachycardia

Atrial flutter

Atrial fibrillation

**Figure 7-1.** Atrial arrhythmias.

ation (morphology) from the sinus P waves (Figure 7-2) because the impulse originates in an ectopic site and follows a different conduction pathway to the AV node. In slower atrial rhythms (premature atrial beats, wandering atrial pacemaker) the P wave is typically visible as a small, pointed, upright waveform, or it may be inverted if the impulse originates in the lower atrium near the AV junction. In faster atrial rhythms the abnormal P wave is either superimposed on the preceding T wave (paroxysmal atrial tachycardia), appears in a sawtooth pattern (atrial flutter), or is seen as a wavy baseline (atrial fibrillation).

When the atrial rate is extremely rapid, as seen in atrial flutter and atrial fibrillation, the AV node blocks some of the atrial impulses from being conducted to the ventricles, thus protecting the ventricle from dangerously high rates. This results in a ventricular rate that is slower than the atrial rate (fewer QRS complexes than P waves). Younger patients and individuals without underlying heart disease may tolerate episodes of rapid heart rate with no serious problems. However, in patients with limited cardiac reserve, increased heart rates can have serious consequences. In atrial rhythms associated with rapid ventricular rates, cardiac output and coronary perfusion may be reduced secondary to decreased diastolic filling time in the ventricles. Treatment depends on the hemodynamic consequences of the arrhythmia.

## Wandering atrial pacemaker

A wandering atrial pacemaker (WAP) (Figure 7-3 and Box 7-1) occurs when the pacemaker site shifts back and forth between the sinus node, other atrial sites, and sometimes the AV node. The P waves change their shape as the pacemaker "wanders" between the multiple sites. WAP is thought to result from multiple pacemaker sites competing with each other for control of the heart. Some feel you should identify at least three different P-wave morphologies before making the diagnosis of WAP. The heart rate is usually normal, but can be slow. The rhythm may be regular or irregular. The PR interval may vary depending on the pacemaker site. The QRS complex is normal in duration. The distinguishing feature of this arrhythmia is the changing P-wave configuration across the rhythm strip.

**Box 7-1.**
### Wandering atrial pacemaker: Identifying ECG features

| | |
|---|---|
| **Rhythm:** | Regular or irregular |
| **Rate:** | Usually normal (60 to 100 beats/minute) but may be slow (less than 60 beats/minute) |
| **P waves:** | Vary in size, shape, and direction across rhythm strip; one P wave precedes each QRS complex |
| **PR interval:** | Usually normal duration, but may vary depending on changing pacemaker locations |
| **QRS complex:** | Normal (0.10 second or less) |

In most cases WAP is caused by increased vagal effect on the sinoatrial (SA) node, slowing the sinus rate and allowing other pacemaker sites an opportunity to compete for control of the heart rate. WAP is a normal phenomenon observed in young healthy hearts (especially those of athletes) and during sleep.

WAP usually isn't clinically significant, and treatment isn't indicated. If the heart rate is slow, medications should be reviewed and discontinued if necessary. Asking the patient to cough may decrease vagal tone and encourage the reappearance of a sinus rhythm.

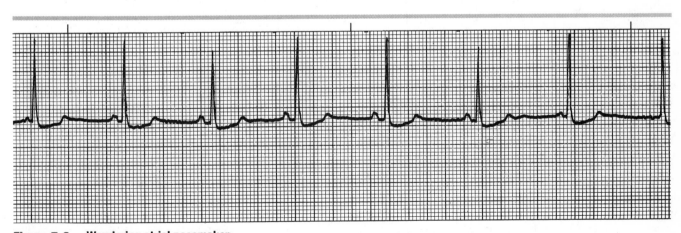

| **Figure 7-3.** | **Wandering atrial pacemaker** |
|---|---|
| **Rhythm:** | Irregular |
| **Rate:** | 60 beats/minute |
| **P waves:** | Vary in size, shape, across rhythm strip |
| **PR interval:** | 0.10 to 0.14 second |
| **QRS complex:** | 0.04 to 0.08 second |

A variant of WAP is multifocal atrial tachycardia (MAT). At rates above 100 beats/minute WAP becomes MAT. MAT is most commonly observed in persons with severe chronic obstructive pulmonary disease (COPD).

## Premature atrial contraction

A premature atrial contraction (PAC) (Figures 7-4 through 7-10 and Box 7-2) is an early beat that occurs when an ectopic site within the atria discharges an impulse before the next sinus node impulse is discharged, thus interrupting the sinus rhythm. The premature beat will occur in addition to an underlying rhythm (usually sinus). PACs may originate from a single ectopic pacemaker site or from multiple sites in the atria. The early beat is characterized by a premature, abnormal (occasionally normal appearing) P wave; a premature QRS complex that's identical or similar to the QRS complex of the normally conducted beats; and is followed by a pause.

The shape of the P wave depends on the location of the ectopic pacemaker site. If the ectopic focus is in the vicinity of the SA node, the P wave may closely resemble the sinus P wave (Figure 7-4). Its sole distinguishing feature may be its prematurity. As a rule, however, the P wave is usually different from the sinus P waves. In lead II it's generally upright and pointed (Figure 7-8), or it may be inverted (Figure 7-5) if the pacemaker site is near the AV junction. If the premature beat occurs very early, the abnormal P wave can be found hidden in the preceding T wave, causing a distortion of the T-wave contour (Figure 7-6).

### Premature atrial contraction (PAC): Identifying ECG features

| | |
|---|---|
| **Rhythm:** | Underlying rhythm usually regular; irregular with PACs |
| **Rate:** | That of underlying rhythm |
| **P waves:** | P wave associated with PAC is premature and abnormal in size, shape, and direction (commonly appears small, upright, and pointed; may be inverted); abnormal P wave commonly found hidden in preceding T wave, distorting the T-wave contour |
| **PR interval:** | Usually normal but can be prolonged; not measurable if hidden in T wave |
| **QRS complex:** | Premature; normal duration (0.10 second or less) |

The PR intervals of the PACs are usually normal, similar to those of the underlying rhythm. Occasionally the PR interval is prolonged if there is a delay in conduction (Figure 7-7).The PR interval will be unmeasurable if the abnormal P wave is obscured in the preceding T wave.

The QRS complex of the PAC usually resembles that of the underlying rhythm because the impulse is conducted normally through the AV node with simultaneous depolarization of the bundle branches and ventricles. If the PAC occurs very early, the impulse may reach the bundle branches before repolarization is complete. The right bundle branch is usually slower to repolarize than the left. Therefore, the left bundle branch and left ventricle are depolarized before the right bundle branch and right ventricle (sequential de-

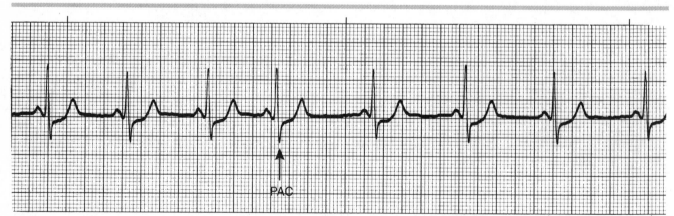

PAC

**Figure 7-4.    Normal sinus rhythm with premature atrial contraction**

| | |
|---|---|
| **Rhythm:** | Basic rhythm regular; irregular with PAC |
| **Rate:** | Basic rhythm rate 72 beats/minute; rate slows to 60 beats/minute following PAC (Temporary rate suppression is common following a pause in the basic rhythm; after several cardiac cycles the rate usually returns to the basic rhythm rate.) |
| **P waves:** | Sinus P waves with basic rhythm; P wave associated with PAC is premature and closely resembles that of the sinus P waves in the underlying rhythm, indicating the ectopic atrial pacemaker site is close to the SA node |
| **PR interval:** | 0.12 second (basic rhythm and PAC) |
| **QRS complex:** | 0.08 second (basic rhythm and PAC) |

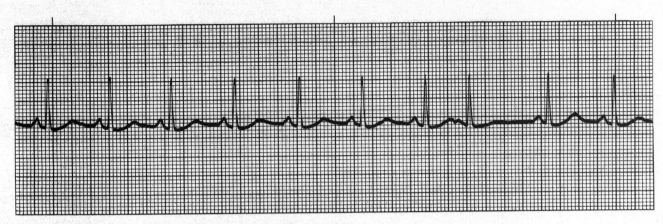

**Figure 7-5.**    **Normal sinus rhythm with premature atrial contraction**
**Rhythm:**        Basic rhythm regular; irregular with PAC
**Rate:**          Basic rhythm rate 88 beats/minute
**P waves:**       Sinus P waves with basic rhythm; premature, inverted P wave with PAC
**PR interval:**   0.14 to 0.16 second (basic rhythm); 0.14 second (PAC)
**QRS complex:**   0.04 to 0.06 second (basic rhythm); 0.06 second (PAC)

polarization). Because of this delay in ventricular depolarization the QRS complex will appear wide (0.12 second or greater). PACs associated with a wide QRS complex are called *aberrantly conducted PACs* (Figure 7-7), indicating that conduction through the ventricle is abnormal (aberrant). This wide complex must be differentiated from a premature ventricular contraction (PVC), especially if the abnormal P wave associated with the PAC is obscured in the preceding T wave. PVCs are discussed in Chapter 9.

The pause associated with the PAC is usually noncompensatory (the measurement from the R wave before the PAC to the R wave after the PAC is less than the sum of two R-R intervals of the underlying regular rhythm (Figure 7-8). This is because premature depolarization of the atria by the PAC results in subsequent premature depolarization of the sinus node, causing the sinus node to reset itself a little earlier than expected. Occasionally, the PAC will occur with a compensatory pause (a pause that is equal to the sum of two R-R intervals), but this is usually seen with the PVC. With the compensatory pause the SA node isn't depolarized by the PAC, its timing isn't reset, and the underlying rhythm

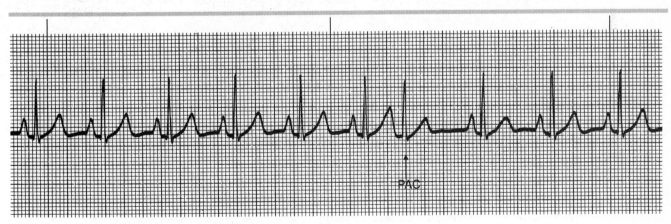

**Figure 7-6.**    **Normal sinus rhythm with premature atrial contraction**
**Rhythm:**        Basic rhythm regular; irregular with PAC
**Rate:**          Basic rhythm rate 84 beats/minute
**P waves:**       Sinus P waves with basic rhythm; premature, abnormal P wave with PAC (The P wave of the PAC is hidden in the preceding
                   T wave, distorting the T wave contour. [T wave is taller and more pointed.])
**PR interval:**   0.12 to 0.14 second (basic rhythm); not measurable with PAC
**QRS complex:**   0.06 to 0.08 second (basic rhythm); 0.06 second (PAC)

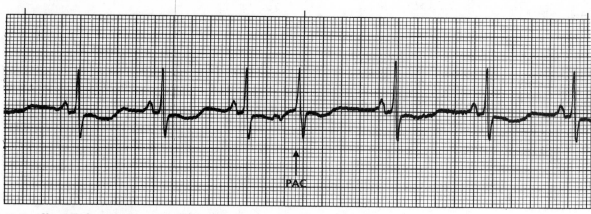

**Figure 7-7.    Normal sinus rhythm with 1 PAC with aberrant ventricular conduction**

**Rhythm:**       Basic rhythm regular; irregular with PAC
**Rate:**         Basic rhythm rate 68 beats/minute
**P waves:**      Sinus in basic rhythm; premature, abnormal P wave with PAC
**PR interval:**  0.16 to 0.18 second (basic rhythm); 0.24 second (PAC)
**QRS complex:**  0.08 second (basic rhythm); 0.12 second (PAC)

appears at the time expected after the pause. Rarely, the PAC may occur with a pause that's longer than compensatory.

PACs may appear as a single beat, every other beat (*bigeminal PACs,* Figure 7-9), every third beat (*trigeminal PACs*), every fourth beat (*quadrigeminal PACs*), in pairs (also called *couplets,* Figure 7-10), or in runs. When PACs occur in consecutive runs of three or more (at a rate of 140 to 250 beats/minute), atrial tachycardia is considered to be present. Frequent PACs may initiate more serious atrial arrhythmias,

such as paroxysmal atrial tachycardia, atrial flutter, or atrial fibrillation.

Premature atrial beats are common. They can occur in individuals with a normal heart or in those with heart disease. In healthy patients PACs are seen with emotional stress (which can increase sympathetic tone and catecholamine release), or ingestion of alcohol, caffeine, or nicotine. Other causes include hypoxia, myocardial ischemia, chronic lung disease, and the administration of sympathomimetics (such as epinephrine, isoproterenol, or theophylline). Be-

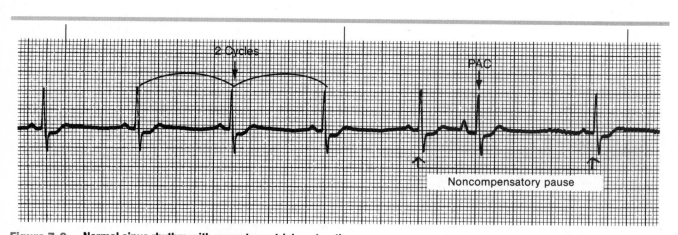

**Figure 7-8.    Normal sinus rhythm with premature atrial contraction**

**Rhythm:**       Basic rhythm regular; irregular with PAC
**Rate:**         Basic rhythm rate 60 beats/minute
**P waves:**      Sinus P waves with basic rhythm; premature, abnormal P wave with PAC
**PR interval:**  0.12 to 0.16 second (basic rhythm); 0.16 second (PAC)
**QRS complex:**  0.08 second (basic rhythm and PAC)
**Comment:**      To determine the type of pause after premature beats, measure from the QRS complex before the premature beat to the QRS complex after the premature beat. If the measurement equals two R-R intervals, the pause is compensatory. If the measurement equals less than two R-R intervals, the pause is noncompensatory. ST-segment depression is present.

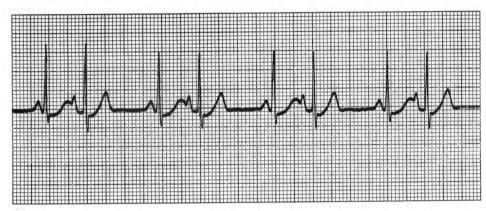

**Figure 7-9.** Bigeminal PACs.

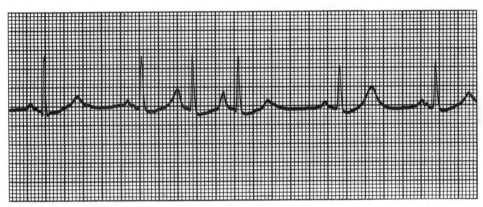

**Figure 7-10.** Paired PACs.

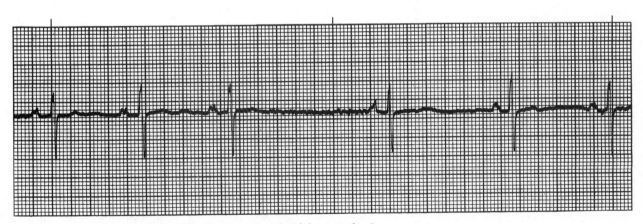

**Figure 7-11. Normal sinus rhythm with sinus arrest and atrial escape beat**

**Rhythm:** Basic rhythm regular; irregular during pause

**Rate:** Basic rhythm rate 63 beats/minute; rate slows to 58 beats/minute after pause due to temporary rate supression (common following pauses in the basic rhythm)

**P waves:** Sinus P waves; P waves are notched in basic rhythm which could be due to left atrial enlargement; peaked P wave with escape beat

**PR interval:** 0.18 to 0.20 second (basic rhythm and escape beat)

**QRS complex:** 0.08 second (basic rhythm); 0.06 second (escape beat)

cause PACs may also result from stretching of the myocardium, they can be a warning sign in the development of heart failure. PACs may also occur without apparent cause.

Infrequent PACs require no treatment. If treatment is needed, the best approach is to eliminate the cause (such as caffeine, alcohol, tobacco, or stress).

On some occasions an ectopic atrial beat will occur late instead of early. These beats are called *atrial escape beats* (Figure 7-11). Atrial escape beats occur when the sinus node slows down (increased vagal effect) or fails to initiate an impulse (sinus arrest), or if conduction of the sinus impulse is blocked for any reason (for example, because of sinus exit block, nonconducted PAC, or second-degree AV block, Mobitz I). This allows another pacemaker site in the atria to spontaneously produce electrical impulses and assume responsibility for pacing the heart. The morphologic characteristics of the late beat will be the same as the PAC. Escape beats are protective mechanisms to maintain the heart rate and require no treatment. It's important, however, to identify the cause of the initiating pause so that appropriate intervention can be started if necessary.

## Nonconducted PAC

A nonconducted PAC (Figures 7-12 through 7-14 and Box 7-3) results when an ectopic atrial focus occurs so early that it finds the AV node refractory and the impulse isn't conducted to the ventricles. This results in a premature, abnormal P wave not accompanied by a QRS complex, but followed by a pause (Figure 7-12).

Like the conducted PAC, the P wave associated with the nonconducted PAC will be premature and abnormal in size,

shape, or direction. The P wave is comonly found hidden in the preceding T waves, distorting the T-wave contour (Figure 7-13), and the pause that follows is usually noncompensatory. The nonconducted PAC is the most common cause of unexpected pauses in a regular sinus rhythm.

### Box 7-3.
### Nonconducted PACs: Identifying ECG features

| | |
|---|---|
| **Rhythm:** | Underlying rhythm usually regular; irregular with nonconducted PACs |
| **Rate:** | That of underlying rhythm |
| **P waves:** | P wave associated with the nonconducted PAC is premature, and abnormal in size, shape, or direction; often found hidden in preceding T wave, distorting the T wave contour |
| **PR interval:** | Absent with nonconducted PAC |
| **QRS complex:** | Absent with nonconducted PAC |

The nonconducted PAC can be confused with sinus arrest or block (especially if the P wave of the PAC occurs early enough to be hidden in the preceding T wave). All three produce a sudden pause in the rhythm without QRS complexes. To differentiate between these rhythms, one must examine and compare T-wave contours (Figure 7-14). The early P wave of the nonconducted PAC will distort the preceding T wave. In sinus arrest or sinus block, no P wave is produced and the T-wave contour remains unchanged.

Nonconducted PACs have the same significance as conducted PACs and may be treated in the same manner.

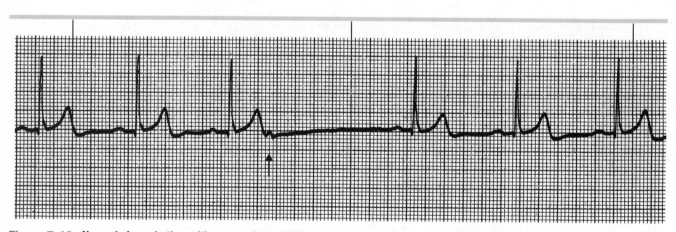

**Figure 7-12.  Normal sinus rhythm with nonconducted PAC**
**Rhythm:**        Basic rhythm regular; irregular with nonconducted PAC
**Rate:**          Basic rate 60 beats/minute; rate slows following nonconducted PAC (Rate suppression can occur following a pause in the basic rhythm; after several cycles, the rate will return to the basic rhythm rate.)
**P waves:**       Sinus P waves with basic rhythm; premature, abnormal P wave with nonconducted PAC
**PR interval:**   0.20 second
**QRS complex:**   0.06 to 0.08 second
**Comment:**       A U wave is present.

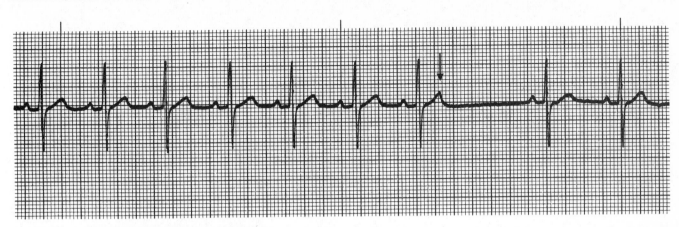

**Figure 7-13. Sinus rhythm with nonconducted PAC**

Rhythm:        Basic rhythm regular; irregular with nonconducted PACs
Rate:          Basic rhythm rate 88 beats/minute
P waves:       Sinus P waves with basic rhythm; P wave of nonconducted PAC is premature, abnormal, and hidden in the preceding T wave
               (T wave is taller and more pointed than those of underlying rhythm.)
PR interval:   0.16 to 0.18 second (basic rhythm); not present with nonconducted PAC
QRS complex:   0.06 to 0.08 second (basic rhythm); not present with nonconducted PAC

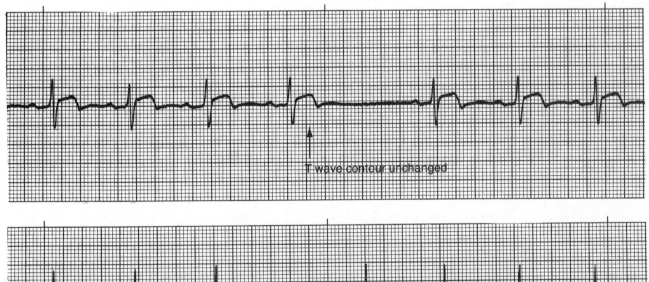

T wave contour unchanged

A

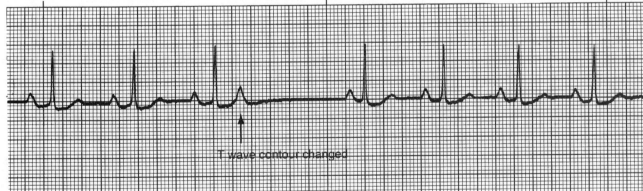

T wave contour changed

B

**Figure 7-14. Differentiation of sinus arrest or block from the nonconducted PAC**

**A  Sinus arrest or block**
1. Sudden pause in the basic rhythm
2. No P wave present
3. T-wave contour occurring during pause remains unchanged

**B  Nonconducted PAC**
1. Sudden pause in the basic rhythm
2. Abnormal, premature P wave present and often found hidden in T wave
3. T wave contour occurring during pause will be different from the contours of the basic rhythm

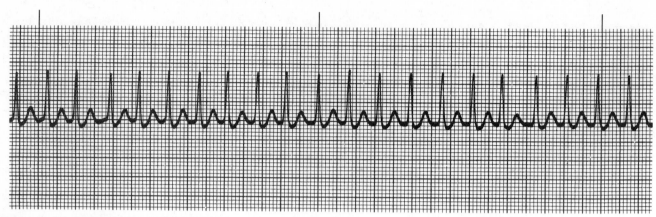

**Figure 7-15.** Paroxysmal atrial tachycardia
Rhythm:        Regular
Rate:          188 beats/minute
P waves:       Hidden
PR interval:   Not measurable
QRS complex:   0.06 to 0.08 second

## Paroxysmal atrial tachycardia

Paroxysmal atrial tachycardia (PAT) (Figures 7-15 and 7-16 and Box 7-4) originates in an ectopic pacemaker site in the atria producing a rapid, regular atrial rhythm between 140 and 250 beats/minute. Atrial tachycardia commonly starts and stops abruptly, occurring in bursts, or paroxysms (thus the name *paroxysmal atrial tachycardia*). PAT is commonly initiated by a PAC. By definition, three or more consecutive PACs (at a rate of 140 to 250 beats/minute) is considered to be atrial tachycardia (Figure 7-16).

The P waves associated with atrial tachycardia are abnormal (commonly pointed), but may be difficult to identify because they're usually hidden in the preceding T wave (the T wave and P wave appear as one deflection called the *T-P wave*). One P wave precedes each QRS complex, unless AV block is present. The PR interval isn't measurable if the P waves are hidden. The duration of the QRS complex is normal.

Atrial tachycardia may occur in persons with healthy hearts as well as those with diseased hearts. As with PACs, atrial tachycardia can be associated with emotional stress

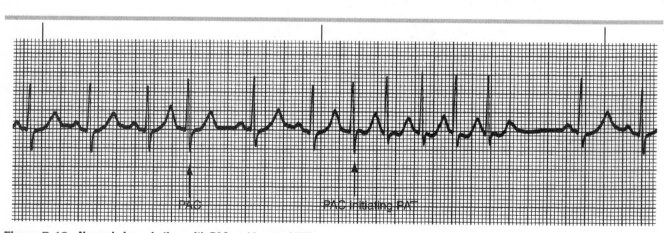

**Figure 7-16.  Normal sinus rhythm with PAC and burst of PAT**
Rhythm:        Basic rhythm regular; irregular with PAC and burst of PAT
Rate:          Basic rhythm rate 94 beats/minute; PAT rate 167 beats/minute
P waves:       Sinus P waves with basic rhythm; premature, pointed P waves with PAC and PAT (P waves are superimposed on preceding
               T waves.)
PR interval:   0.16 second
QRS complex:   0.08 second
Comment:       A run of three or more consecutive PACs is considered PAT.

and ingestion of caffeine, tobacco, or alcohol. Other causes include COPD and digitalis toxicity.

## Box 7-4.
## Atrial tachycardia: identifying ECG features

| | |
|---|---|
| **Rhythm:** | Regular |
| **Rate:** | 140 to 250 beats/minute |
| **P waves:** | Abnormal (commonly pointed); usually hidden in preceding T wave, making T wave and P wave appear as one wave deflection (T-P wave); one P wave to each QRS complex unless AV block is present |
| **PR interval:** | Usually not measurable |
| **QRS complex:** | Normal (0.10 second or less) |

During an episode of PAT many individuals can feel the rapid heart rate (palpitations), and this is a source of nervousness and anxiety. When the ventricular rate is rapid the ventricles are unable to fill completely during diastole, resulting in a significant reduction in cardiac output. In addition, a rapid heart rate increases myocardial oxygen requirements and cardiac workload. Treatment of atrial tachycardia is directed toward controlling the ventricular rate and converting the rhythm.

Priorities of treatment depend on the patient's tolerance of the rhythm. Electrical cardioversion is the initial treatment of choice in patients whose condition is hemodynamically unstable. If the patient's condition is hemodynamically stable (systolic blood pressure 90 mm Hg or above, normal level of consciousness, skin warm and dry, and free from chest pain, dyspnea, and signs of heart failure) try sedation first. In addition to relieving the anxiety that commonly accompanies tachyarrhythmias, sedation can reduce sympathetic tone and might convert the arrhythmia to a sinus rhythm. If sedation doesn't convert the rhythm, vagal maneuvers should be tried next. Vagal maneuvers work by slowing the heart rate through increasing parasympathetic tone. The most common of these measures include carotid sinus massage and the Valsalva maneuver ("bearing down"). If vagal maneuvers fail, administer a 6-mg bolus of I.V. adenosine rapidly over 1 to 2 seconds, followed by a rapid 20-ml flush of saline or plain I.V. fluid. If the initial dose is ineffective after 2 minutes, administer a 12-mg bolus of I.V. adenosine rapidly over 1 to 2 seconds, followed by a rapid 20-ml flush of saline or plain I.V. fluid. If the second dose is ineffective after 2 minutes, repeat a 12-mg dose of adenosine in the same manner.

If the patient doesn't respond to vagal maneuvers or the administration of adenosine, attempt rate control first using a calcium channel blocker, such as diltiazem, or a beta blocker. These drugs act primarily on nodal tissue either to slow the ventricular response by blocking conduction through the AV node or to terminate the reentry mechanism that depends on conduction through the AV node. In the setting of significantly impaired left ventricular (LV) function (clinical evidence of congestive heart failure or moderately to severly reduced LV ejection fraction), caution should be exercised in administering drugs with negative inotropic effects. These include beta-blockers and calcium channel blockers with the exception of diltiazem, a calcium channel blocker that exhibits less depression of contractility when compared with similar drugs.

When AV nodal agents are unsuccessful in terminating the rhythm, strong consideration should be given to electrical cardioversion. If electrical cardioversion is not feasible, or is unsuccessful, the rhythm may be treated with an antiarrhythmic such as amiodarone. Radiofrequency catheter ablation of the ectopic focus or reentry circuit may be necessary for recurrent PAT unresponsive to oral therapy.

## Atrial flutter

Atrial flutter (Figures 7-17 through 7-19 and Box 7-5) originates in an ectopic pacemaker site in the atria typically depolarizing at a rate between 250 and 400 beats/minute. The atrial muscles respond to this rapid stimulation by producing waveforms that resemble the teeth of a saw. The sawtooth deflections are called *flutter waves* (*F waves*). The typical atrial flutter wave consists of an initial negative component followed by a positive component producing V-shaped waveforms with a sawtooth appearance. The sawtooth waves affect the whole baseline to such a degree that there is no isoelectric line between the F waves, and the T wave is partially or completely obscured by the flutter waves. Atrial flutter is primarily recognized by this sawtooth baseline. The QRS complexes are usually narrow as long as conduction through the ventricles is normal.

The AV node is bombarded by the rapid atrial impulses but will only conduct some impulses to the ventricles. Usually, the AV node blocks at least half of the impulses to protect the ventricles from excessive rates. The AV node conducts the impulses in various ratios. For example, the AV node might allow every second impulse to travel through the AV junction to the ventricles, resulting in a 2:1 AV conduction ratio (a 2:1 conduction ratio indicates that for every two flutter waves, only one is followed by a QRS complex). Even ratios (2:1, 4:1) are more common than odd ratios (3:1, 5:1). If the conduction ratio remains constant (for example, 2:1), the ventricular rhythm will be regular, and the rhythm is described as atrial flutter with 2:1 AV conduction. If the conduction ratio varies (from 4:1 to 2:1 to 6:1, for example), the ventricular rhythm will be irregular, and the rhythm is described as atrial flutter with variable AV conduction. In atrial flutter the ventricular rate is slower than the atrial rate, with the rate depending on the number of impulses conducted through the AV node to the ventricles.

Because atrial flutter usually occurs at a rate of 300 beats/minute and the AV node usually blocks at least half of these impulses, a ventricular rate of 150 beats/minute is common

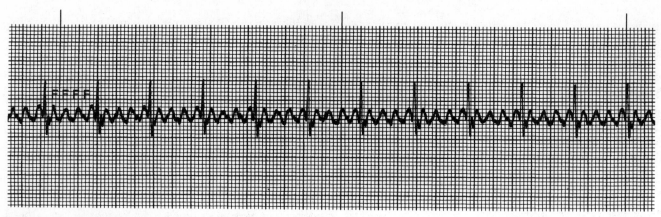

**Figure 7-17. Atrial flutter with 4:1 AV conduction**

| | |
|---|---|
| Rhythm: | Regular |
| Rate: | Atrial: 428 beats/minute |
| | Ventricular: 107 beats/minute |
| | *Note:* If the ventricular rate is regular, multiply the number of flutter waves before each QRS × the ventricular rate to determine atrial rate. |
| P waves: | Four flutter waves before each QRS (marked as F waves above) |
| PR interval: | Not measurable |
| QRS complex: | 0.06 to 0.08 second |

(a 2:1 conduction ratio). Atrial flutter, with a ventricular rate of 150 beats per minute, can be difficult to differentiate from atrial tachycardia with a ventricular rate of 150 beats/minute. These two arrhythmias can be differentiated by closely examining the baseline. In atrial tachycardia an isoelectric line can usually be seen, whereas in atrial flutter the isoelectric line is absent.

**Box 7-5.**
## Atrial flutter: Identifying ECG features

| | |
|---|---|
| Rhythm: | Regular or irregular (depends on AV conduction ratios) |
| Rate: | Atrial rate: 250 to 400 beats/minute |
| | Ventricular rate: Varies with number of impulses conducted through AV node (will be less than the atrial rate) |
| P waves: | Sawtooth deflections called flutter waves (F waves) affecting entire baseline |
| PR interval: | Not measurable |
| QRS complex: | Normal (0.10 second or less) |

Atrial flutter is rarely seen in people with a normal heart. Atrial flutter can be observed in patients with valvular heart disease, hypertensive heart disease, cardiomyopathy, heart failure, chronic lung disease, and pulmonary emboli. This arrhythmia is common after cardiac surgery.

Like PAT, the ventricular rate in atrial flutter may be rapid, increasing myocardial oxygen requirements and cardiac workload and decreasing cardiac output. In addition, the rapidly contracting atria don't contract strongly enough to empty all their contents. This results not only in a loss of the "atrial kick" but also in a stasis of blood, which may form clots in the atria (mural thrombi), leading to a risk of arterial or pulmonary emboli.

Priorities of treatment include controlling the ventricular rate, assessing anticoagulation needs, and restoring sinus rhythm. As with atrial tachycardia, controlling the ventricular rate should be attempted first using a calcium channel blocker, such as diltiazem, or a beta-blocker, using caution in those patients with impaired left ventricular function. Before attempting conversion of the rhythm it's essential to know the approximate onset of the arrhythmia. If atrial flutter has been present for less than 48 hours, it's safe to convert the rhythm with electrical cardioversion or amiodarone. If atrial flutter has been present for more than 48 hours (or the onset is unknown), systemic embolization with conversion to sinus rhythm is a risk, unless the patient has been adequately anticoagulated. In this situation attempts to convert the rhythm with cardioversion or an antiarrhythmic should be delayed until the patient is adequately anticoagulated.

One method of anticoagulation involves placing the patient on an oral anticoagulant for 3 weeks, cardioverting the rhythm, and having the patient take an oral anticoagulant for an additional 4 weeks. Some physicians prefer a more aggressive approach, using I.V. heparin or subcutaneous lovenox, use of transesophageal echocardiography to rule out mural thrombi, and cardioversion within 24 hours, followed by anticoagulants for 4 more weeks.

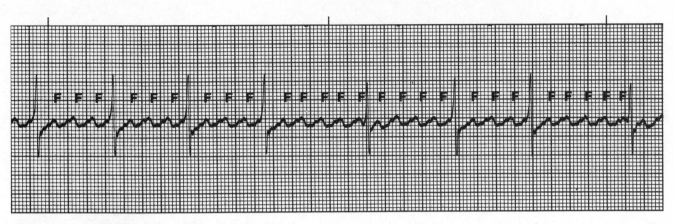

**Figure 7-18. Atrial flutter with variable AV conduction**

| | |
|---|---|
| **Rhythm:** | Irregular |
| **Rate:** | Atrial: 250 beats/minute |
| | Ventricular: 60 beats/minute |
| | *Note:* If the ventricular rate is irregular, count the number of flutter waves in a 6-second strip and multiply × 10 to obtain atrial rate. |
| **P waves:** | Flutter waves before each QRS (varying ratios) |
| **PR interval:** | Not measurable |
| **QRS complex:** | 0.08 second |

Hemodynamically unstable, rapid atrial flutter should immediately be treated with cardioversion, regardless of the duration of the arrhythmia. Figure 7-19 is an example of atrial flutter converting to sinus rhythm after electrical shock (cardioversion).

Radiofrequency catheter ablation of the ectopic atrial focus or reentry circuit may be a treatment option for chronic or recurrent atrial flutter.

## Atrial fibrillation

Atrial fibrillation (Figures 7-20 through 7-22 and Box 7-6) arises from an ectopic pacemaker site in the atria, depolar-izing at a rate greater than 400 beats/minute. These impulses are so rapid that they cause the atria to quiver instead of contract regularly, producing irregular, wavy deflections. These wavy deflections are called *fibrillatory waves* (*f waves*). If the waves are large, they're described as *coarse fibrillatory waves*. If the waves are small, they're described as *fine fibrillatory waves*. Sometimes the f waves are so small (Figure 7-22) that they appear to be almost a flat line between the QRS complexes. As in atrial flutter, the wavy deflections seen in atrial fibrillation affect the whole baseline. Flutter waves are sometimes seen mixed with the fibrillatory waves. This mixed rhythm is commonly called *fib-flutter*. The QRS complexes are usually narrow as long as conduction through

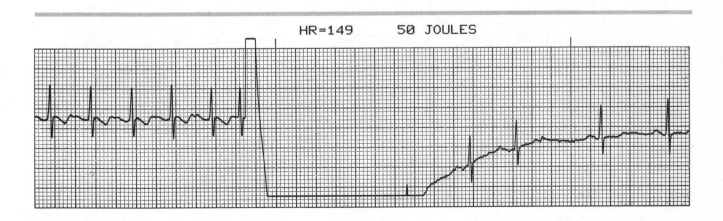

**Figure 7-19.** Cardioversion of atrial flutter with 2:1 atrioventricular conduction to normal sinus rhythm using 50 joules electrical energy.

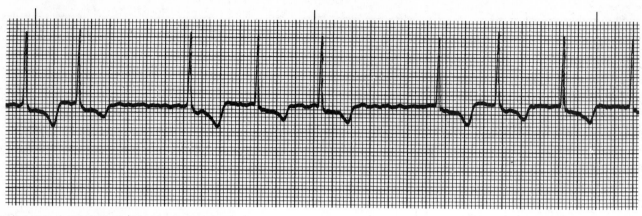

**Figure 7-20. Atrial fibrillation (Controlled rate)**

| | |
|---|---|
| Rhythm: | Irregular |
| Rate: | Ventricular rate 70 beats/minute |
| P waves: | Fibrillatory waves present |
| PR interval: | Not measurable |
| QRS complex: | 0.04 to 0.06 second |
| Comment: | ST segment depression and T wave inversion are present. |

the ventricles is normal. As in atrial flutter the AV node is being bombarded by these rapid atrial impulses, but the AV node (the "gatekeeper" of the ventricles) blocks most of the impulses to protect the ventricles from excessive rates. Characteristically, the ventricular rate is grossly irregular because the AV junction is being stimulated in an apparently random fashion by the rapidly fibrillating atria. The ventricular rate is slower than the atrial rate and depends on the number of impulses conducted through the AV node to the ventricles. When the ventricular rate is less than 100 beats/minute, the rhythm is called *controlled atrial fibrillation*. When the ventricular rate is greater than 100 beats/

minute, the rhythm is called *uncontrolled atrial fibrillation*, or *atrial fibrillation with a rapid ventricular response*. Atrial fibrillation is primarily recognized by the wavy baseline and the grossly irregular ventricular rhythm (Figure 7-20) — that is, unless the ventricular rate is rapid, in which case the rhythm becomes more regular (Figure 7-21).

Atrial fibrillation is the most common rhythm next to sinus rhythm. Atrial fibrillation can occur in normal individuals or in those with heart disease. In normal individuals the rhythm is usually temporary and may be associated with emotional stress or excessive alcohol consumption ("holiday heart syndrome"). In many patients this type of atrial

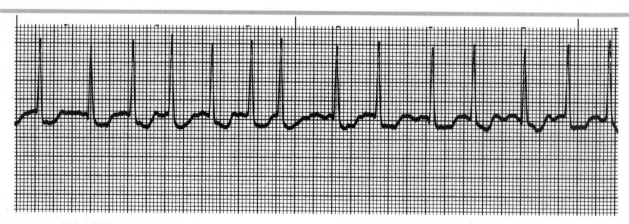

**Figure 7-21. Atrial fibrillation (Uncontrolled rate)**

| | |
|---|---|
| Rhythm: | Irregular |
| Rate: | Ventricular rate 130 beats/minute |
| P waves: | Fibrillatory waves present |
| PR interval: | Not measurable |
| QRS complex: | 0.06 to 0.08 second |
| Comment: | ST segment depression is present. |

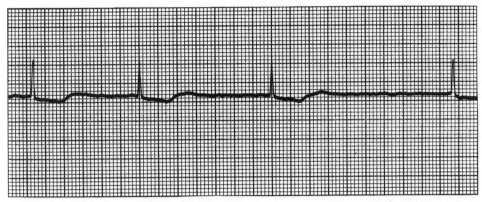

**Figure 7-22.** Atrial fibrillation with f waves so small they appear to be almost a flat line beteen QRS complexes.

fibrillation spontaneously reverts to sinus rhythm or is easily converted with drug therapy alone. In other individuals the rhythm is chronic and may persist indefinitely. Chronic atrial fibrillation is commonly caused by valvular heart disease, particularly when the mitral valve is involved. Other conditions associated with atrial fibrillation include hypertensive heart disease, coronary artery disease, pulmonary emboli, and hyperthyroidism. Atrial fibrillation is common after cardiac surgery.

The clinical consequences of atrial fibrillation are similar to those of atrial flutter. The ventricular rate may be rapid, increasing myocardial oxygen demands and cardiac workload and decreasing cardiac output. With atrial fibrillation, normal atrial depolarization is lost and the atria fibrillate (quiver) instead of contracting synchronously. In this circumstance, the normal "atrial kick" is lost, further compromising cardiac output. Decreased cardiac output is especially marked in patients with underlying cardiac impairment and in the elderly, who appear to be more dependent on atrial contraction for filling of the ventricles. Thus, decreased cardiac output in atrial fibrillation is related to the rapid ventricular rate as well as to the loss of the "atrial kick."

The noncontracting atria also tend to pool blood in the atrial chamber, increasing the potential for thrombus formation. These clots (mural thrombi) may dislodge into the pulmonary circulation and cause pulmonary emboli, or enter the arterial circulation and cause a stroke or an occlusion of the blood supply to the legs, intestines, or kidneys.

Treatment of atrial fibrillation includes controlling the heart rate, providing anticoagulation as a prophylaxis for thromboembolism, and returning the atria to a sinus rhythm. The treatment protocols for atrial fibrillation are the same as those for atrial flutter. Rate control should be achieved first, using a calcium channel blocker, such as diltiazem, or a beta-blocker, using caution in those patients with impaired left ventricular function. After rate control, electrical cardioversion or an antiarrhythmic such as amiodarone can be used in an attempt to restore the rhythm to a sinus rhythm if the atrial fibrillation is less than 48 hours old. If atrial fibrillation has been present for more than 48 hours, the patient must be adequately anticoagulated (refer to anticoagulation protocols for atrial flutter) before attempts to restore sinus rhythm using electrical cardioversion or an antiarrhythmic. Hemodynamically unstable atrial fibrillation should be electrically cardioverted immediately, regardless of the duration of the arrhythmia. Patients with chronic atrial fibrillation (present for months or years) may not convert to sinus rhythm with any therapy. Treatment of these patients should be directed at controlling the ventricular rate and providing anticoagulation.

A summary of the identifying ECG features of atrial arrhythmias can be found in Table 7-1.

## Box 7-6.
## Atrial fibrillation: Identifying ECG features

| | |
|---|---|
| **Rhythm:** | Grossly irregular (unless the ventricular rate is very rapid, in which case the rhythm becomes more regular) |
| **Rate:** | Atrial rate: 400 beats/minute or more; not measurable on surface ECG<br>Ventricular rate: Varies with number of impulses conducted through AV node to the ventricles (will be less than the atrial rate) |
| **P waves:** | Irregular wave deflections called fibrillatory waves (f waves) affecting entire baseline |
| **PR interval:** | Not measurable |
| **QRS complex:** | Normal (0.10 second or less) |

**Table 7-1.**

## Atrial arrhythmias: Summary of identifying ECG features

| Name | Rhythm | Rate (beats/minute) | P waves (lead II) | PR interval | QRS complex |
|---|---|---|---|---|---|
| Wandering atrial pacemaker | Regular or irregular | Normal (60 to 100) or slow (< 60) | Vary in size, shape, and direction; one P wave precedes each QRS complex | Usually normal duration, but may vary depending on changing pacemaker location | Normal (0.10 second or less) |
| Premature atrial pacemaker | Basic rhythm usually regular; irregular with premature atrial contraction (PAC) | That of basic rhythm | P wave associated with PAC is premature and abnormal in size, shape, or direction (commonly small, upright, and pointed; may be inverted); commonly found hidden in preceding T wave, distorting T-wave contour | Usually normal, but may be prolonged; not measurable if hidden in preceding T wave | Premature; normal duration (0.10 second or less) |
| Nonconducted premature atrial contraction | Basic rhythm usually regular; irregular with nonconducted PAC | That of basic rhythm | Premature P wave that is abnormal in size, shape, or direction; commonly found in preceding T wave, distorting T-wave contour | Absent with nonconducted PAC | Absent with nonconducted PAC |
| Paroxysmal atrial tachycardia (PAT) | Regular | 140 to 250 | Abnormal P wave (commonly pointed); usually hidden in preceding T wave so that T and P wave appear as one wave deflection (T-P wave); one P wave to each QRS complex unless AV block is present | Usually not measurable | Normal (0.10 second or less) |
| Atrial flutter | Regular or irregular (depends on atrioventricular [AV] conduction ratios) | Atrial: 250 to 400 Ventricular: varies with number of impulses conducted through AV node (will be less than atrial rate) | Sawtooth deflections affecting entire baseline | Not measurable | Normal (0.10 second or less) |
| Atrial fibrillation | Grossly irregular (unless ventricular rate is rapid, in which case rhythm becomes more regular) | Atrial: 400 or more (can't be counted) Ventricular: varies with number of impulses conducted through AV node (will be less than atrial rate; controlled if rate < 100, uncontrolled if > 100) | Wavy deflections affecting entire baseline | Not measurable | Normal (0.10 second or less) |

# Rhythm strip practice: Atrial arrhythmias

For each of the following rhythm strips:
- determine the rhythm regularity, the ventricular rate, and the atrial rate (that is, if it differs from the ventricular rate)
- identify and examine P waves
- measure the duration of the PR interval and the QRS complex
- interpret the rhythm.

All rhythm strips are lead II unless otherwise noted. Check your answers with the answer key in the appendix.

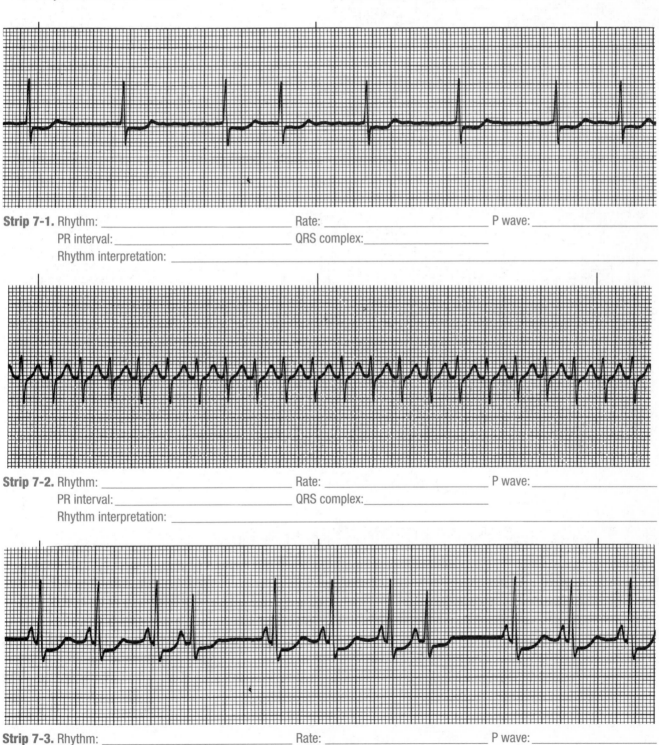

**Strip 7-1.** Rhythm: _____ Rate: _____ P wave: _____

PR interval: _____ QRS complex: _____

Rhythm interpretation: _____

**Strip 7-2.** Rhythm: _____ Rate: _____ P wave: _____

PR interval: _____ QRS complex: _____

Rhythm interpretation: _____

**Strip 7-3.** Rhythm: _____ Rate: _____ P wave: _____

PR interval: _____ QRS complex: _____

Rhythm interpretation: _____

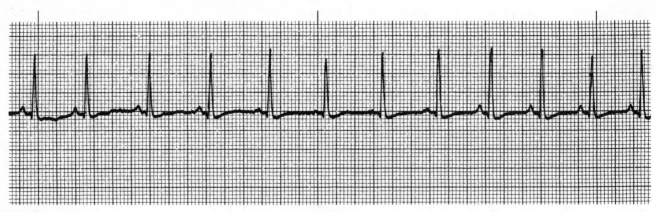

**Strip 7-4.** Rhythm: _____ Rate: _____ P wave: _____

PR interval: _____ QRS complex: _____

Rhythm interpretation: _____

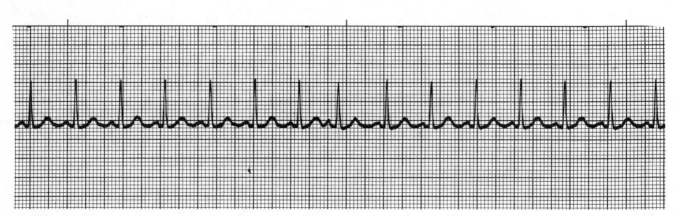

**Strip 7-5.** Rhythm: _____ Rate: _____ P wave: _____

PR interval: _____ QRS complex: _____

Rhythm interpretation: _____

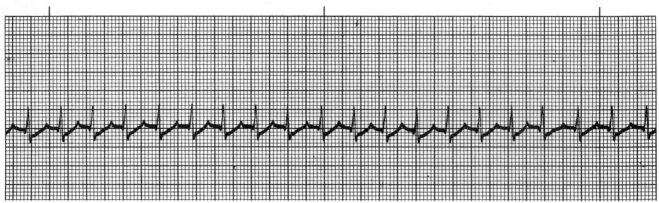

**Strip 7-6.** Rhythm: _____ Rate: _____ P wave: _____

PR interval: _____ QRS complex: _____

Rhythm interpretion: _____

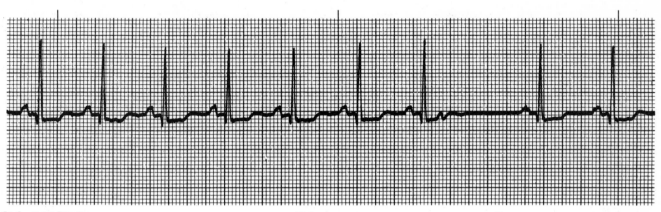

**Strip 7-7.** Rhythm: _____ Rate: _____ P wave: _____

PR interval: _____ QRS complex: _____

Rhythm interpretation: _____

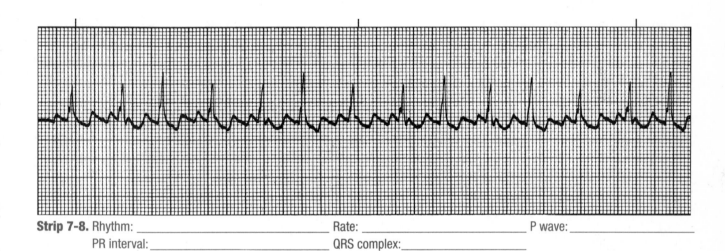

**Strip 7-8.** Rhythm: _____ Rate: _____ P wave: _____

PR interval: _____ QRS complex: _____

Rhythm interpretation: _____

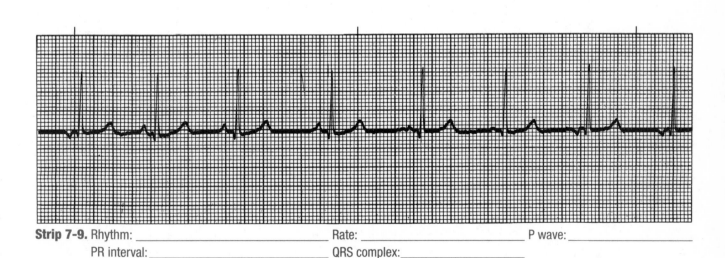

**Strip 7-9.** Rhythm: _____ Rate: _____ P wave: _____

PR interval: _____ QRS complex: _____

Rhythm interpretation: _____

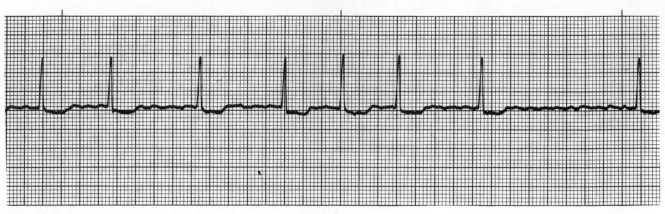

**Strip 7-10.** Rhythm:_____ Rate:_____ P wave:_____
PR interval:_____ QRS complex:_____
Rhythm interpretation:_____

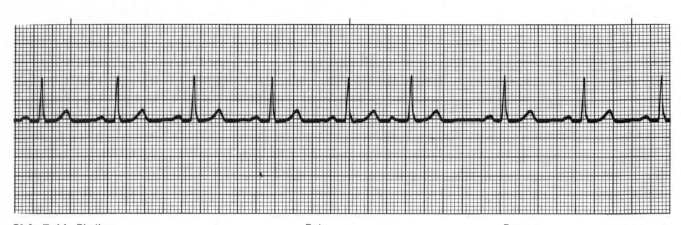

**Strip 7-11.** Rhythm:_____ Rate:_____ P wave:_____
PR interval:_____ QRS complex:_____
Rhythm interpretation:_____

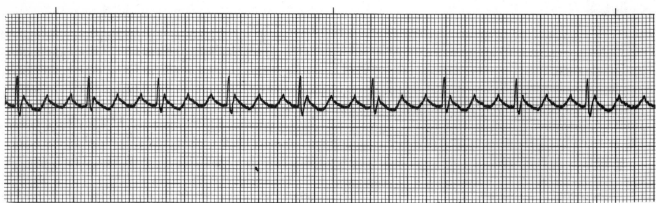

**Strip 7-12.** Rhythm:_____ Rate:_____ P wave:_____
PR interval:_____ QRS complex:_____
Rhythm interpretation:_____

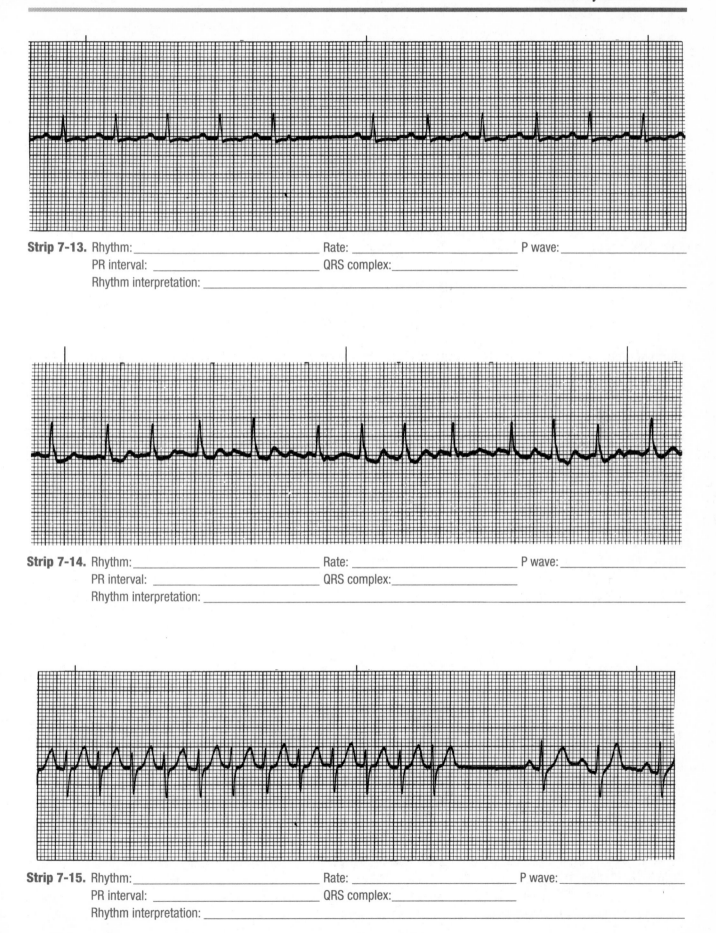

**Strip 7-13.** Rhythm:_____ Rate:_____ P wave:_____

PR interval:_____ QRS complex:_____

Rhythm interpretation:_____

**Strip 7-14.** Rhythm:_____ Rate:_____ P wave:_____

PR interval:_____ QRS complex:_____

Rhythm interpretation:_____

**Strip 7-15.** Rhythm:_____ Rate:_____ P wave:_____

PR interval:_____ QRS complex:_____

Rhythm interpretation:_____

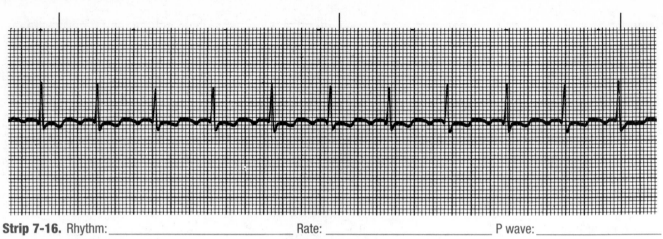

**Strip 7-16.** Rhythm:_____ Rate:_____ P wave:_____

PR interval:_____ QRS complex:_____

Rhythm interpretation:_____

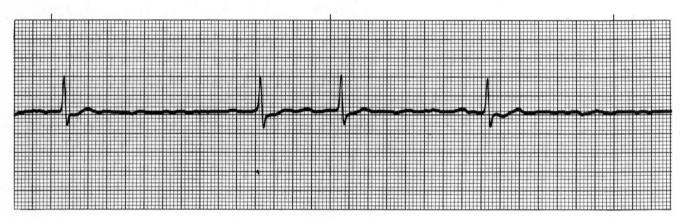

**Strip 7-17.** Rhythm:_____ Rate:_____ P wave:_____

PR interval:_____ QRS complex:_____

Rhythm interpretation:_____

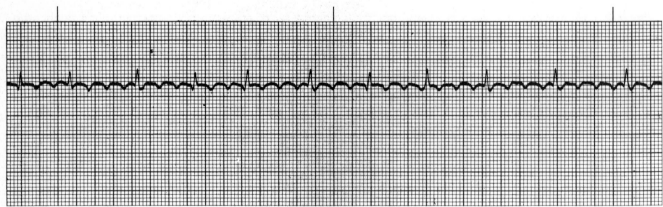

**Strip 7-18.** Rhythm:_____ Rate:_____ P wave:_____

PR interval:_____ QRS complex:_____

Rhythm interpretation:_____

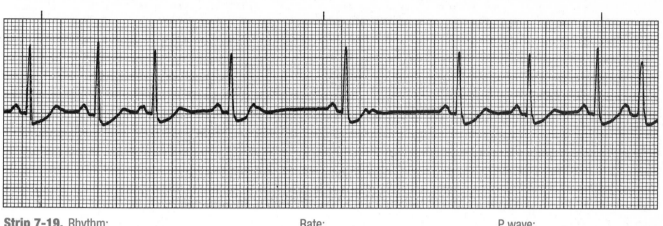

**Strip 7-19.** Rhythm:_____ Rate: _____ P wave:_____
PR interval: _____ QRS complex:_____
Rhythm interpretation: _____

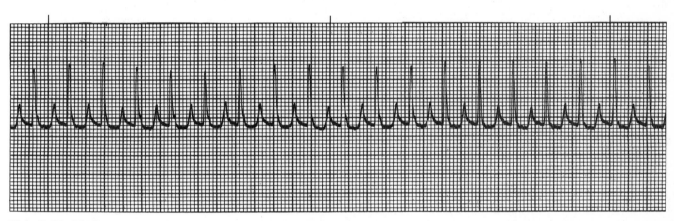

**Strip 7-20.** Rhythm:_____ Rate: _____ P wave:_____
PR interval: _____ QRS complex:_____
Rhythm interpretation: _____

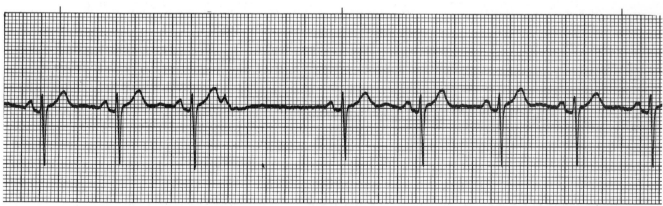

**Strip 7-21.** Rhythm:_____ Rate: _____ P wave:_____
PR interval: _____ QRS complex:_____
Rhythm interpretation: _____

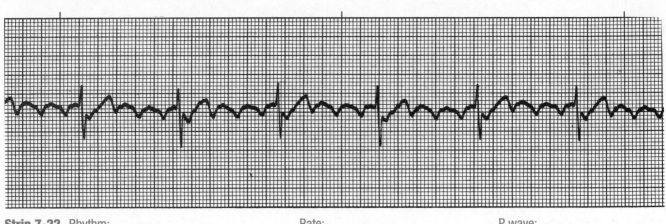

**Strip 7-22.** Rhythm:_____ Rate: _____ P wave:_____

PR interval: _____ QRS complex:_____

Rhythm interpretation: _____

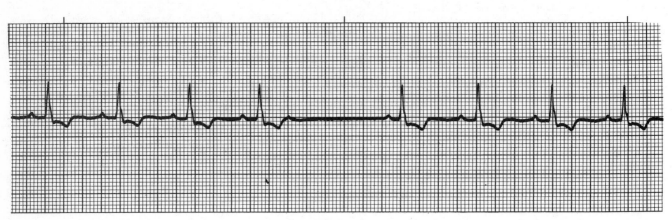

**Strip 7-23.** Rhythm:_____ Rate: _____ P wave:_____

PR interval: _____ QRS complex:_____

Rhythm interpretation: _____

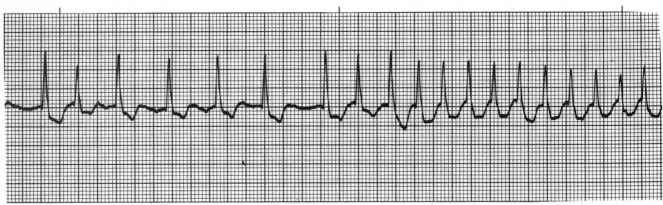

**Strip 7-24.** Rhythm:_____ Rate: _____ P wave:_____

PR interval: _____ QRS complex:_____

Rhythm interpretation: _____

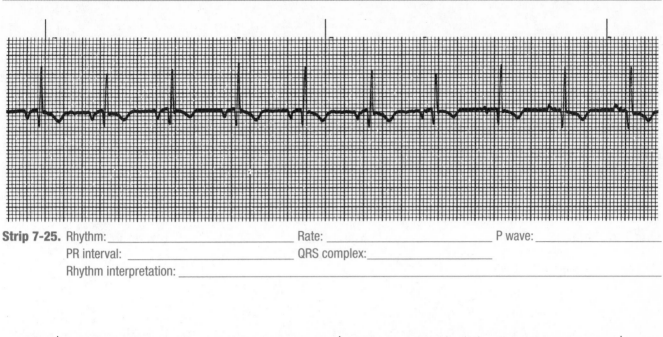

**Strip 7-25.** Rhythm:_____ Rate:_____ P wave:_____
PR interval:_____ QRS complex:_____
Rhythm interpretation:_____

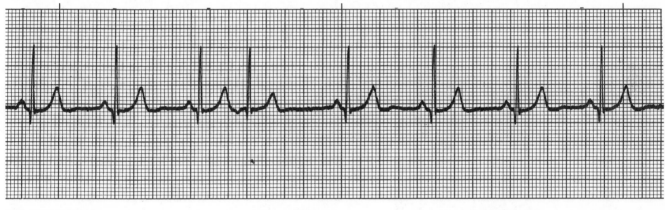

**Strip 7-26.** Rhythm:_____ Rate:_____ P wave:_____
PR interval:_____ QRS complex:_____
Rhythm interpretation:_____

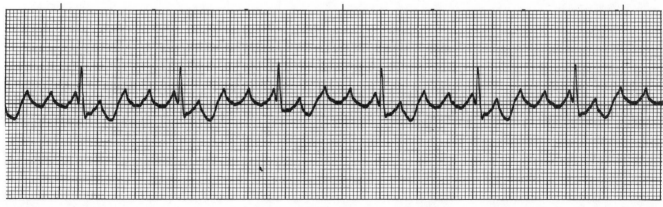

**Strip 7-27.** Rhythm:_____ Rate:_____ P wave:_____
PR interval:_____ QRS complex:_____
Rhythm interpretation:_____

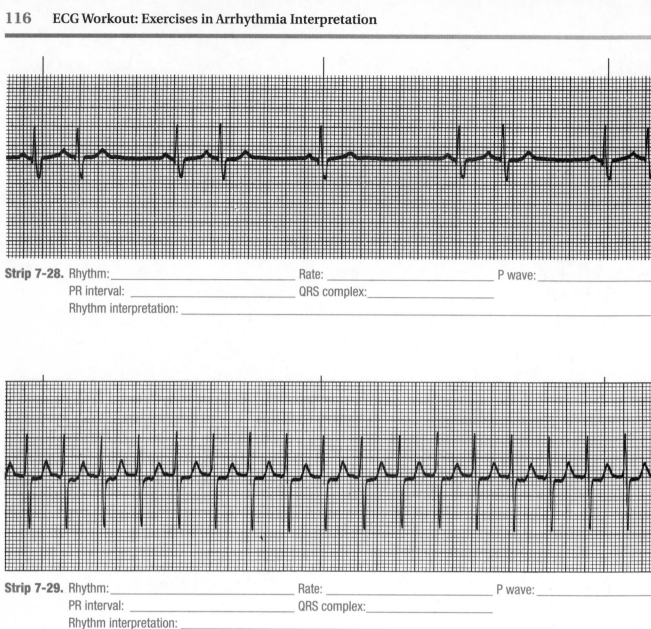

**Strip 7-28.** Rhythm:_____ Rate:_____ P wave:_____

PR interval:_____ QRS complex:_____

Rhythm interpretation:_____

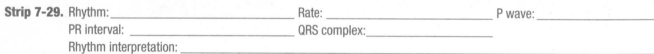

**Strip 7-29.** Rhythm:_____ Rate:_____ P wave:_____

PR interval:_____ QRS complex:_____

Rhythm interpretation:_____

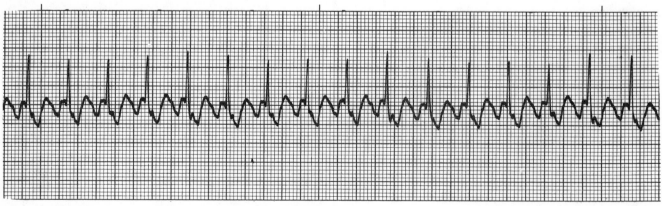

**Strip 7-30.** Rhythm:_____ Rate:_____ P wave:_____

PR interval:_____ QRS complex:_____

Rhythm interpretation:_____

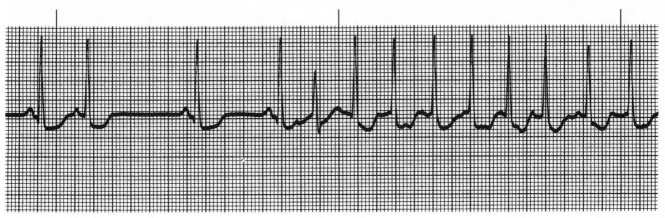

**Strip 7-31.** Rhythm:_____ Rate:_____ P wave:_____

PR interval:_____ QRS complex:_____

Rhythm interpretation:_____

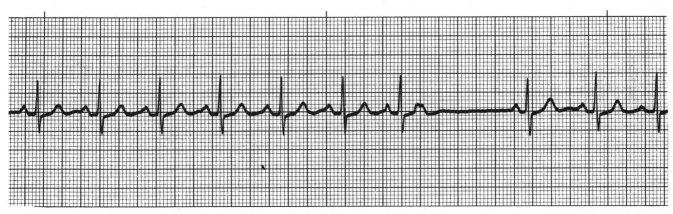

**Strip 7-32.** Rhythm:_____ Rate:_____ P wave:_____

PR interval:_____ QRS complex:_____

Rhythm interpretation:_____

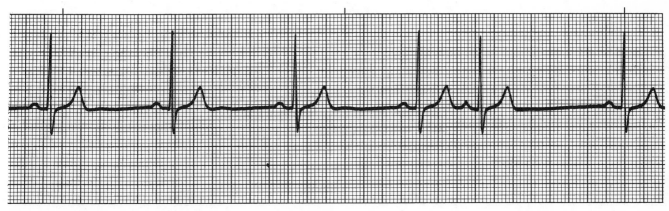

**Strip 7-33.** Rhythm:_____ Rate:_____ P wave:_____

PR interval:_____ QRS complex:_____

Rhythm interpretation:_____

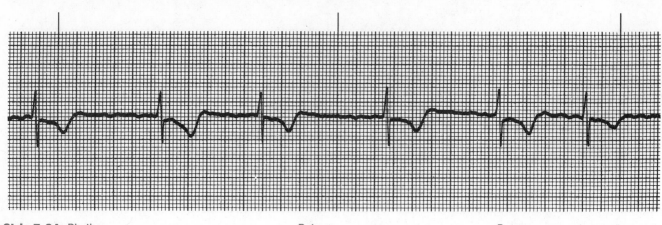

**Strip 7-34.** Rhythm: _____ Rate: _____ P wave: _____

PR interval: _____ QRS complex: _____

Rhythm interpretation: _____

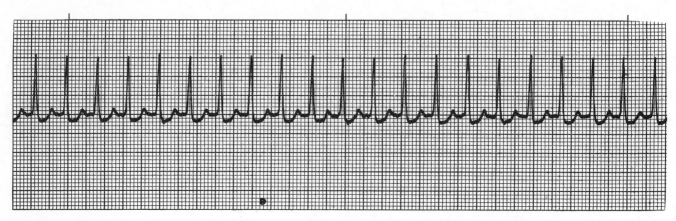

**Strip 7-35.** Rhythm: _____ Rate: _____ P wave: _____

PR interval: _____ QRS complex: _____

Rhythm interpretation: _____

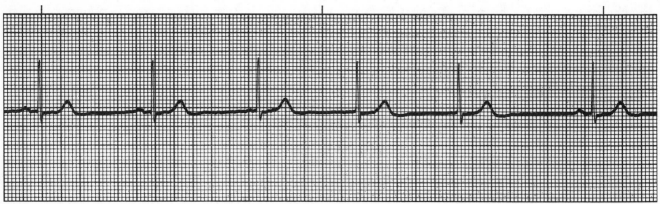

**Strip 7-36.** Rhythm: _____ Rate: _____ P wave: _____

PR interval: _____ QRS complex: _____

Rhythm interpretation: _____

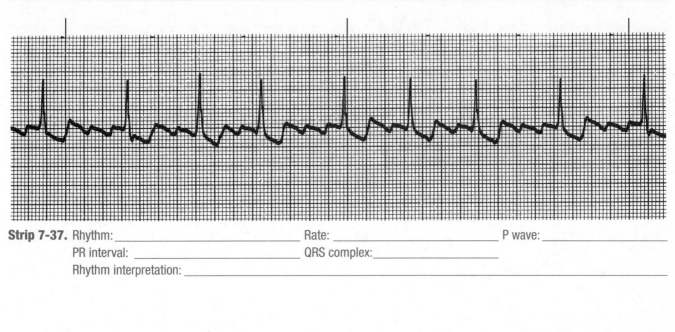

**Strip 7-37.** Rhythm:_____ Rate:_____ P wave:_____

PR interval:_____ QRS complex:_____

Rhythm interpretation:_____

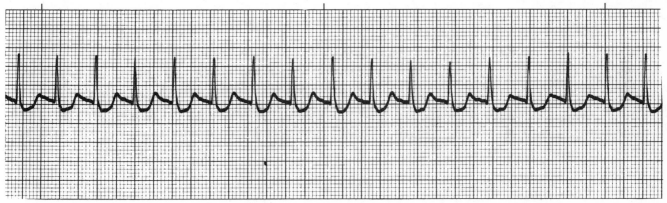

**Strip 7-38.** Rhythm:_____ Rate:_____ P wave:_____

PR interval:_____ QRS complex:_____

Rhythm interpretation:_____

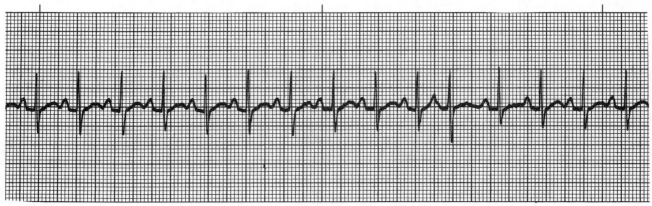

**Strip 7-39.** Rhythm:_____ Rate:_____ P wave:_____

PR interval:_____ QRS complex:_____

Rhythm interpretation:_____

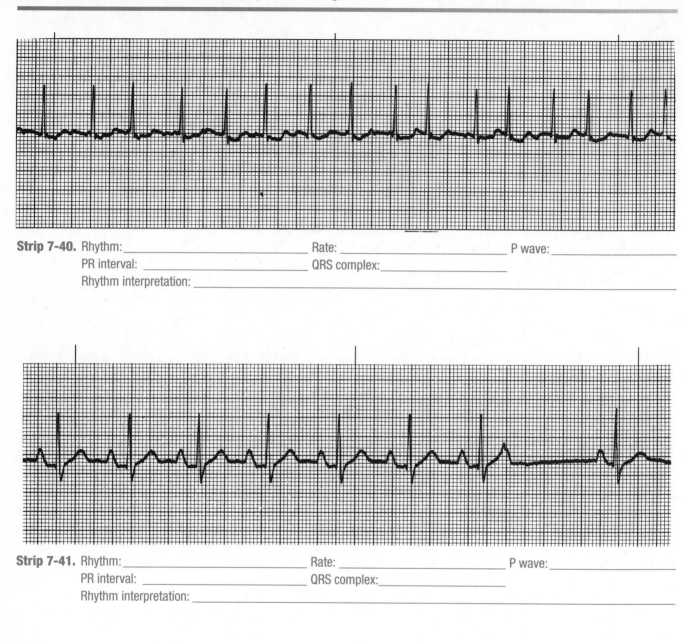

**Strip 7-40.** Rhythm: _____ Rate: _____ P wave: _____

PR interval: _____ QRS complex: _____

Rhythm interpretation: _____

**Strip 7-41.** Rhythm: _____ Rate: _____ P wave: _____

PR interval: _____ QRS complex: _____

Rhythm interpretation: _____

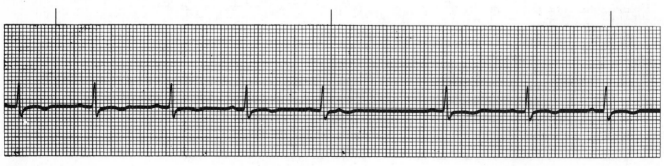

**Strip 7-42.** Rhythm: _____ Rate: _____ P wave: _____

PR interval: _____ QRS complex: _____

Rhythm interpretation: _____

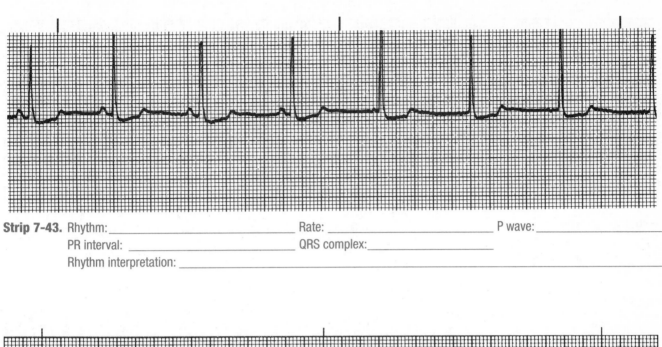

**Strip 7-43.** Rhythm:_____ Rate:_____ P wave:_____
PR interval:_____ QRS complex:_____
Rhythm interpretation:_____

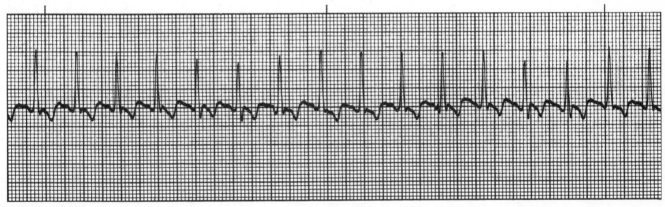

**Strip 7-44.** Rhythm:_____ Rate:_____ P wave:_____
PR interval:_____ QRS complex:_____
Rhythm interpretation:_____

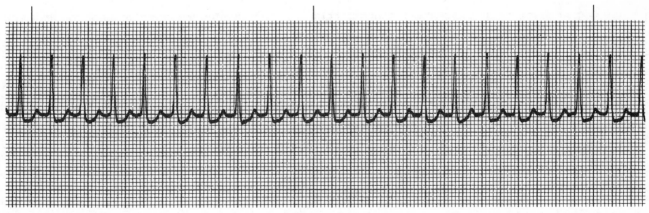

**Strip 7-45.** Rhythm:_____ Rate:_____ P wave:_____
PR interval:_____ QRS complex:_____
Rhythm interpretation:_____

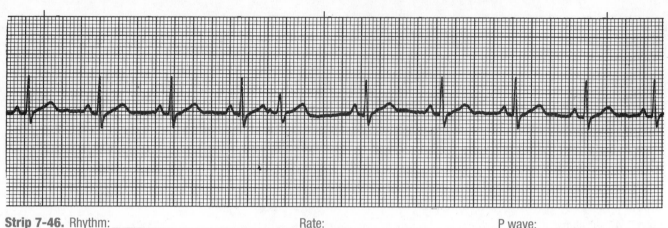

**Strip 7-46.** Rhythm: _____ Rate: _____ P wave: _____

PR interval: _____ QRS complex: _____

Rhythm interpretation: _____

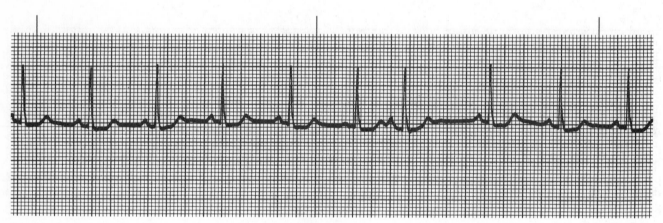

**Strip 7-47.** Rhythm: _____ Rate: _____ P wave: _____

PR interval: _____ QRS complex: _____

Rhythm interpretation: _____

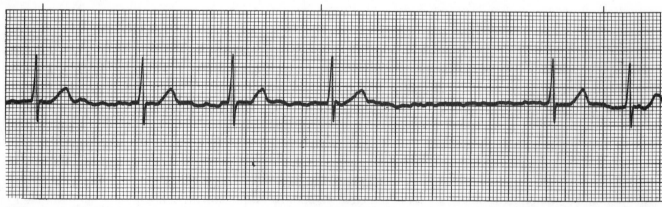

**Strip 7-48.** Rhythm: _____ Rate: _____ P wave: _____

PR interval: _____ QRS complex: _____

Rhythm interpretation: _____

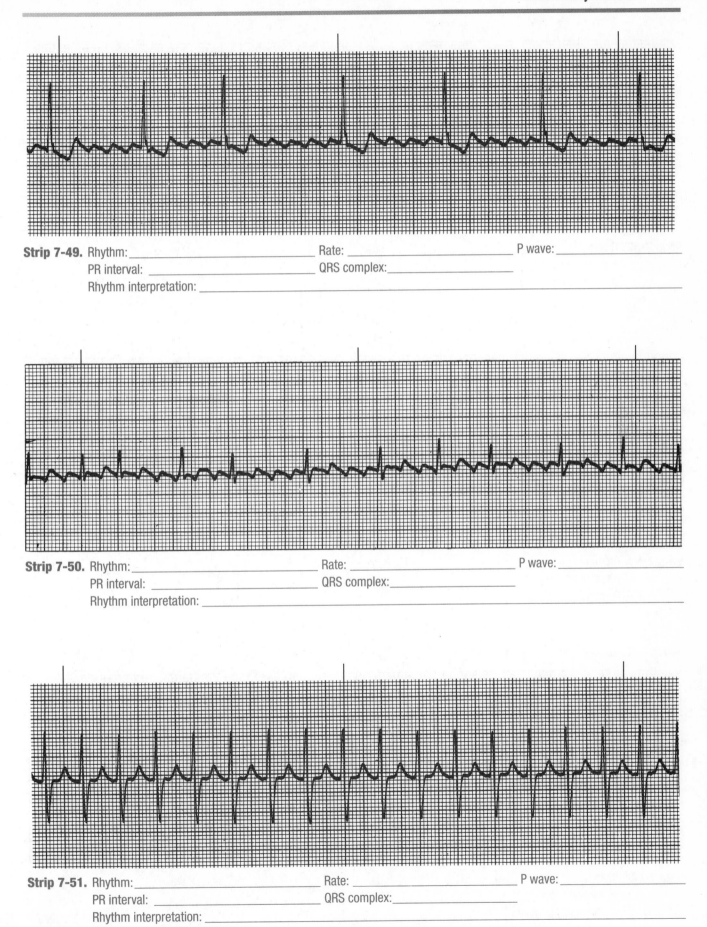

**Strip 7-49.** Rhythm:_____ Rate:_____ P wave:_____
PR interval:_____ QRS complex:_____
Rhythm interpretation:_____

**Strip 7-50.** Rhythm:_____ Rate:_____ P wave:_____
PR interval:_____ QRS complex:_____
Rhythm interpretation:_____

**Strip 7-51.** Rhythm:_____ Rate:_____ P wave:_____
PR interval:_____ QRS complex:_____
Rhythm interpretation:_____

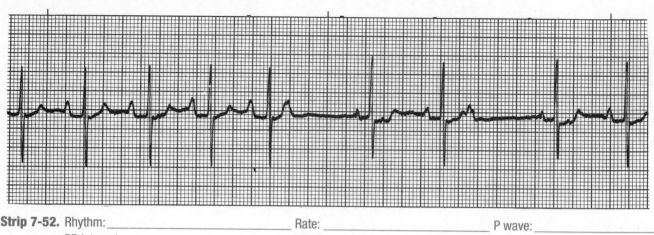

**Strip 7-52.** Rhythm:_____ Rate:_____ P wave:_____

PR interval:_____ QRS complex:_____

Rhythm interpretation:_____

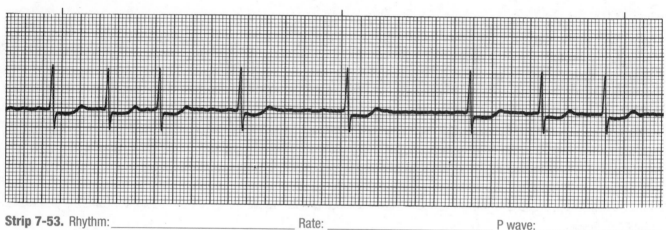

**Strip 7-53.** Rhythm:_____ Rate:_____ P wave:_____

PR interval:_____ QRS complex:_____

Rhythm interpretation:_____

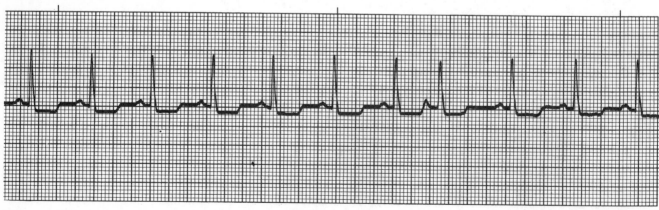

**Strip 7-54.** Rhythm:_____ Rate:_____ P wave:_____

PR interval:_____ QRS complex:_____

Rhythm interpretation:_____

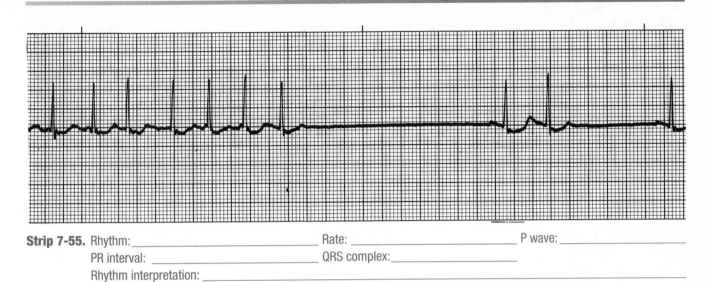

**Strip 7-55.** Rhythm:_____ Rate:_____ P wave:_____

PR interval:_____ QRS complex:_____

Rhythm interpretation:_____

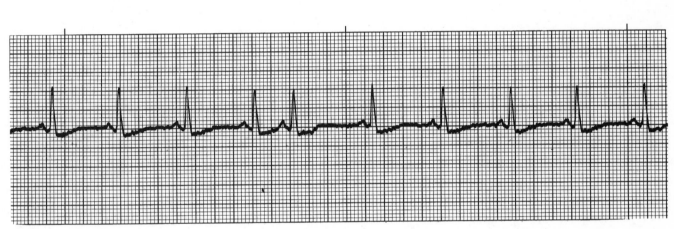

**Strip 7-56.** Rhythm:_____ Rate:_____ P wave:_____

PR interval:_____ QRS complex:_____

Rhythm interpretation:_____

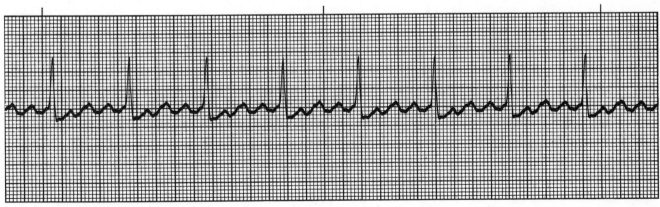

**Strip 7-57.** Rhythm:_____ Rate:_____ P wave:_____

PR interval:_____ QRS complex:_____

Rhythm interpretation:_____

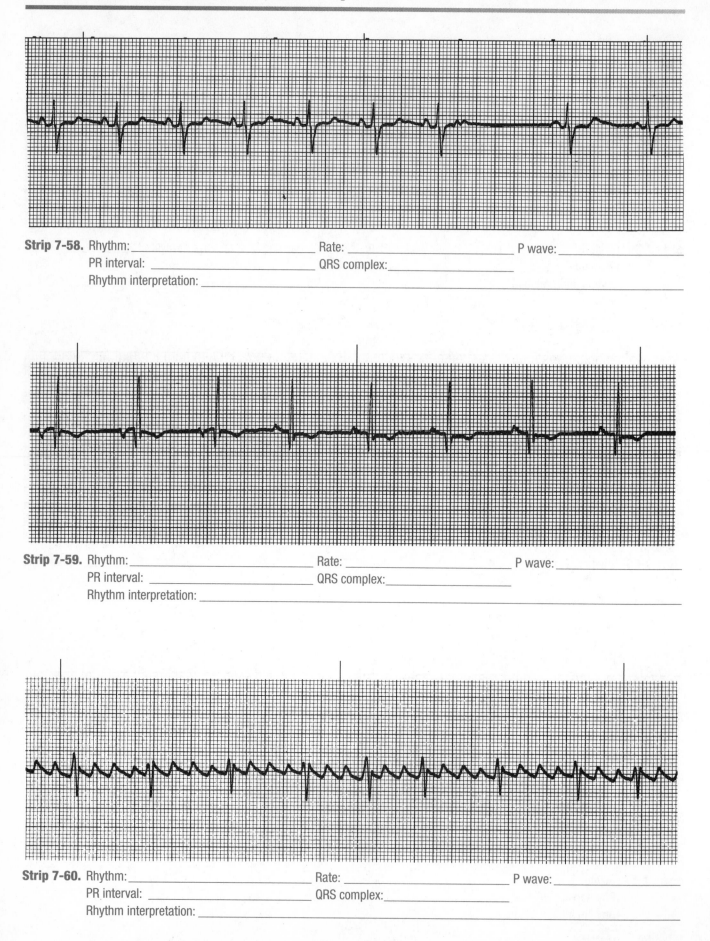

**Strip 7-58.** Rhythm:_____ Rate:_____ P wave:_____

PR interval: _____ QRS complex:_____

Rhythm interpretation: _____

**Strip 7-59.** Rhythm:_____ Rate:_____ P wave:_____

PR interval: _____ QRS complex:_____

Rhythm interpretation: _____

**Strip 7-60.** Rhythm:_____ Rate:_____ P wave:_____

PR interval: _____ QRS complex:_____

Rhythm interpretation: _____

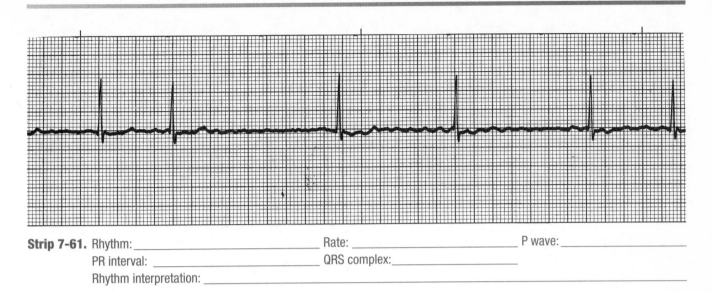

**Strip 7-61.** Rhythm:_____ Rate: _____ P wave:_____

PR interval: _____ QRS complex:_____

Rhythm interpretation: _____

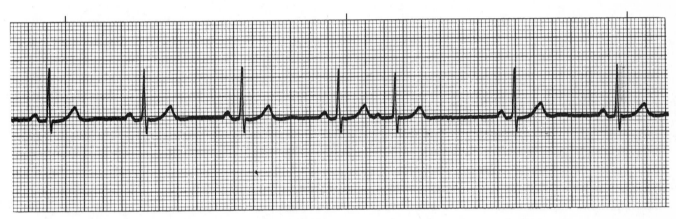

**Strip 7-62.** Rhythm:_____ Rate: _____ P wave:_____

PR interval: _____ QRS complex:_____

Rhythm interpretation: _____

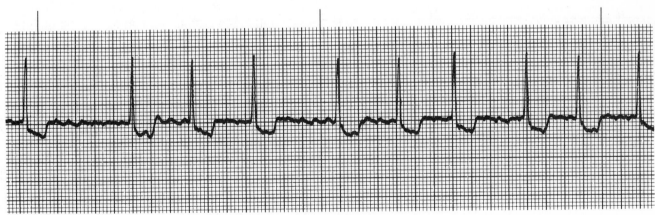

**Strip 7-63.** Rhythm:_____ Rate: _____ P wave:_____

PR interval: _____ QRS complex:_____

Rhythm interpretation: _____

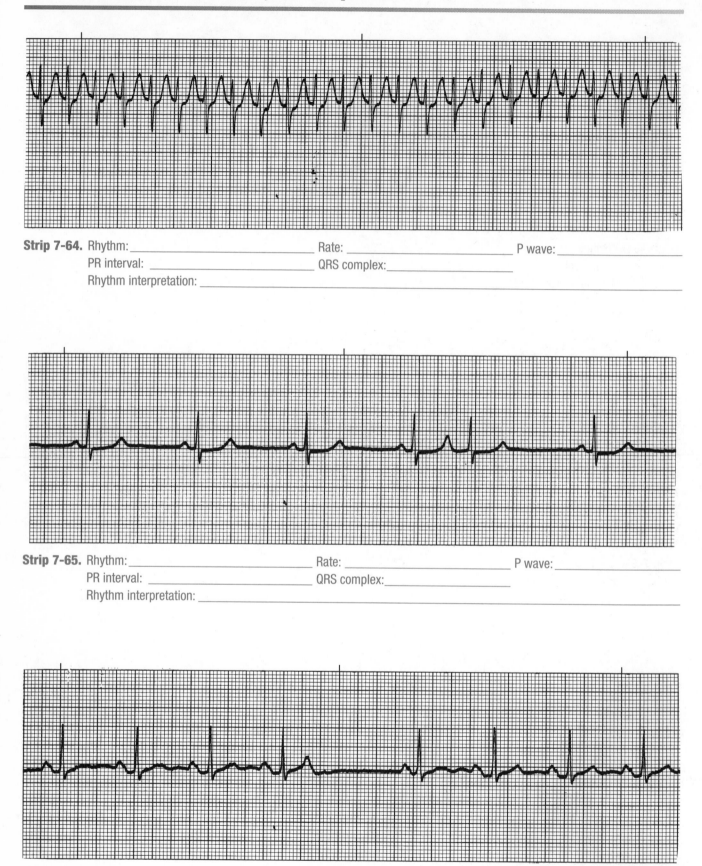

**Strip 7-64.** Rhythm: _____ Rate: _____ P wave: _____
PR interval: _____ QRS complex: _____
Rhythm interpretation: _____

**Strip 7-65.** Rhythm: _____ Rate: _____ P wave: _____
PR interval: _____ QRS complex: _____
Rhythm interpretation: _____

**Strip 7-66.** Rhythm: _____ Rate: _____ P wave: _____
PR interval: _____ QRS complex: _____
Rhythm interpretation: _____

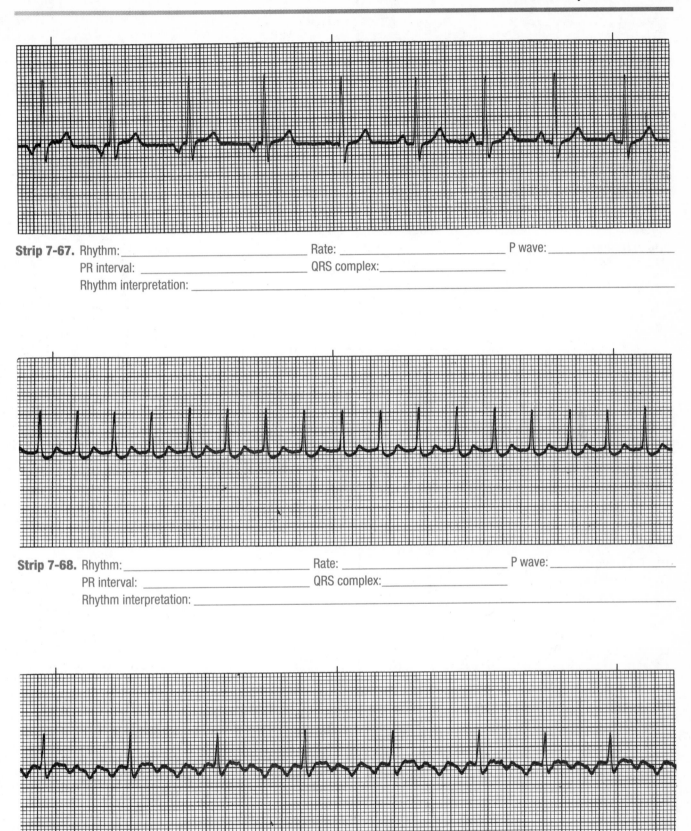

**Strip 7-67.** Rhythm: _____ Rate: _____ P wave: _____
PR interval: _____ QRS complex: _____
Rhythm interpretation: _____

**Strip 7-68.** Rhythm: _____ Rate: _____ P wave: _____
PR interval: _____ QRS complex: _____
Rhythm interpretation: _____

**Strip 7-69.** Rhythm: _____ Rate: _____ P wave: _____
PR interval: _____ QRS complex: _____
Rhythm interpretation: _____

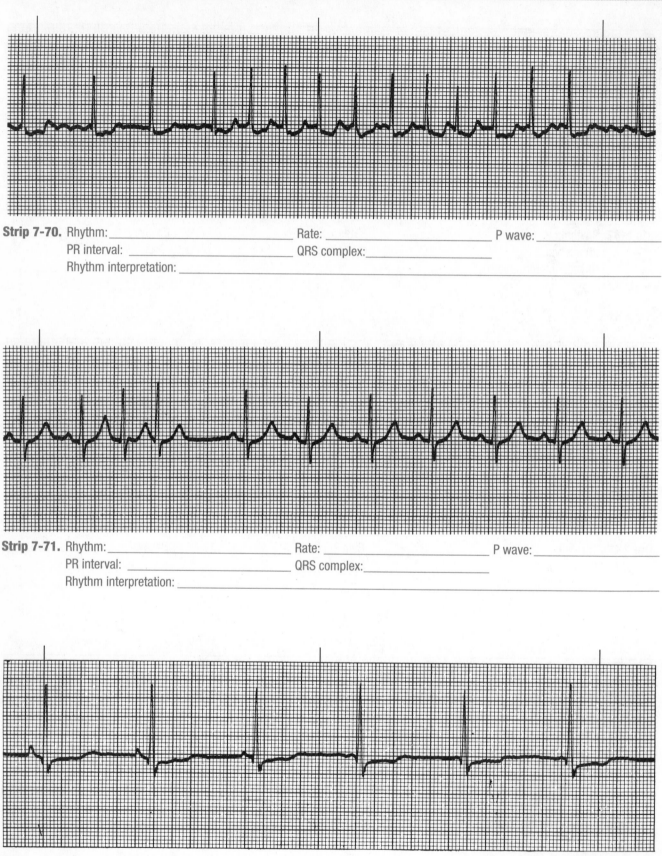

**Strip 7-70.** Rhythm:_____ Rate:_____ P wave:_____

PR interval:_____ QRS complex:_____

Rhythm interpretation:_____

**Strip 7-71.** Rhythm:_____ Rate:_____ P wave:_____

PR interval:_____ QRS complex:_____

Rhythm interpretation:_____

**Strip 7-72.** Rhythm:_____ Rate:_____ P wave:_____

PR interval:_____ QRS complex:_____

Rhythm interpretation:_____

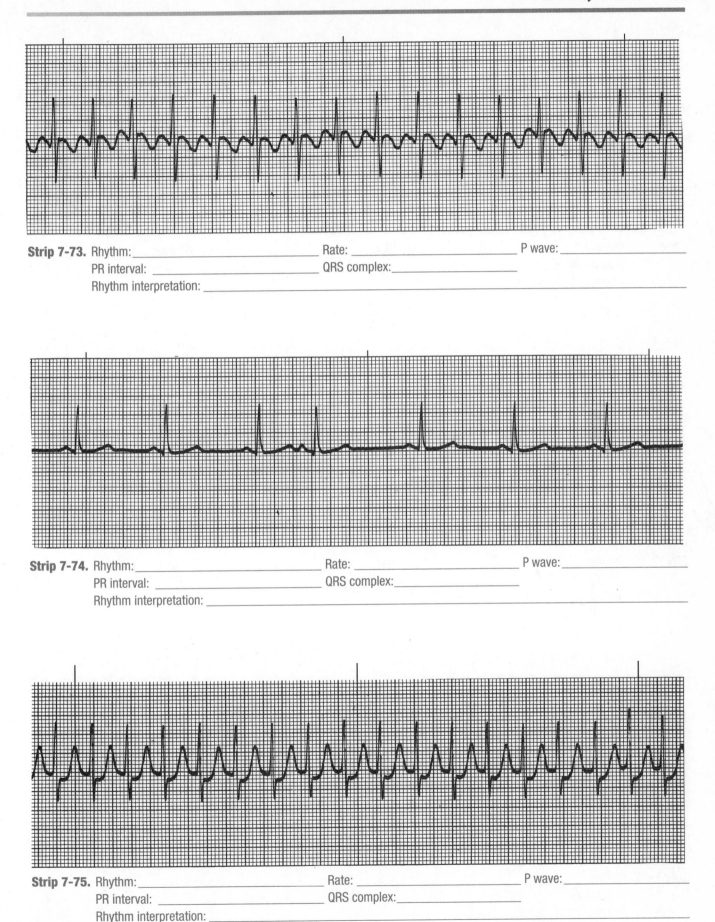

**Strip 7-73.** Rhythm:_____ Rate:_____ P wave:_____
PR interval:_____ QRS complex:_____
Rhythm interpretation:_____

**Strip 7-74.** Rhythm:_____ Rate:_____ P wave:_____
PR interval:_____ QRS complex:_____
Rhythm interpretation:_____

**Strip 7-75.** Rhythm:_____ Rate:_____ P wave:_____
PR interval:_____ QRS complex:_____
Rhythm interpretation:_____

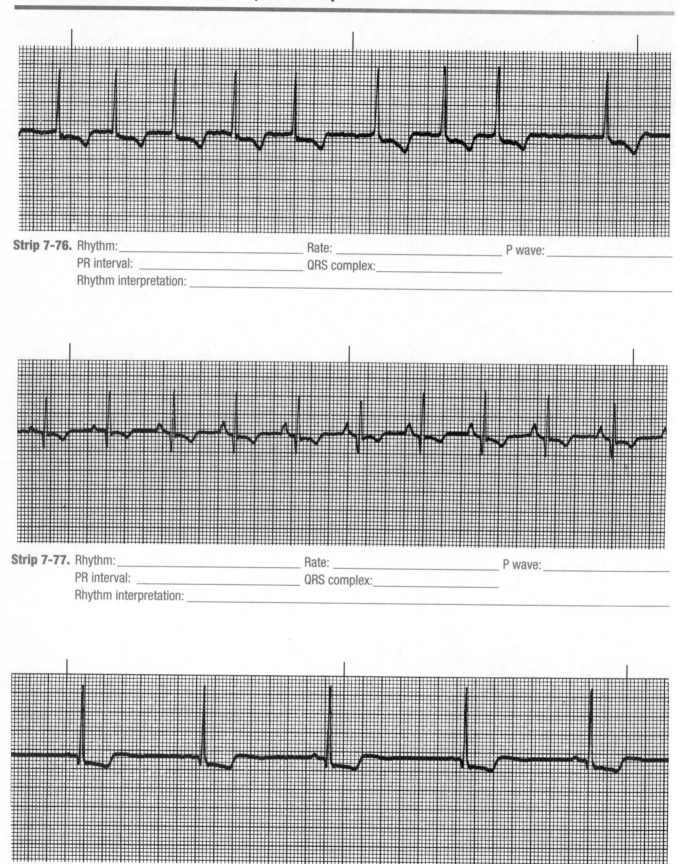

**Strip 7-76.** Rhythm:_____ Rate:_____ P wave:_____

PR interval:_____ QRS complex:_____

Rhythm interpretation:_____

**Strip 7-77.** Rhythm:_____ Rate:_____ P wave:_____

PR interval:_____ QRS complex:_____

Rhythm interpretation:_____

**Strip 7-78.** Rhythm:_____ Rate:_____ P wave:_____

PR interval:_____ QRS complex:_____

Rhythm interpretation:_____

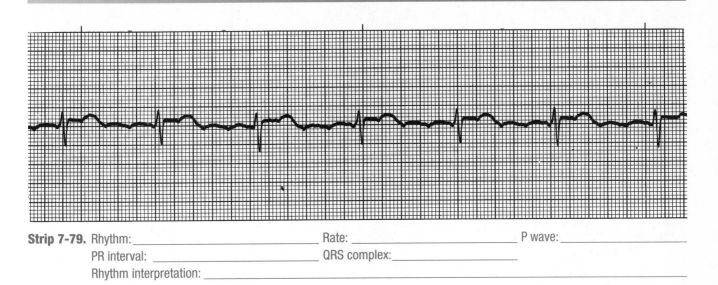

**Strip 7-79.** Rhythm:_____ Rate: _____ P wave:_____

PR interval: _____ QRS complex:_____

Rhythm interpretation: _____

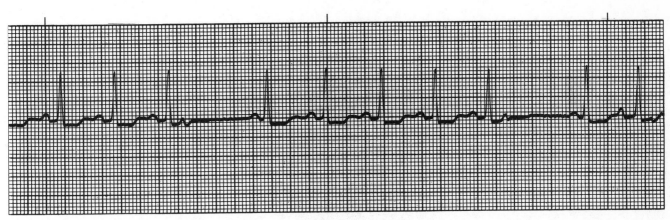

**Strip 7-80.** Rhythm:_____ Rate: _____ P wave:_____

PR interval: _____ QRS complex:_____

Rhythm interpretation: _____

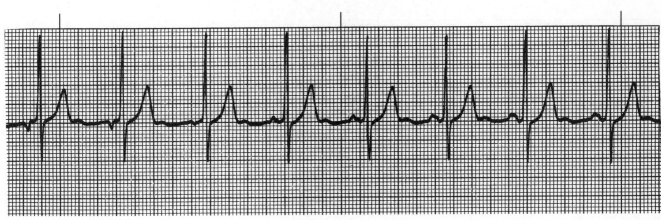

**Strip 7-81.** Rhythm:_____ Rate: _____ P wave:_____

PR interval: _____ QRS complex:_____

Rhythm interpretation: _____

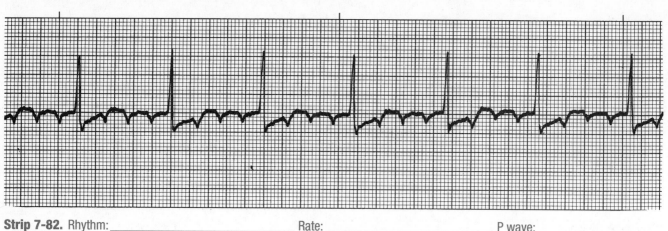

**Strip 7-82.** Rhythm:_____ Rate: _____ P wave:_____

PR interval: _____ QRS complex:_____

Rhythm interpretation: _____

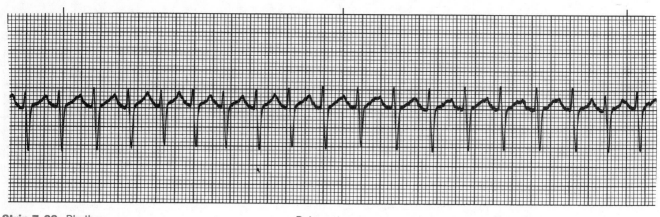

**Strip 7-83.** Rhythm:_____ Rate: _____ P wave:_____

PR interval: _____ QRS complex:_____

Rhythm interpretation: _____

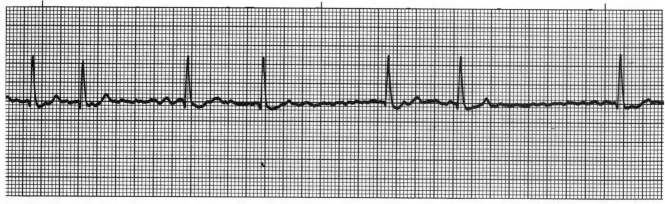

**Strip 7-84.** Rhythm:_____ Rate: _____ P wave:_____

PR interval: _____ QRS complex:_____

Rhythm interpretation: _____

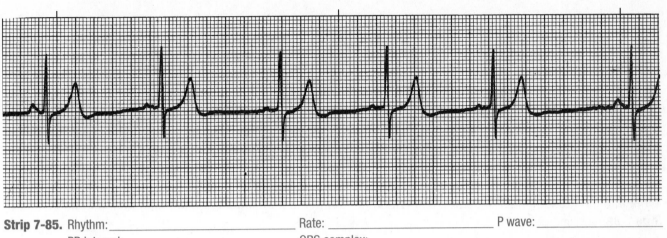

**Strip 7-85.** Rhythm:_____ Rate: _____ P wave: _____

PR interval: _____ QRS complex:_____

Rhythm interpretation: _____

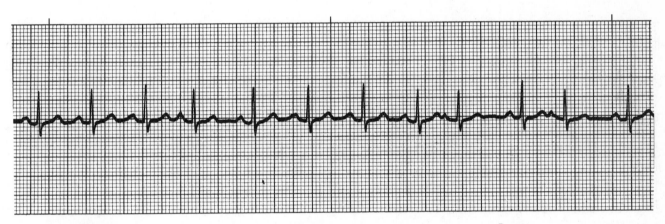

**Strip 7-86.** Rhythm:_____ Rate: _____ P wave: _____

PR interval: _____ QRS complex:_____

Rhythm interpretation: _____

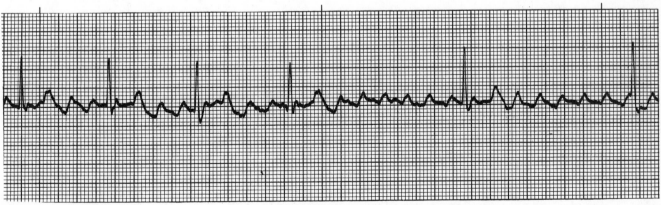

**Strip 7-87.** Rhythm:_____ Rate: _____ P wave: _____

PR interval: _____ QRS complex:_____

Rhythm interpretation: _____

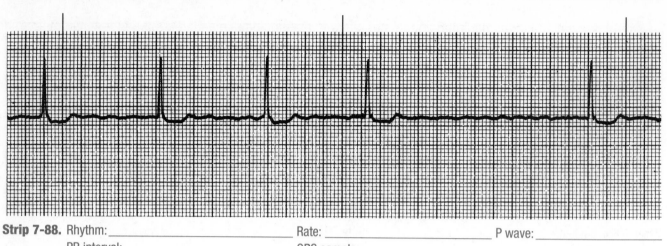

**Strip 7-88.** Rhythm:_____ Rate:_____ P wave:_____

PR interval:_____ QRS complex:_____

Rhythm interpretation:_____

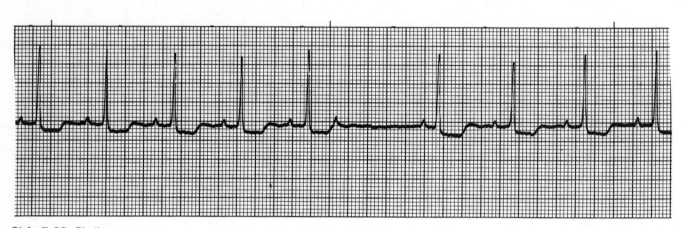

**Strip 7-89.** Rhythm:_____ Rate:_____ P wave:_____

PR interval:_____ QRS complex:_____

Rhythm interpretation:_____

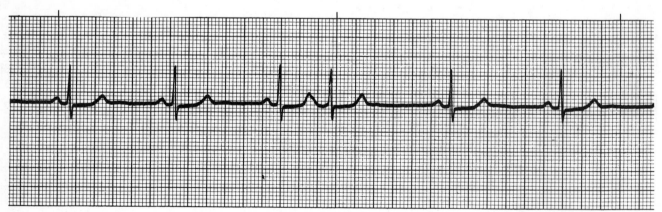

**Strip 7-90.** Rhythm:_____ Rate:_____ P wave:_____

PR interval:_____ QRS complex:_____

Rhythm interpretation:_____

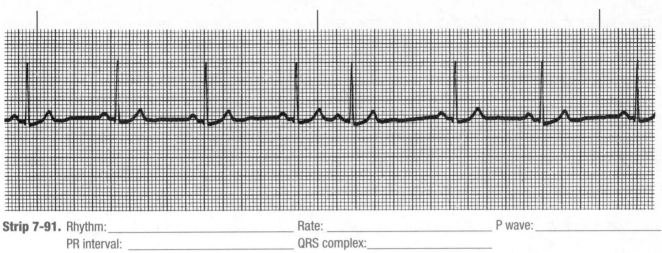

**Strip 7-91.** Rhythm:_____ Rate:_____ P wave:_____
PR interval:_____ QRS complex:_____
Rhythm interpretation:_____

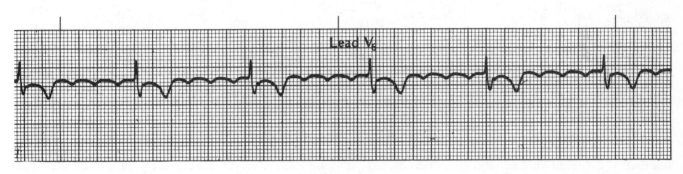

**Strip 7-92.** Rhythm:_____ Rate:_____ P wave:_____
PR interval:_____ QRS complex:_____
Rhythm interpretation:_____

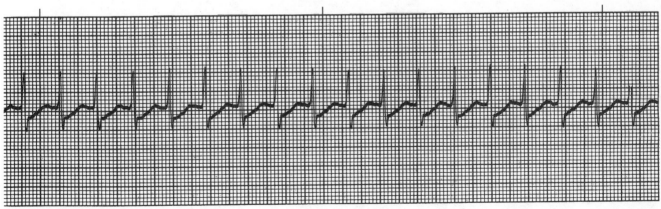

**Strip 7-93.** Rhythm:_____ Rate:_____ P wave:_____
PR interval:_____ QRS complex:_____
Rhythm interpretation:_____

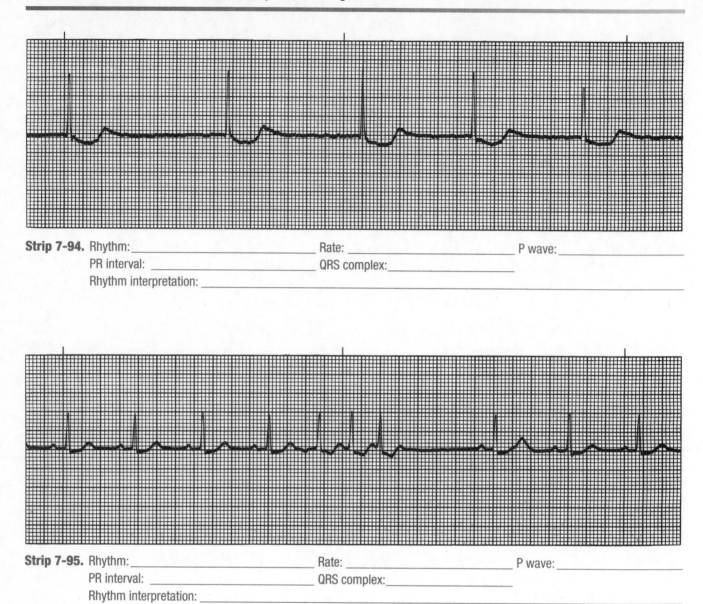

**Strip 7-94.** Rhythm:_____ Rate:_____ P wave:_____

PR interval: _____ QRS complex:_____

Rhythm interpretation: _____

**Strip 7-95.** Rhythm:_____ Rate:_____ P wave:_____

PR interval: _____ QRS complex:_____

Rhythm interpretation: _____

# 8

# AV junctional arrhythmias and AV blocks

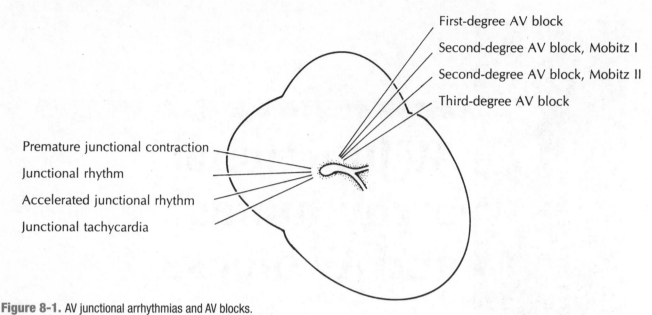

**Figure 8-1.** AV junctional arrhythmias and AV blocks.

## Overview

Atrioventricular (AV) junctional arrhythmias (Figure 8-1) originate in the area of the AV junction. The AV junction consists of the AV node and the bundle of His; it includes three regions: the atrial-nodal or upper junctional region, the nodal or middle junctional region, and the nodal-His or lower junctional region. The middle nodal region is where the electrical impulses are slowed down in their progression from the atria to the ventricles. This region doesn't contain pacemaker cells. The upper and lower junctional regions possess pacemaker cells, which can spontaneously generate electrical impulses and assume the role as a secondary pacemaker site if the sinoatrial (SA) node fails or slows below its normal range.

The inherent firing rate of the junctional pacemaker cells is 40 to 60 beats/minute. A rhythm occurring at this rate is called a *junctional rhythm*. Junctional rhythm is the normal response of the AV junction if the sinus rate falls below the AV junctional rate or if the sinus impulse fails to reach the AV junction. Other arrhythmias originating in the AV junctional area include premature junctional contractions, accelerated junctional rhythm, and junctional tachycardia. The electrophysiologic mechanisms thought to be responsible for the junctional arrhythmias are altered automaticity, triggered activity, or a reentry circuit.

When the AV node is functioning as the pacemaker of the heart, the electrical impulse produces a wave of depolarization that spreads backward (retrograde) into the atria as well as forward (antegrade) into the ventricles. The location of the P wave relative to the QRS complex depends on the speed of antegrade and retrograde conduction:

■ If the electrical impulse from the AV junction depolarizes the atria first and then depolarizes the ventricles, the P wave will be in front of the QRS complex.

■ If the electrical impulse from the AV junction depolarizes the ventricles first and then depolarizes the atria, the P wave will be after the QRS complex.

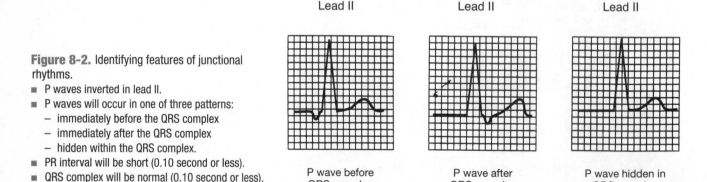

**Figure 8-2.** Identifying features of junctional rhythms.
■ P waves inverted in lead II.
■ P waves will occur in one of three patterns:
  – immediately before the QRS complex
  – immediately after the QRS complex
  – hidden within the QRS complex.
■ PR interval will be short (0.10 second or less).
■ QRS complex will be normal (0.10 second or less).

Lead II — P wave before QRS complex

Lead II — P wave after QRS complex

Lead II — P wave hidden in QRS complex

- If the electrical impulse from the AV junction depolarizes both the atria and the ventricles simultaneously, the P wave will be hidden in the QRS complex.

Retrograde stimulation of the atria is just opposite the direction of atrial depolarization when normal sinus rhythm is present, and produces negative P waves (instead of upright) in lead II. The PR interval is short (0.10 second or less). The ventricles are depolarized normally, resulting in a narrow QRS complex. Identifying features of AV junctional rhythms are shown in Figure 8-2.

## Premature junctional contractions

A premature junctional contraction (PJC) (Figures 8-3 through 8-7 and Box 8-1) is an early beat that originates in an ectopic pacemaker site in the AV junction. Like the PAC, the premature junctional beat is characterized by a premature, abnormal P wave; a premature QRS complex that's identical or similar to the QRS complex of the normally conducted beats; and is followed by a pause that is usually noncompensatory. Some differences do exist, however. Because atrial depolarization occurs in a retrograde fashion with the PJC, the P wave associated with the premature beat will be negative (inverted) in lead II and will occur immediately before or after the QRS complex, or will be hidden within the QRS complex. The PR interval will be short (0.10 second or less). Inverted P waves in lead II may also occur with PACs arising from the lower atria, but the associated PR interval will not be short. If difficulty is encountered in differentiating PJCs from PACs, keep the following in mind—PACs are much more common than PJCs. As a result, narrow complex premature beats probably shouldn't be interpreted as PJCs unless P waves are definitely absent or the P wave is inverted in lead II with a short PR interval.

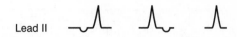

Lead II

**Figure 8-3.** Premature junctional contractions will appear as a single beat in any of the above three patterns.

PJCs occur in addition to the underlying rhythm. They occur in the same patterns as PACs: as a single beat, in pairs (Figure 8-7), or in bigeminal, trigeminal, or quadrigeminal patterns. A series of three or more consecutive junctional beats is considered a rhythm (that is, a junctional rhythm, an accelerated junctional rhythm, or a junctional tachycardia). Differentiation of the rhythm depends on the heart rate.

### Box 8-1.
### Premature junctional contraction: Identifying ECG features

| | |
|---|---|
| **Rhythm:** | Underlying rhythm usually regular; irregular with PJC |
| **Rate:** | That of the underlying rhythm |
| **P waves:** | P waves associated with the PJC will be premature, inverted in lead II, and will occur immediately before or after the QRS complex, or will be hidden within the QRS complex |
| **PR interval:** | Short (0.10 second or less) |
| **QRS complex:** | Premature; normal duration (0.10 second or less) |

Some causes of premature junctional contractions include digitalis toxicity, enhanced automaticity of the AV junction, coronary artery disease, heart failure, and valvular disease. PJCs may also occur without apparent cause.

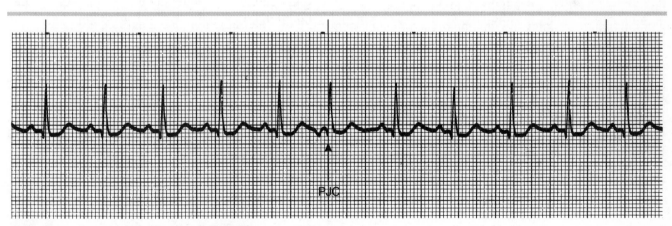

**Figure 8-4.    Normal sinus rhythm with one PJC**
| | |
|---|---|
| **Rhythm:** | Basic rhythm regular; irregular with PJC |
| **Rate:** | Basic rhythm rate 94 beats/minute |
| **P waves:** | Sinus P waves with basic rhythm; inverted P wave with PJC |
| **PR interval:** | 0.14 to 0.16 second (basic rhythm); 0.08 second (PJC) |
| **QRS complex:** | 0.08 second |
| **Comment:** | ST segment depression is present. |

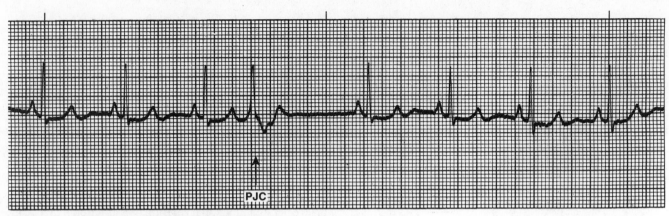

**Figure 8-5.   Normal sinus rhythm with one PJC**

| | |
|---|---|
| **Rhythm:** | Basic rhythm regular; irregular with PJC |
| **Rate:** | Basic rhythm rate 72 beats/minute |
| **P waves:** | Sinus P waves with basic rhythm; inverted P wave after PJC (4th QRS complex) |
| **PR interval:** | 0.14 to 0.16 second (basic rhythm); 0.06 to 0.08 second (PJC) |
| **QRS complex:** | 0.06 to 0.08 second (basic rhythm); 0.08 second (PJC) |
| **Comment:** | A U wave is present. |

PJCs don't normally require treatment. Frequent PJCs may initiate more serious junctional arrhythmias.

Occasionally, an ectopic junctional beat will occur late instead of early. These are called *junctional escape beats* (Figure 8-8). Escape beats are more likely to occur as a result of increased vagal effect on the SA node rather than to enhanced automaticity (a common cause of premature junctional beats). Junctional escape beats are common after a pause in the underlying rhythm (for example, sinus arrest or block, nonconducted PACs, or type I second-degree AV block). The morphologic characteristics of the late beat are the same as that of the PJC. Escape beats are protective mechanisms to maintain the heart rate and require no treatment. It's important, however, to identify the cause of the initiating pause so that appropriate intervention can be started if necessary.

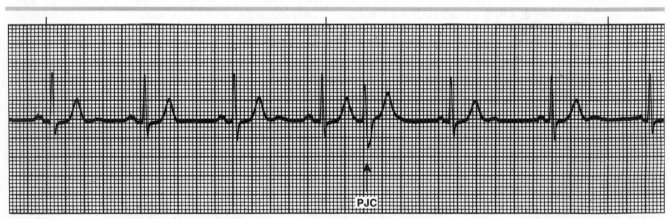

**Figure 8-6.   Normal sinus rhythm with one PJC**

| | |
|---|---|
| **Rhythm:** | Basic rhythm regular; irregular with PJC |
| **Rate:** | Basic rhythm rate 63 beats/minute; rate slows to 56 beats/minute following PJC due to rate suppression (common following a pause in the basic rhythm) |
| **P waves:** | Sinus P waves with basic rhythm; P wave associated with PJC is hidden in the QRS complex |
| **PR interval:** | 0.16 to 0.18 second (basic rhythm) |
| **QRS complex:** | 0.06 to 0.08 second (basic rhythm); 0.10 second (PJC) |
| **Comment:** | A U wave is present. |

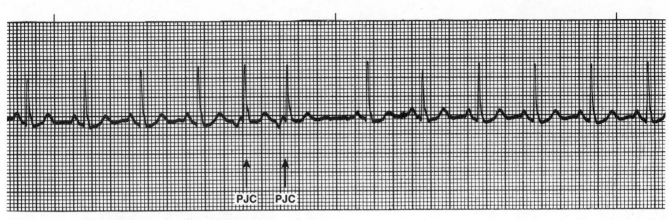

**Figure 8-7.** **Normal sinus rhythm with paired PJCs**

| | |
|---|---|
| **Rhythm:** | Basic rhythm regular; irregular following paired PJCs |
| **Rate:** | Basic rhythm rate 100 beats/minute |
| **P waves:** | Sinus P waves with basic rhythm; inverted P waves with PJCs |
| **PR interval:** | 0.12 to 0.14 second (basic rhythm); 0.08 second (with PJCs) |
| **QRS complex:** | 0.06 to 0.08 second (basic rhythm and PJCs). |

## Junctional rhythm

Junctional rhythm (Figures 8-9 through 8-12 and Box 8-2) is an arrhythmia originating in the AV junction with a rate between 40 to 60 beats/minute. This rhythm is commonly referred to as *junctional escape rhythm* because it usually only appears ("escapes") secondary to depression of the higher pacing center of the heart, the SA node. Junctional rhythm is the normal response of the AV junction when the rate of the dominant pacemaker (usually the SA node) becomes less than the rate of the AV node or when the electrical impulses from the SA node fail to reach the AV node. When an electrical impulse fails to reach the AV junction within 1 to 1½ seconds, the escape pacemaker in the AV junction begins to generate electrical impulses at its inherent firing rate of 40 to 60 beats/minute. The result could be a junctional escape beat or junctional escape rhythm.

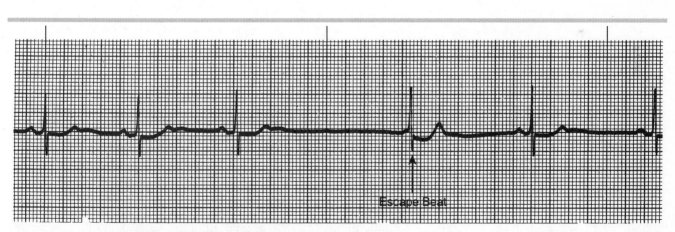

**Figure 8-8.** **Normal sinus rhythm with sinus arrest and junctional escape beat**

| | |
|---|---|
| **Rhythm:** | Basic rhythm regular; irregular with escape beat |
| **Rate:** | Basic rhythm 60 beats/minute; rate slows to 45 beats/minute after escape beat (Rate suppression can occur following any pause in the basic rhythm. After several cycles the rate will return to the basic rate.) |
| **P waves:** | Sinus P waves with basic rhythm; hidden P wave with escape beat |
| **PR interval:** | 0.16 second |
| **QRS complex:** | 0.06 second |
| **Comment:** | ST segment depression and a U wave are present. |

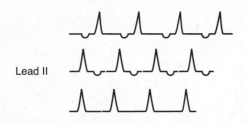

Lead II

**Figure 8-9.** Junctional rhythm will appear as a continuous rhythm at a rate of 40 to 60 beats/minute in either of the above three patterns.

### Box 8-2.
### Junctional rhythm: Identifying ECG features

| | |
|---|---|
| Rhythm: | Regular |
| Rate: | 40 to 60 beats/minute |
| P waves: | Inverted in lead II and occurs immediately before the QRS complex, immediately after the QRS complex, or is hidden within the QRS complex |
| PR interval: | Short (0.10 second or less) |
| QRS complex: | Normal (0.10 second or less) |

Retrograde stimulation of the atria by the AV node impulse produces a rhythm with the following characteristics:
■ P waves that are inverted in lead II and that occur immediately before or after the QRS complex or are hidden within the QRS complex
■ a short PR interval (0.10 second or less)

■ a normal QRS complex (0.10 second or less).

Junctional rhythm is a continuous rhythm, usually temporary in nature, with the same electrocardiogram (ECG) characteristics as accelerated junctional rhythm and junctional tachycardia. This rhythm is differentiated from the other junctional rhythms by the heart rate (40 to 60 beats/minute).

A junctional rhythm may be caused by disease of the SA node, increased vagal effect on the SA node, an acute myocardial infarction (MI) (especially an inferior wall MI), or drug effects (for example, from digitalis, quinidine, a beta-blocker, or a calcium channel blocker). Junctional rhythm may also occur with complete heart block.

The slow rate and loss of normal atrial depolarization ("atrial kick") associated with junctional rhythm may cause a decrease in cardiac output. Treatment for symptomatic junctional rhythm includes increasing the heart rate (for example, with atropine or transcutaneous or transvenous pacing) and reversing the consequences of reduced cardiac output. Treatment should also be directed at identifying and correcting the underlying cause of the rhythm if possible. All medications should be reviewed and discontinued if indicated.

## Accelerated junctional rhythm

Accelerated junctional rhythm (Figures 8-13 through 8-15 and Box 8-3) is an arrhythmia originating in the AV junction with a rate between 60 and 100 beats/minute. The term *accelerated* denotes a rhythm that occurs at a rate that exceeds the inherent junctional escape rate of 40 to

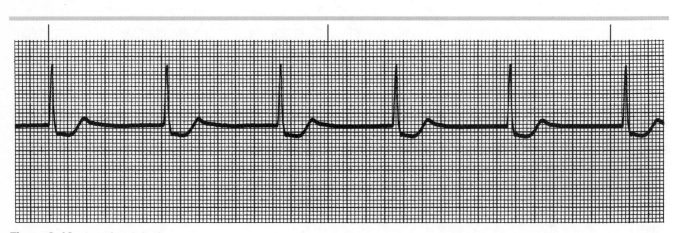

**Figure 8-10. Junctional rhythm**

| | |
|---|---|
| Rhythm: | Regular |
| Rate: | 50 beats/minute |
| P waves: | Hidden in QRS complex |
| PR interval: | Not measurable |
| QRS complex: | 0.06 to 0.08 second |
| Comment: | ST segment depression is present. |

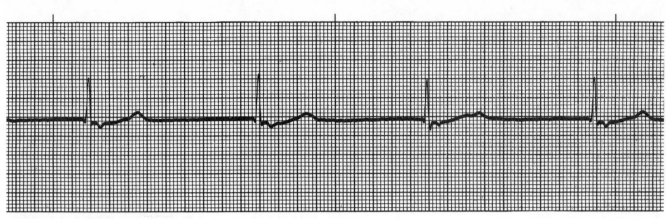

**Figure 8-11. Junctional rhythm**

| | |
|---|---|
| **Rhythm:** | Regular |
| **Rate:** | 33 beats/minute |
| **P waves:** | Inverted after QRS complex |
| **PR interval:** | 0.08 to 0.10 second |
| **QRS complex:** | 0.08 to 0.10 second |

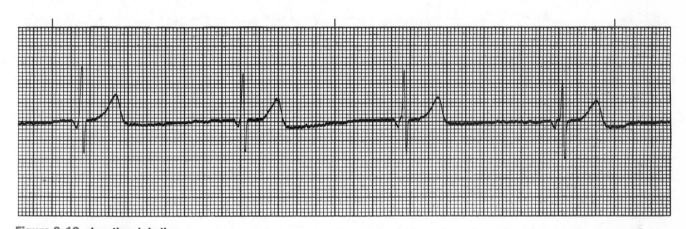

**Figure 8-12. Junctional rhythm**

| | |
|---|---|
| **Rhythm:** | Regular |
| **Rate:** | 35 beats/minute |
| **P waves:** | Inverted before the QRS |
| **PR interval:** | 0.06 to 0.08 second |
| **QRS complex:** | 0.06 to 0.08 second |

60 beats/minute, but isn't fast enough to be junctional tachycardia.

Retrograde stimulation of the atria by the AV node impulse produces a rhythm with the following characteristics:

■ P waves that are inverted in lead II and that occur immediately before or after the QRS complex or are hidden within the QRS complex

■ a short PR interval (0.10 second or less)

■ a normal QRS complex (0.10 second or less).

Accelerated junctional rhythm is a continuous rhythm, usually temporary in nature, with the same ECG charac-

**Box 8-3.**

## Accelerated junctional rhythm: Identifying ECG features

| | |
|---|---|
| **Rhythm:** | Regular |
| **Rate:** | 60 to 100 beats/minute |
| **P waves:** | Inverted in lead II and occurs immediately before the QRS complex, immediately after the QRS complex, or is hidden within the QRS complex |
| **PR interval:** | Short (0.10 second or less) |
| **QRS complex:** | Normal (0.10 second or less) |

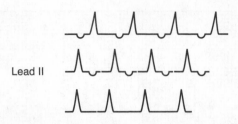

Lead II

**Figure 8-13.** Accelerated junctional rhythm will appear as a continuous rhythm at a rate of 60 to 100 beats/minute in any of the above three patterns.

teristics as junctional rhythm and junctional tachycardia. This rhythm is differentiated from the other junctional rhythms by the heart rate (60 to 100 beats/minute).

Accelerated junctional rhythm can result from enhanced automaticity secondary to digitalis toxicity. Other causes include damage to the AV node secondary to an acute inferior wall MI, heart failure, acute rheumatic fever, myocarditis, valvular heart disease, and cardiac surgery (especially valve surgery).

As a rule, the heart rate associated with accelerated junctional rhythm isn't a problem because it corresponds to that of the sinus node (60 to 100 beats/minute). Problems are more likely to occur from the loss of normal atrial depolar-

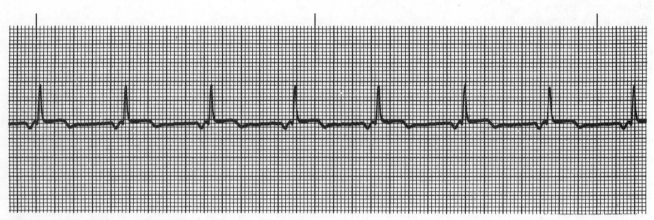

**Figure 8-14.  Accelerated junctional rhythm**
**Rhythm:**      Regular
**Rate:**        65 beats/minute
**P waves:**     Inverted before each QRS complex
**PR interval:**  0.08 to 0.10 second
**QRS complex:** 0.08 second
**Comment:**     ST segment elevation and T wave inversion are present.

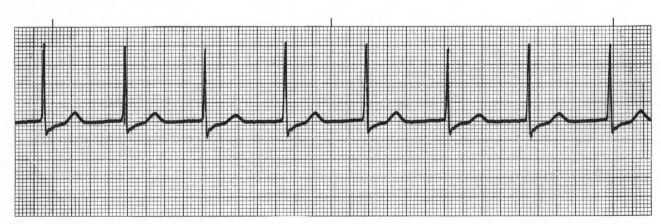

**Figure 8-15.  Accelerated junctional rhythm**
**Rhythm:**      Regular
**Rate:**        68 beats/minute
**P waves:**     Hidden in QRS complex
**PR interval:**  Not measurable
**QRS complex:** 0.06 to 0.08 second

ization ("atrial kick") resulting in a decrease in cardiac output. Treatment is directed at reversing the consequences of reduced cardiac output as well as identifying and correcting the underlying cause of the rhythm. All medications should be reviewed and discontinued if indicated.

## Paroxysmal junctional tachycardia

Paroxysmal junctional tachycardia (PJT) (Figures 8-16 and 8-17 and Box 8-4) is an arrhythmia originating in the AV junction with a heart rate that exceeds 100 beats/minute. Like PAT, junctional tachycardia is regular and commonly starts and ends abruptly in a paroxysmal manner.

### Box 8-4.
### Paroxysmal junctional tachycardia: Identifying ECG features

| | |
|---|---|
| Rhythm: | Regular |
| Rate: | Greater than 100 beats/minute |
| P waves: | Inverted in lead II and occurs immediately before the QRS complex, immediately after the QRS complex, or is hidden within the QRS complex |
| PR interval: | Short (0.10 second or less) |
| QRS complex: | Normal (0.10 second or less) |

Retrograde stimulation of the atria by the AV node impulse produces a rhythm with the following characteristics:
- P waves that are inverted in lead II and that occur immediately before or after the QRS complex or are hidden within the QRS complex
- a short PR interval (0.10 second or less)

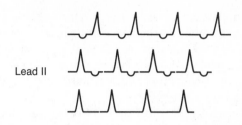

Lead II

**Figure 8-16.** Paroxysmal junctional tachycardia will appear as a continuous rhythm at a rate exceeding 100 beats/minute in any of the above three patterns.

- a normal QRS complex (0.10 second or less).

Junctional tachycardia has the same ECG characteristics as junctional rhythm and accelerated junctional rhythm. This rhythm is differentiated from the other junctional rhythms by the heart rate (greater than 100 beats/minute).

It may be difficult at times to distinguish PJT from PAT electrocardiographically. The P waves are commonly hidden in both rhythms—in PAT the P wave is hidden in the preceding T wave, and in PJT the P wave may be hidden in the QRS complex. If one can't be differentiated from the other, the term *paroxysmal supraventricular tachycardia* may be used. This term implies that the tachycardia is paroxysmal in nature (either PAT or PJT) and has a supraventricular origin (above the bifurcation of the bundle of His) with a narrow QRS complex. The term shouldn't be confused with the general term *supraventricular,* which refers to any rhythm above the bifurcation of the bundle of His. In adults, true junctional tachycardia is rare. PAT is much more common than PJT. Therefore, if the tachycardia is supraventricular and paroxysmal in nature, the rhythm is most likely PAT.

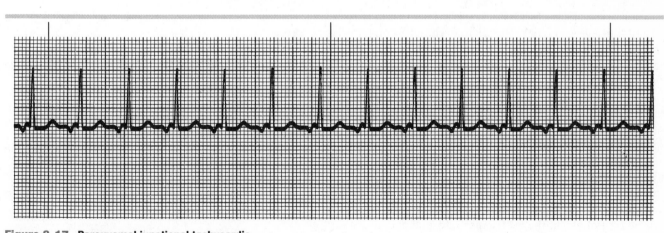

**Figure 8-17. Paroxysmal junctional tachycardia**

| | |
|---|---|
| Rhythm: | Regular |
| Rate: | 115 beats/minute |
| P waves: | Inverted before each QRS complex |
| PR interval: | 0.08 second |
| QRS complex: | 0.06 to 0.08 second |

Junctional tachycardia is usually a manifestation of digitalis toxicity or of catecholamine or theophylline infusion. Other causes include damage to the AV node secondary to an acute inferior MI, heart failure, acute rheumatic fever, myocarditis, valvular heart disease, and cardiac surgery (especially valve surgery).

Junctional tachycardia may lead to a decrease in cardiac output from the faster rate as well as the loss of normal atrial depolarization ("atrial kick"). Treatment is directed at reversing the consequences of reduced cardiac output as well as identifying and correcting the underlying cause of the rhythm. If no apparent cause is identified, symptomatic junctional tachycardia may respond to diltiazem or beta blockers (use beta-blockers with caution in pulmonary disease or congestive heart failure). Electrical cardioversion is not likely to be effective for treatment of junctional tachycardia.

## AV heart blocks

The term *heart block* is used to describe arrhythmias in which there is delayed or failed conduction of supraventricular impulses through the AV node into the ventricles. The site of pathology is at the AV junction, the bundle of His, or in the bundle branches. The conduction disturbance may be temporary or permanent.

Normally, the AV node acts as a bridge between the atria and the ventricles. The PR interval is primarily a measure of conduction between the initial stimulation of the atria and the initial stimulation of the ventricles. As mentioned previously the normal PR interval measures 0.12 to 0.20 second.

AV heart blocks are classified into first-degree, second-degree (type I and type II), and third-degree. The classification system is based on the degree (type) of block and the location of the block. The PR interval is the key to differentiating the degree of block. The width of the QRS complex and the ventricular rate are keys to differentiating the location of the block (the lower the location of the block in the conduction system, the wider the QRS complex and the slower the ventricular rate). In first-degree AV block (the mildest form), the electrical impulses are delayed in the AV node longer than normal, but all impulses are conducted to the ventricles. In second-degree AV block, some impulses are conducted to the ventricles and some are blocked. The most extreme form of heart block is third-degree AV block, in which no impulses are conducted from the atria to the ventricles. The clinical significance of an AV block depends on the type of block, the ventricular rate, and patient response.

The ability to accurately diagnose AV blocks depends on the use of a systematic approach. The following steps are suggested:
- Assess the regularity of the rhythm (both atrial and ventricular).
- Identify the P wave (or P waves if more than one is present).
- Assess the width of the QRS complex—Is it narrow or wide?
- Assess the relationship between the P waves and the QRS complexes—Is the PR interval consistent or does it vary? Remember, *the PR interval is the key to identifying the degree (type) of block present.*

## First-degree AV block

In first-degree AV block (Figure 8-18 and Box 8-5), the sinus impulse is normally conducted to the AV node, where it's delayed longer than usual before being conducted to the ventricles. This delay in the AV node results in a prolonged PR interval (greater than 0.20 second in duration). This rhythm is reflected on the ECG by a regular rhythm (both atrial and ventricular), one P wave preceding each QRS complex, a consistent but prolonged PR interval, and a narrow QRS complex. Anatomically, this conduction disorder is located at the level of the AV node (thus the narrow QRS complex) and isn't a serious form of heart block. First-degree heart block is simply a normal sinus rhythm with a prolonged PR interval.

First-degree AV block may occur from drug therapy (for example, from digitalis, a beta-blocker, a calcium channel blocker, or amiodarone), increased vagal tone, hyperkalemia, acute rheumatic fever or myocarditis, an MI (especially an inferior wall MI), degeneration of the conducting pathways associated with aging, or an idiopathic cause.

**Box 8-5.**
### First-degree AV block: Identifying ECG features

| | |
|---|---|
| **Rhythm:** | Regular |
| **Rate:** | That of the underlying sinus rhythm; both atrial and ventricular rates will be the same |
| **P waves:** | Sinus; one P wave to each QRS complex |
| **PR interval:** | Prolonged (greater than 0.20 second); remains constant |
| **QRS complex:** | Normal (0.10 second or less) |

First-degree AV block produces no symptoms and requires no treatment. Because first-degree heart block can progress

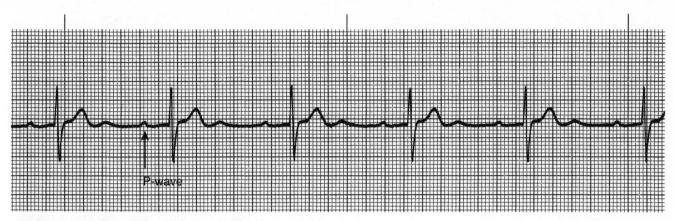

**Figure 8-18. Sinus bradycardia with first-degree AV block**

| | |
|---|---|
| **Rhythm:** | Regular |
| **Rate:** | 48 beats/minute |
| **P waves:** | Sinus P waves present; one P wave to each QRS complex |
| **PR interval:** | 0.28 to 0.32 second (remains constant) |
| **QRS complex:** | 0.08 to 0.10 second |
| **Note:** | A U wave is present. |

to a higher degree of AV block under certain conditions, the rhythm should continue to be monitored until the block resolves or stabilizes. Drugs causing AV block should be reviewed and discontinued if indicated.

## Second-degree AV block, type I (Mobitz I or Wenckebach)

Second-degree AV block, type I (commonly known as *Mobitz I* or *Wenckebach*) (Figures 8-19 and 8-20 and Box 8-6) is characterized by a failure of some of the sinus impulses to be conducted to the ventricles. In this rhythm, the sinus impulse is normally conducted to the AV node, but each successive impulse has more and more difficulty passing through the AV node, until finally an impulse does not pass through (isn't conducted). This rhythm is reflected on the ECG by P waves that occur at regular intervals across the rhythm strip and PR intervals that progressively lengthen from beat to beat until a P wave appears that is not followed by a QRS complex but instead by a pause. The missing QRS complex (dropped beat) causes the ventricular rhythm to be irregular. After each dropped beat the cycle repeats itself. The overall appearance of the rhythm demonstrates group beating (groups of beats separated by pauses) and is a distinguishing characteristic of Mobitz I. Escape beats (atrial, junctional, or ventricular) can occur during the pause in the ventricular rhythm and may obscure the diagnosis because they interrupt the group beating pattern. The location of the conduction disturbance is at the level of the AV node and therefore the QRS complex will be narrow.

**Box 8-6.**
### Second-degree AV block (Mobitz I): Identifying ECG features

| | |
|---|---|
| **Rhythm:** | Regular atrial rhythm; irregular ventricular rhythm |
| **Rate:** | Atrial: That of the underlying sinus rhythm |
| | Ventricular: Varies depending on number of impulses conducted through AV node (will be less than the atrial rate) |
| **P waves:** | Sinus |
| **PR interval:** | Varies; progressively lengthens until a P wave isn't conducted (P wave occurs without the QRS complex); a pause follows the dropped QRS complex |
| **QRS complex:** | Normal (0.10 second or less) |

Mobitz I can be confused with the nonconducted PAC (Figure 8-21). Both rhythms have P waves not followed by a QRS complex but instead by a pause. To differentiate between the two rhythms, one must examine the configuration of the P waves and measure the P-P regularity. The nonconducted PAC will have an abnormal P wave and will occur prematurely. In Mobitz I the P wave configuration remains the same as the sinus beats and the P wave occurs on schedule, not prematurely.

Second-degree AV block, type I is common following an acute inferior wall MI, but it is usually temporary and resolves spontaneously. Other causes include drug effects (for example, from digitalis, a beta-blocker, a calcium channel blocker, or amiodarone), increased vagal tone, hyperkalemia, acute rheumatic fever, and myocarditis. Mobitz I may also

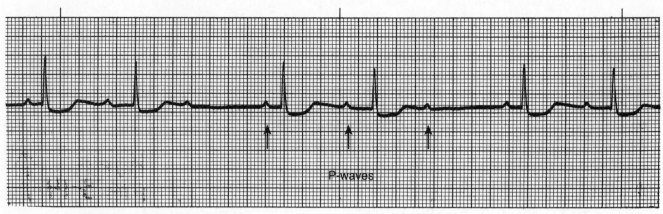

**Figure 8-19. Second-degree AV block, Mobitz I**

| | |
|---|---|
| **Rhythm:** | Regular atrial rhythm; irregular ventricular rhythm |
| **Rate:** | Atrial: 72 beats/minute |
| | Ventricular: 50 beats/minute |
| **P waves:** | Sinus P waves present |
| **PR interval:** | Progressively lengthens from 0.20 to 0.30 second |
| **QRS complex:** | 0.06 to 0.08 second |
| **Note:** | ST segment depression is present. |

occur as a normal variant in athletes at rest because of a physiologic increase in vagal tone.

Mobitz I is seldom a serious form of heart block, although, infrequently, it can progress to a higher degree of AV block. Clinically, patients with Mobitz I AV block are usually without symptoms unless the ventricular rate is slow. If hemodynamic status is compromised because of bradycardia, atropine may be effective in improving AV conduction. Pace-

maker therapy is rarely needed. Drugs causing AV block should be reviewed and discontinued if indicated.

## Second-degree AV block, type II (Mobitz II)

Like Mobitz I, second-degree AV block, type II (or *Mobitz II*) (Figures 8-22 and 8-23 and Box 8-7) is characterized by a

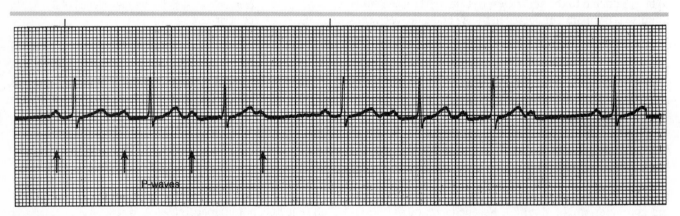

**Figure 8-20. Second-degree AV block, Mobitz I**

| | |
|---|---|
| **Rhythm:** | Regular atrial rhythm; irregular ventricular rhythm |
| **Rate:** | Atrial: 75 beats/minute |
| | Ventricular: 60 beats/minute |
| **P waves:** | Sinus P waves present |
| **PR interval:** | Progressively lengthens from 0.24 to 0.38 second |
| **QRS complex:** | 0.08 second |
| **Comment:** | Good example of group beating |

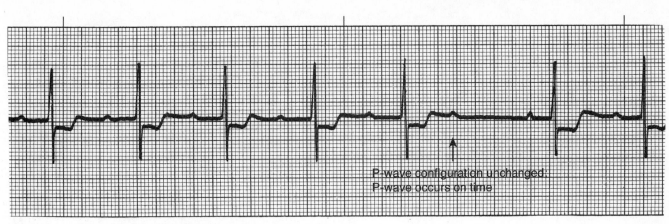

**MOBITZ I**
- Pause in basic ventricular rhythm
- P-P regularity unchanged (P wave occurs on time)
- P wave configuration same as sinus beats
- PR interval of basic rhythm varies

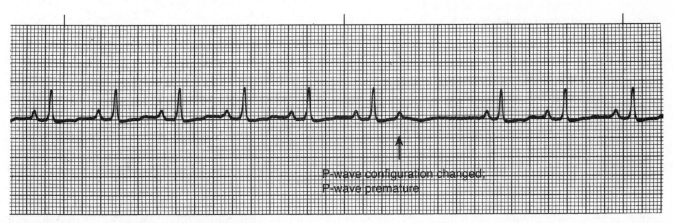

**Nonconducted PAC**
- Pause in basic ventricular rhythm
- P-P regularity interrupted (P wave occurs prematurely)
- P wave configuration different from sinus beats
- PR interval of basic rhythm remains constant

**Figure 8-21.** Differentiation of the nonconducted PAC from Mobitz I.

failure of some of the sinus impulses to be conducted to the ventricles. There are some differences, however, in the anatomic location and severity of the conduction disturbance, as well as in the ECG features. In Mobitz II, there's more than one P wave before each QRS complex (usually two or three, but sometimes more), with only one of the impulses being conducted to the ventricles. The P waves are identical and occur regularly. The PR interval of the conducted beat may be normal or prolonged and remains constant. The ventricular rhythm is usually regular unless the AV conduction ratio varies (alternating between 2:1, 3:1, 4:1, and so on). The location of the conduction disturbance is below the AV node in the bundle of His or bundle branches. As a result the QRS complex may be narrow (if located in the bundle of His) or wide (if located in the bundle branches). The most common location is the bundle branches.

Like Mobitz II, a 2:1 conduction ratio may occasionally occur with Mobitz I (two P waves before each QRS complex

with every other QRS complex dropped). Because every other impulse isn't conducted, Mobitz I with 2:1 conduction doesn't exhibit the lengthening PR intervals that characterize classic Mobitz I. As a rule, if Mobitz I is present, an occasional Wenkebach pattern will usually assert itself when a longer rhythm strip is viewed. However, when a patient presents with a 2:1 conduction ratio, it's sometimes impossible to determine whether the block is Mobitz I or Mobitz II (especially if the QRS complex is of normal duration) without intracardiac recordings. For this reason the AV block rhythm strips with 2:1 conduction, consistent PR intervals, and a narrow QRS complex have been interpreted in the answer keys as Mobitz II, with a notation that clinical correlation is necessary to determine a definite diagnosis.

Mobitz II is commonly associated with an anterior wall MI and, unlike Mobitz I, not the result of increased vagal tone or drug toxicity. Other causes include acute myocarditis

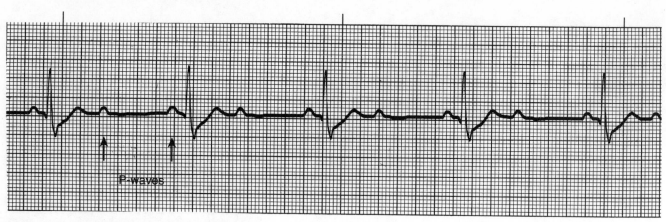

**Figure 8-22. Second-degree AV block, Mobitz II**

| | |
|---|---|
| **Rhythm:** | Regular atrial and ventricular rhythm |
| **Rate:** | Atrial: 82 beats/minute |
| | Ventricular: 41 beats/minute |
| **P waves:** | Two sinus P waves to each QRS complex |
| **PR interval:** | 0.16 second (remains constant) |
| **QRS complex:** | 0.14 second |

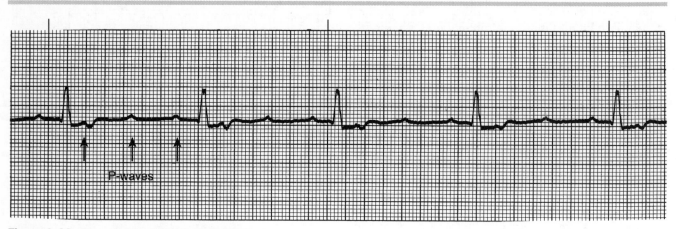

**Figure 8-23. Second-degree AV block, Mobitz II**

| | |
|---|---|
| **Rhythm:** | Regular atrial and ventricular rhythm |
| **Rate:** | Atrial: 123 beats/minute |
| | Ventricular: 41 beats/minute |
| **P waves:** | Three sinus P waves to each QRS complex |
| **PR interval:** | 0.24 to 0.26 second (remains constant) |
| **QRS complex:** | 0.12 second |

and degeneration of the electrical conduction system, which is usually age-related.

Mobitz II is less common but more serious than Mobitz I. Because the anatomic location of the block is lower in the conduction system, Mobitz II has the potential to progress suddenly to third-degree AV block or ventricular standstill with little or no warning. Because of the unpredictable nature of this rhythm, a temporary transvenous pacemaker should be inserted as soon as the rhythm is recognized. If the patient is symptomatic and a transvenous pacemaker is not readily available, a transcutaneous pacemaker may be used in the interim. Atropine must be used with great caution (if at all) for treatment of second-degree AV block of the

Mobitz II type (especially Mobitz II with wide QRS complexes). Administration of atropine increases sinus node discharge, but usually doesn't improve conduction through the AV node. Acceleration of the atrial rate may result in paradoxical slowing of the ventricular rate. This paradoxical response is particularly likely to occur in patients with Mobitz II type second-degree AV block. If significant hypotension is present, start a dopamine infusion at 5 to 20 mcg/kg/minute or, if symptoms are severe, go directly to an epinephrine infusion at 2 to 10 mcg/minute. If the rhythm doesn't resolve, permanent pacing may be necessary.

**Box 8-7.**

## Second-degree AV block (Mobitz II): Identifying ECG features

| | |
|---|---|
| Rhythm: | Atrial: Regular |
| | Ventricular: Usually regular but may be irregular if AV conduction ratios vary |
| Rate: | Atrial: That of the underlying sinus rhythm |
| | Ventricular: Varies depending on number of impulses conducted through AV node (will be less than the atrial rate) |
| P waves: | Sinus; two or three P waves (sometimes more) before each QRS complex |
| PR interval: | May be normal or prolonged; remains constant |
| QRS complex: | Normal if block located at level of bundle of His; wide if block located in bundle branches |

## Third-degree AV block (complete heart block)

Third-degree AV block (Figures 8-24 and 8-25 and Box 8-8) represents complete absence of conduction between the atria and ventricles. This rhythm is also called *complete heart block*. With third-degree heart block, the atria and ventricles beat independently of each other and there's no relationship between atrial activity and ventricular activity (AV dissociation). The atria continue to be paced by the sinus node at its inherent rate of 60 to 100 beats/minute, whereas the ventricles are either paced by an escape pacemaker located in the AV junction at the rate of 40 to 60 beats/minute or in the ventricles at the rate of 30 to 40 beats/minute (sometimes less). The P waves appear at one rate and the QRS complexes at a slower rate, resulting in P waves that march through QRS complexes (hiding at times inside the QRS complex and within the T wave) and PR intervals that vary greatly. Although independent beating between the atria and the ventricles is occurring, both the atrial rhythm and the ventricular rhythm are usually regular. Both the width of the QRS complex and the ventricular rate reflect the location of the blockage. If the block is at the level of the AV node or bundle of His, the QRS complex will be narrow and the heart rate between 40 and 60 beats/minute. If the blockage is in the bundle branches, the QRS complex will be wide and the heart rate much slower (40 beats/minute or less). As a general rule, complete heart block with wide QRS complexes tend to be less stable than complete heart block with narrow QRS complexes.

**Box 8-8.**

## Third-degree AV block (complete heart block): Identifying ECG features

| | |
|---|---|
| Rhythm: | Atrial: Regular |
| | Ventricular: Regular |
| Rate: | Atrial: That of the underlying sinus rhythm |
| | Ventricular: 40 to 60 beats/minute if paced by AV junction; 30 to 40 beats/minute (or less) if paced by ventricles; will be less than the atrial rate |
| P waves: | Sinus P waves with no constant relationship to the QRS complex; P waves can be found hidden in QRS complexes and T waves |
| PR interval: | Varies greatly |
| QRS complex: | Normal if block located at level of AV node or bundle of His; wide if block located at level of bundle branches |

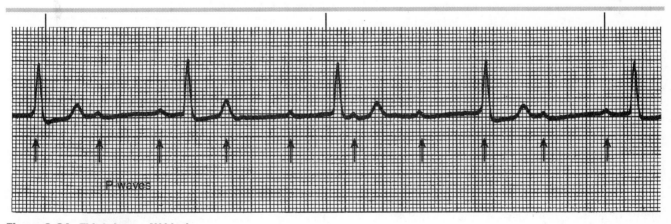

**Figure 8-24. Third-degree AV block**

| | |
|---|---|
| Rhythm: | Regular atrial and ventricular rhythm |
| Rate: | Atrial: 88 beats/minute |
| | Ventricular: 38 beats/minute |
| P waves: | Sinus (bear no relationship to QRS complex; found hidden in QRS complex and T waves) |
| PR interval: | Varies greatly |
| QRS complex: | 0.08 to 0.10 second |

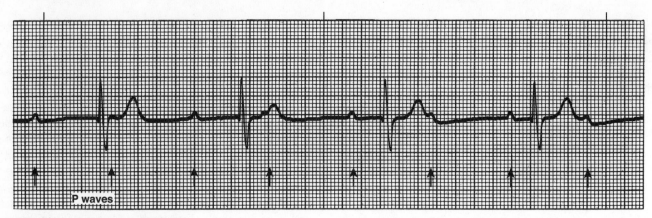

**Figure 8-25. Third-degree AV block**

Rhythm:        Regular atrial and ventricular rhythm
Rate:          Atrial: 72 beats/minute
               Ventricular: 40 beats/minute
P waves:       Sinus P waves present (bear no constant relationship to QRS complexes; found hidden in QRS complexes and T waves)
PR interval:   Varies greatly
QRS complex:   0.12 second

Complete heart block may be temporary or permanent and may occur for a number of reasons. Temporary (reversible) third-degree AV block is usually associated with narrow QRS complexes and can result from an inferior wall MI, ischemic heart disease, increased vagal tone, drug effects (for example, from digitalis, a beta-blocker, a calcium channel blocker, or amiodarone), hyperkalemia, acute rheumatic fever, or myocarditis. Permanent (chronic) third-degree heart block is usually associated with wide QRS complexes and can result from an acute anterior MI or chronic degenerative changes in the electrical conduction system seen in the elderly. Chronic third-degree AV block usually doesn't occur as a result of increased vagal tone or drug toxicity.

Regardless of its cause, complete heart block is a serious and potentially life-threatening arrhythmia. Like Mobitz II, complete heart block can progress to ventricular standstill suddenly, with little or no warning. If third-degree AV block occurs gradually, as seen in age-related degeneration of the electrical conduction system, the patient may have no significant symptoms and may only require cardiac monitoring with a transcutaneous pacemaker on standby until a permanent pacemaker is implanted. However, if complete heart block occurs suddenly (usually as a complication of an acute MI), the patient may become symptomatic (for example, with hypotension, chest pain, dyspnea, a decrease in urine output, or fainting) from reduced cardiac output secondary to the slow ventricular rate and loss of the "atrial kick." The fainting spells associated with complete heart block are called *Stokes-Adams attacks* or *Stokes-Adams syncope.*

Once the rhythm is recognized, a transcutaneous pacemaker should be applied while preparations are made for insertion of a temporary transvenous pacemaker. Atropine may be effective in accelerating the sinus rate and AV node conduction in narrow complex third-degree heart block (AV node level), but has little or no effect on wide complex third-degree heart block (bundle-branch level). For significant hypotension, start a dopamine infusion at 5 to 20 mcg/kg/minute or, if symptoms are severe, go directly to an epinephrine infusion at 2 to 10 mcg/minute. Unresolved third-degree AV block requires a permanent pacemaker.

Table 8-1 compares the ECG characteristics of each type of AV block. A summary of the identifying ECG features of junctional arrhythmias and AV blocks can be found in Table 8-2.

**Table 8-1.**

## AV block comparisons

| PR constant <br> *(First-degree)* | PR varies <br> *(Second-degree, Mobitz I)* |
|---|---|
| PR constant | PR varies |
| PR prolonged <br> One P wave to each QRS | PR progressively gets longer until a QRS is dropped |
| Regular atrial rhythm; regular ventricular rhythm | Regular atrial rhythm; irregular ventricular rhythm |
| *(Second-degree, Mobitz II)* | *(Third-degree)* |
| PR constant | PR varies |
| PR normal or prolonged <br> Two or three P waves (possibly more) to each QRS | P waves have no constant relationship to QRS (found hidden in QRS complexes and T waves) |
| Regular atrial rhythm; regular ventricular rhythm (unless conduction ratios vary) | Regular atrial rhythm; regular ventricular rhythm |

Table 8-2.

## Junctional arrhythmias and AV blocks: Summary of identifying ECG features

| Name | Rhythm | Rate (beats/minute) | P waves (lead II) | PR interval | QRS complex |
|---|---|---|---|---|---|
| Premature junctional contraction (PJC) | Basic rhythm usually regular; irregular with PJC | That of basic rhythm | Premature P wave; inverted in lead II and will occur immediately before or after the QRS complex, or will be hidden within the QRS complex | 0.10 second or less | Premature QRS complex; normal duration (0.10 second or less) |
| Junctional rhythm | Regular | 40 to 60 | Inverted in lead II and will occur immediately before or after the QRS complex, or will be hidden within the QRS complex | Short (0.10 second or less) | Normal (0.10 second or less) |
| Accelerated junctional rhythm | Regular | 60 to 100 | Inverted in lead II and will occur immediately before or after the QRS complex, or will be hidden within the QRS complex | Short (0.10 second or less) | Normal (0.10 second or less) |
| Junctional tachycardia | Regular | > 100 | Inverted in lead II and will occur immediately before or after the QRS complex, or will be hidden within the QRS complex | Short (0.10 second or less) | Normal (0.10 second or less) |
| First-degree atrioventricular (AV) block | Regular | That of underlying sinus rhythm; both atrial and ventricular rates will be the same | Sinus origin; one P wave to each QRS complex | Prolonged (more than 0.20 second); remains constant | Normal (0.10 second or less) |
| Second-degree AV block, Mobitz I | Atrial: regular Ventricular: irregular | Atrial: that of underlying sinus rhythm Ventricular: depends on number of impulses conducted through AV node; will be less than atrial late | Sinus origin | Varies; progressively lengthens until a P wave isn't conducted (P wave occurs without the QRS complex); a pause follows the dropped QRS complex | Normal (0.10 second or less) |
| Second-degree AV block, Mobitz II | Atrial: regular Ventricular: usually regular, but may be irregular if conductions ratios vary | Atrial: that of underlying sinus rhythm Ventricular: depends on number of impulses conducted through AV node; will be less than atrial late | Sinus origin; two or three P waves (sometimes more) before each QRS complex | Normal or prolonged; remains constant | Normal if block at level of bundle of His; wide if block in bundle branches |
| Third-degree AV block | Atrial: regular Ventricular: regular | Atrial: that of underlying sinus rhythm Ventricular: 40 to 60 if paced by AV junction; 30 to 40 (sometimes less) if paced by ventricles; will be less than atrial rate | Sinus P waves with no constant relationship to the QRS complex; P waves found hidden in QRS complexes and T waves | Varies greatly | Normal if block at level of AV node or bundle of His; wide if block in bundle branches |

# Rhythm strip practice: AV junctional arrhythmias and AV blocks

For each of the following rhythm strips:
- determine the rhythm regularity, the ventricular rate, and the atrial rate (that is, if it differs from the ventricular rate)
- identify and examine P waves

- measure the duration of the PR interval and the QRS complex
- interpret the rhythm.

All rhythm strips are lead II unless otherwise noted. Check your answers with the answer key in the appendix.

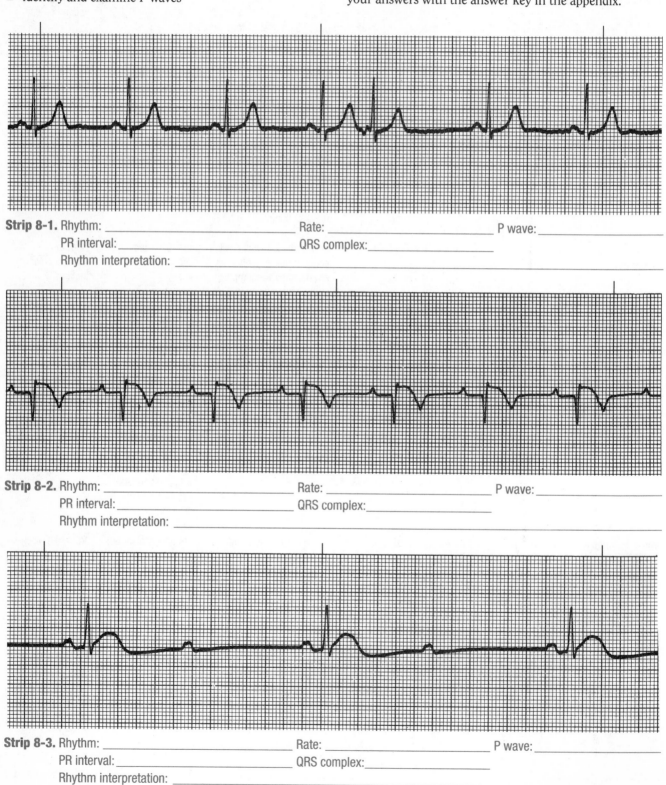

**Strip 8-1.** Rhythm: _____ Rate: _____ P wave: _____
PR interval: _____ QRS complex: _____
Rhythm interpretation: _____

**Strip 8-2.** Rhythm: _____ Rate: _____ P wave: _____
PR interval: _____ QRS complex: _____
Rhythm interpretation: _____

**Strip 8-3.** Rhythm: _____ Rate: _____ P wave: _____
PR interval: _____ QRS complex: _____
Rhythm interpretation: _____

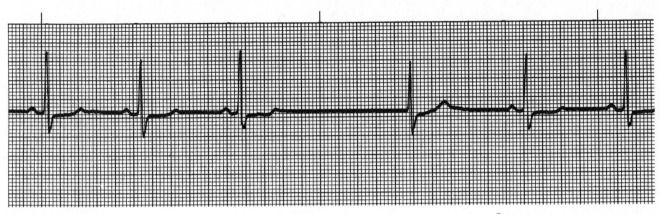

**Strip 8-4.** Rhythm: _____ Rate: _____ P wave: _____
PR interval: _____ QRS complex: _____
Rhythm interpretation: _____

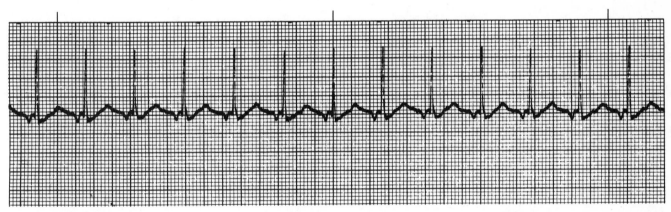

**Strip 8-5.** Rhythm: _____ Rate: _____ P wave: _____
PR interval: _____ QRS complex: _____
Rhythm interpretation: _____

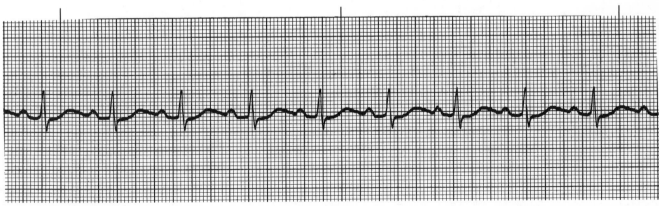

**Strip 8-6.** Rhythm: _____ Rate: _____ P wave: _____
PR interval: _____ QRS complex: _____
Rhythm interpretation: _____

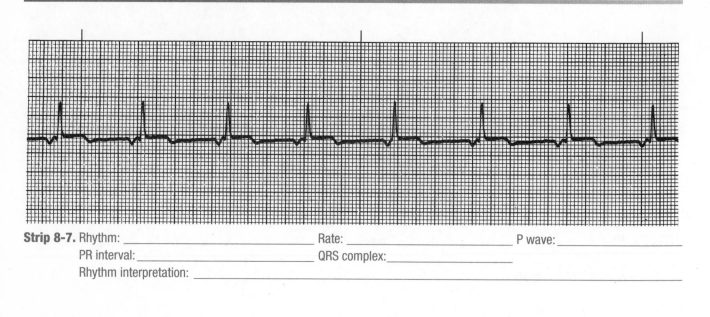

**Strip 8-7.** Rhythm: _____ Rate: _____ P wave: _____

PR interval: _____ QRS complex: _____

Rhythm interpretation: _____

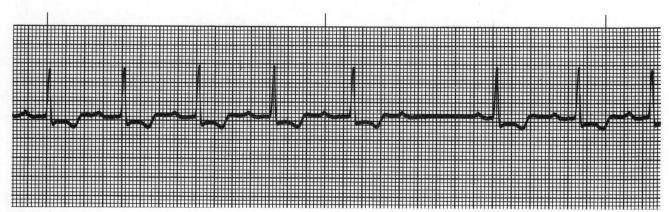

**Strip 8-8.** Rhythm: _____ Rate: _____ P wave: _____

PR interval: _____ QRS complex: _____

Rhythm interpretation: _____

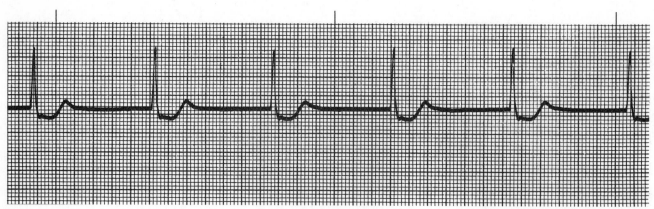

**Strip 8-9.** Rhythm: _____ Rate: _____ P wave: _____

PR interval: _____ QRS complex: _____

Rhythm interpretation: _____

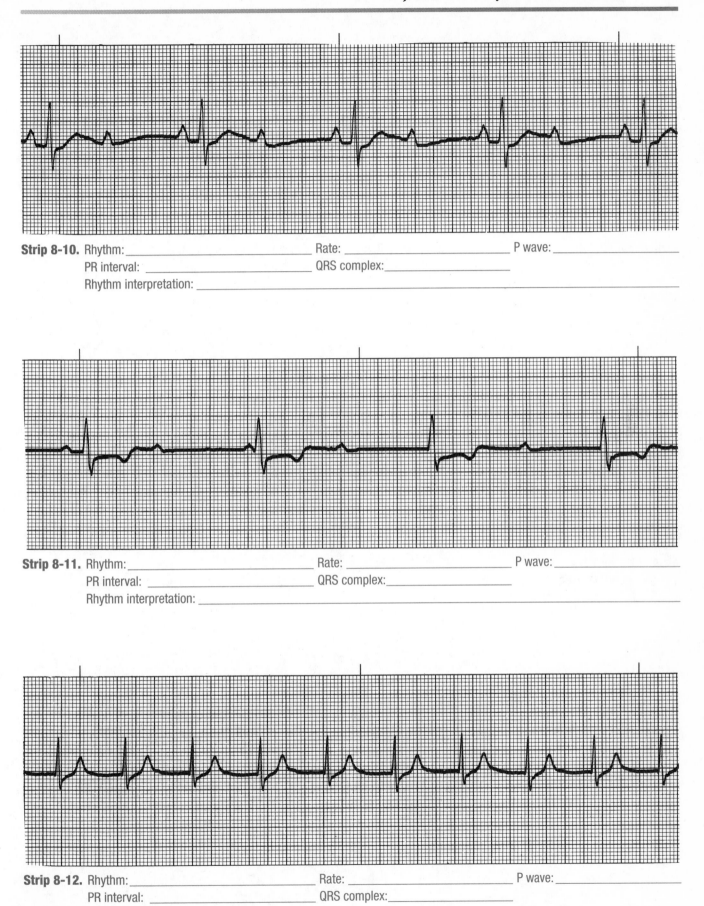

**Strip 8-10.** Rhythm:_____ Rate: _____ P wave: _____

PR interval: _____ QRS complex:_____

Rhythm interpretation: _____

**Strip 8-11.** Rhythm:_____ Rate: _____ P wave: _____

PR interval: _____ QRS complex:_____

Rhythm interpretation: _____

**Strip 8-12.** Rhythm:_____ Rate: _____ P wave: _____

PR interval: _____ QRS complex:_____

Rhythm interpretation: _____

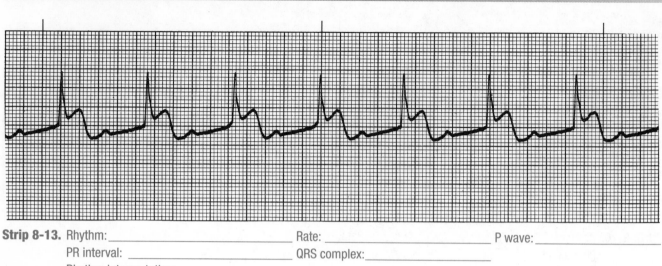

**Strip 8-13.** Rhythm: _____ Rate: _____ P wave: _____

PR interval: _____ QRS complex: _____

Rhythm interpretation: _____

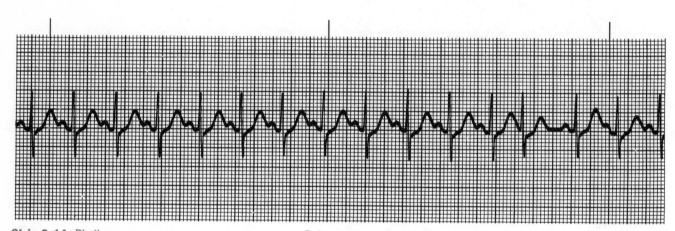

**Strip 8-14.** Rhythm: _____ Rate: _____ P wave: _____

PR interval: _____ QRS complex: _____

Rhythm interpretation: _____

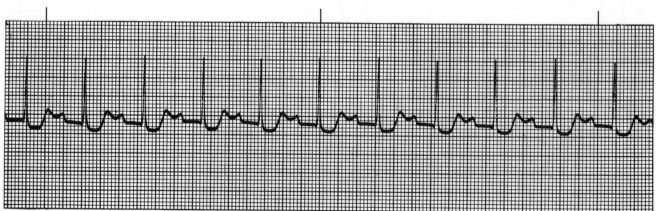

**Strip 8-15.** Rhythm: _____ Rate: _____ P wave: _____

PR interval: _____ QRS complex: _____

Rhythm interpretation: _____

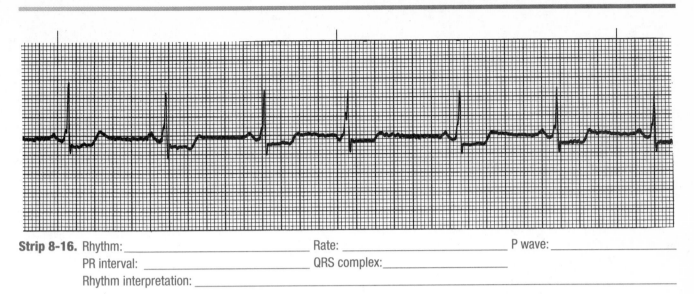

**Strip 8-16.** Rhythm: _____ Rate: _____ P wave: _____

PR interval: _____ QRS complex: _____

Rhythm interpretation: _____

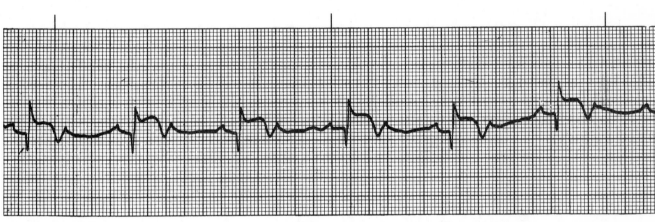

**Strip 8-17.** Rhythm: _____ Rate: _____ P wave: _____

PR interval: _____ QRS complex: _____

Rhythm interpretation: _____

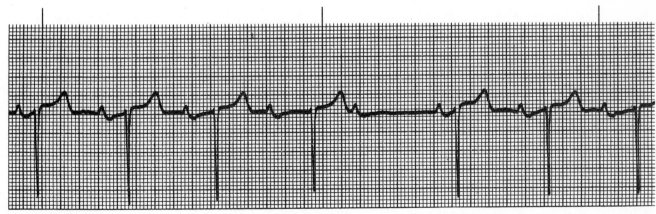

**Strip 8-18.** Rhythm: _____ Rate: _____ P wave: _____

PR interval: _____ QRS complex: _____

Rhythm interpretation: _____

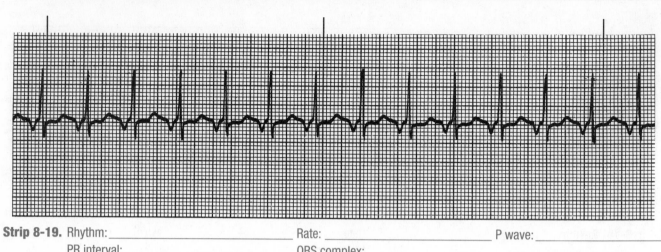

**Strip 8-19.** Rhythm:_____ Rate: _____ P wave: _____

PR interval: _____ QRS complex:_____

Rhythm interpretation: _____

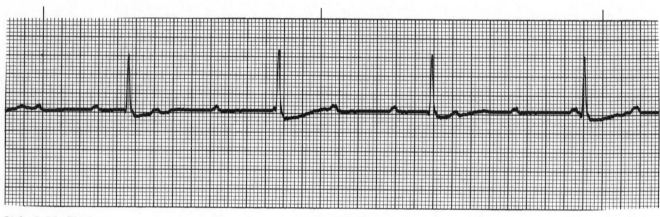

**Strip 8-20.** Rhythm:_____ Rate: _____ P wave: _____

PR interval: _____ QRS complex:_____

Rhythm interpretation: _____

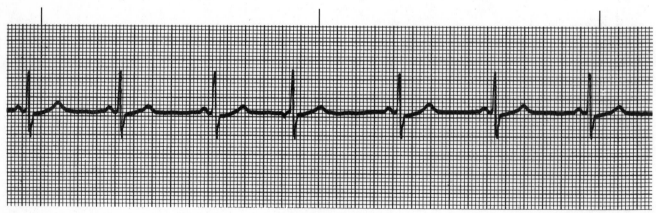

**Strip 8-21.** Rhythm:_____ Rate: _____ P wave: _____

PR interval: _____ QRS complex:_____

Rhythm interpretation: _____

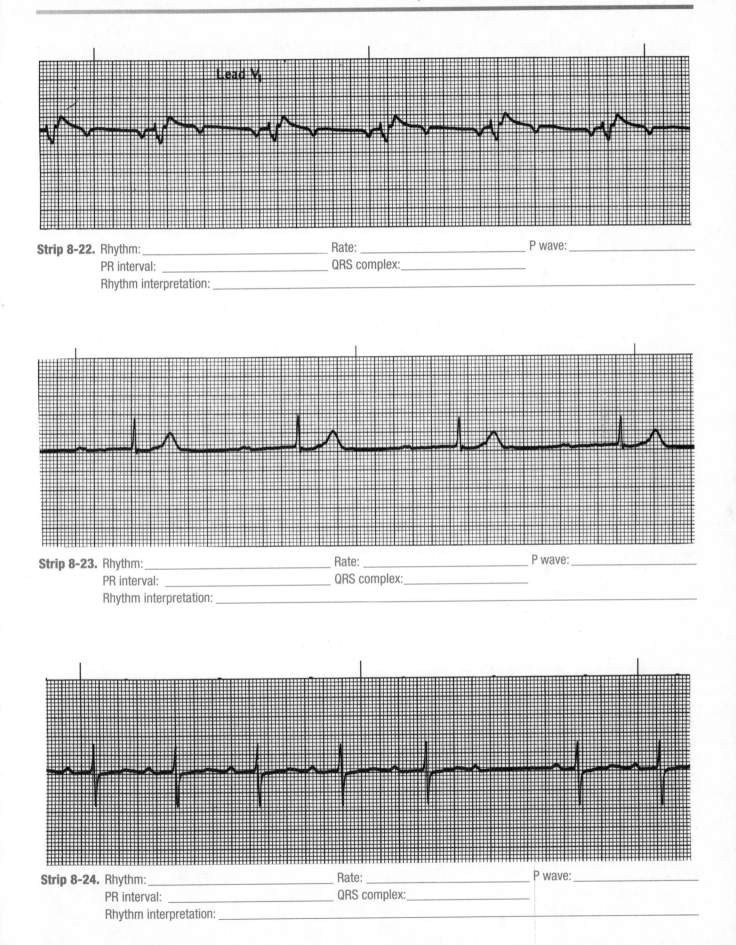

**Lead V₁**

**Strip 8-22.** Rhythm: _____    Rate: _____    P wave: _____
PR interval: _____    QRS complex: _____
Rhythm interpretation: _____

**Strip 8-23.** Rhythm: _____    Rate: _____    P wave: _____
PR interval: _____    QRS complex: _____
Rhythm interpretation: _____

**Strip 8-24.** Rhythm: _____    Rate: _____    P wave: _____
PR interval: _____    QRS complex: _____
Rhythm interpretation: _____

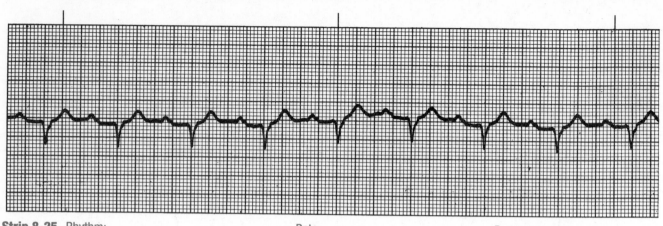

**Strip 8-25.** Rhythm:_____ Rate:_____ P wave:_____

PR interval:_____ QRS complex:_____

Rhythm interpretation:_____

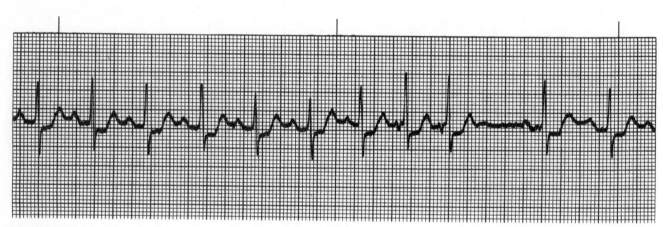

**Strip 8-26.** Rhythm:_____ Rate:_____ P wave:_____

PR interval:_____ QRS complex:_____

Rhythm interpretation:_____

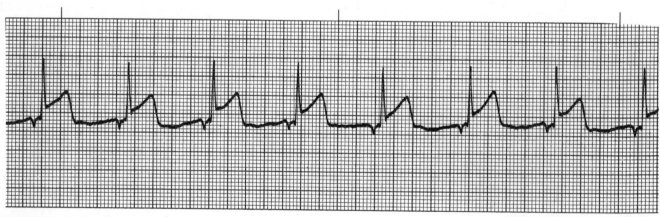

**Strip 8-27.** Rhythm:_____ Rate:_____ P wave:_____

PR interval:_____ QRS complex:_____

Rhythm interpretation:_____

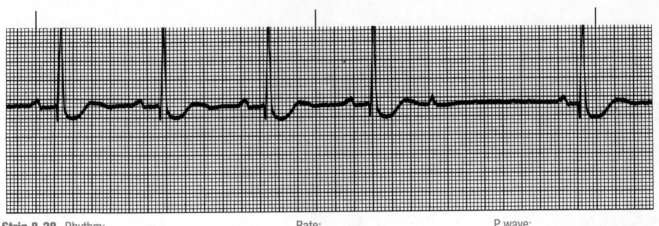

**Strip 8-28.** Rhythm: _____ Rate: _____ P wave: _____
PR interval: _____ QRS complex: _____
Rhythm interpretation: _____

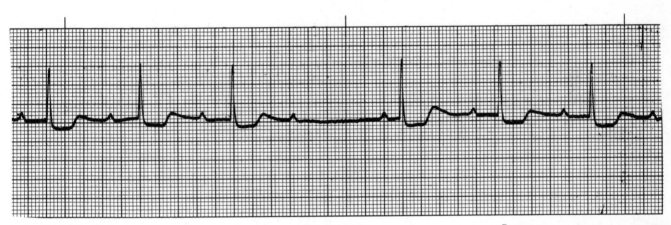

**Strip 8-29.** Rhythm: _____ Rate: _____ P wave: _____
PR interval: _____ QRS complex: _____
Rhythm interpretation: _____

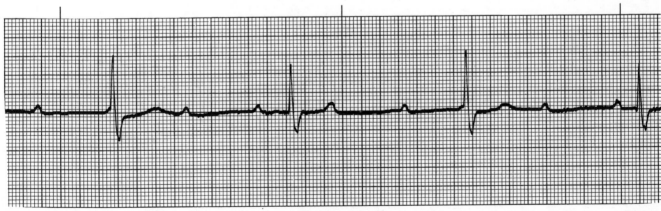

**Strip 8-30.** Rhythm: _____ Rate: _____ P wave: _____
PR interval: _____ QRS complex: _____
Rhythm interpretation: _____

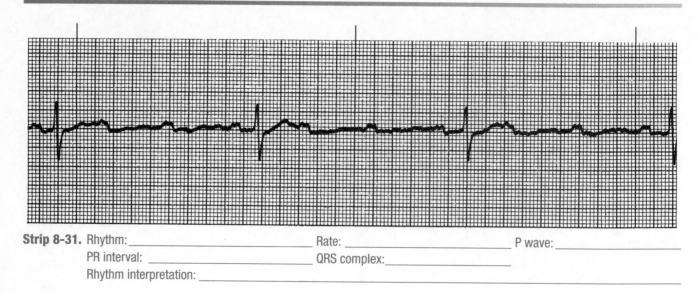

**Strip 8-31.** Rhythm:_____ Rate:_____ P wave:_____

PR interval: _____ QRS complex:_____

Rhythm interpretation: _____

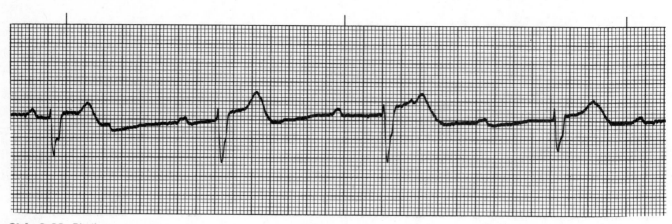

**Strip 8-32.** Rhythm:_____ Rate:_____ P wave:_____

PR interval: _____ QRS complex:_____

Rhythm interpretation: _____

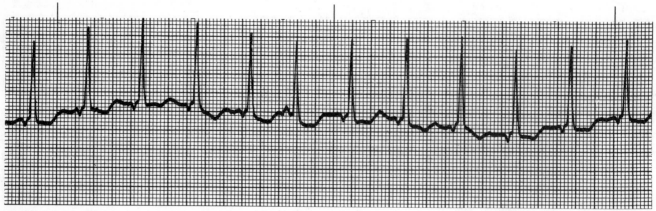

**Strip 8-33.** Rhythm:_____ Rate:_____ P wave:_____

PR interval: _____ QRS complex:_____

Rhythm interpretation: _____

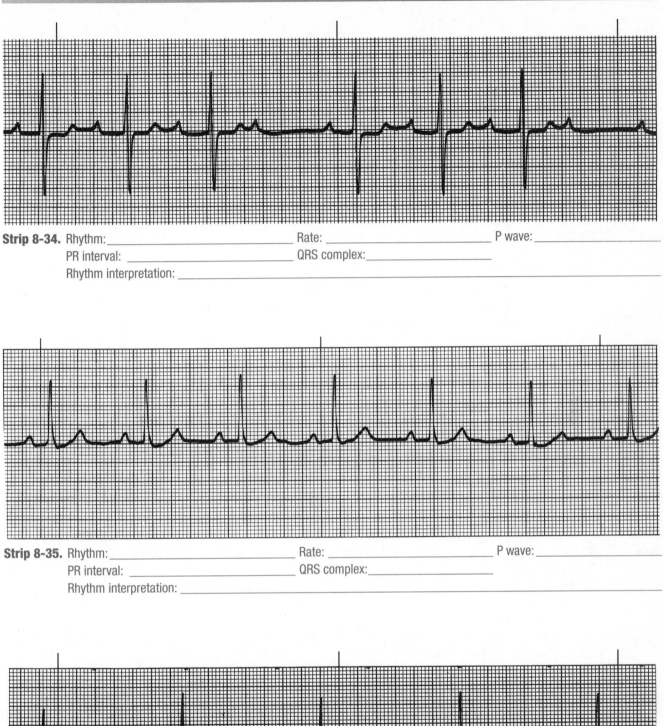

**Strip 8-34.** Rhythm:_____ Rate:_____ P wave:_____

PR interval:_____ QRS complex:_____

Rhythm interpretation:_____

**Strip 8-35.** Rhythm:_____ Rate:_____ P wave:_____

PR interval:_____ QRS complex:_____

Rhythm interpretation:_____

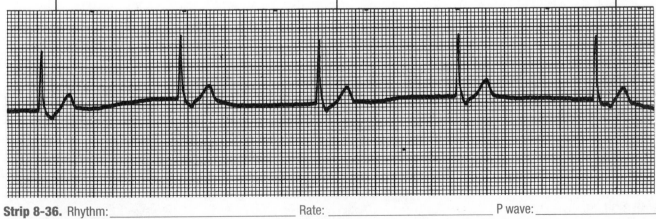

**Strip 8-36.** Rhythm:_____ Rate:_____ P wave:_____

PR interval:_____ QRS complex:_____

Rhythm interpretation:_____

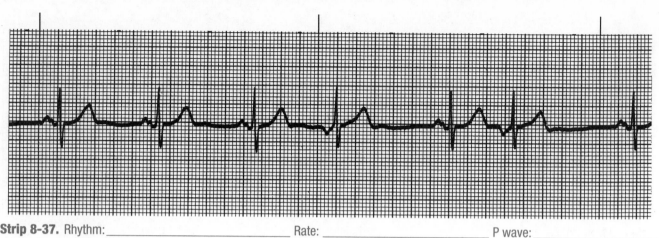

**Strip 8-37.** Rhythm:_____ Rate:_____ P wave:_____

PR interval: _____ QRS complex:_____

Rhythm interpretation: _____

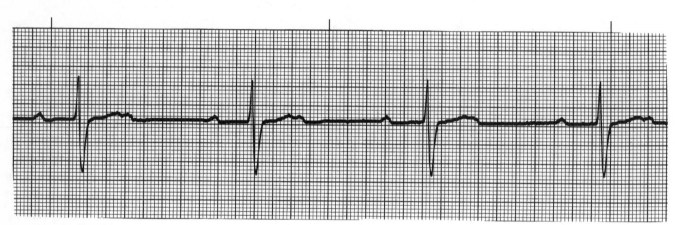

**Strip 8-38.** Rhythm:_____ Rate:_____ P wave:_____

PR interval: _____ QRS complex:_____

Rhythm interpretation: _____

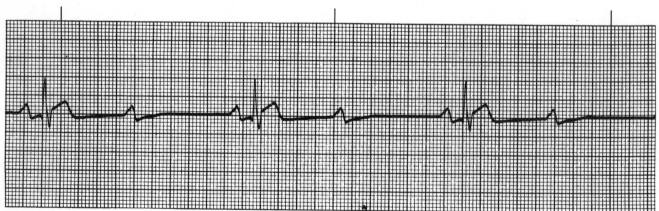

**Strip 8-39.** Rhythm:_____ Rate:_____ P wave:_____

PR interval: _____ QRS complex:_____

Rhythm interpretation: _____

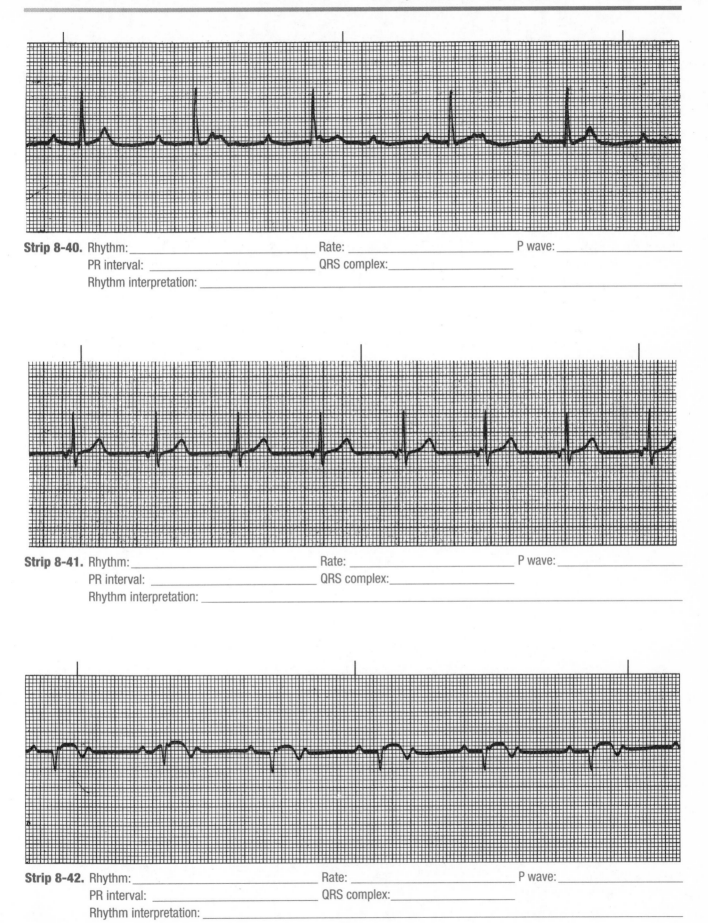

**Strip 8-40.** Rhythm:_____ Rate:_____ P wave:_____

PR interval:_____ QRS complex:_____

Rhythm interpretation:_____

**Strip 8-41.** Rhythm:_____ Rate:_____ P wave:_____

PR interval:_____ QRS complex:_____

Rhythm interpretation:_____

**Strip 8-42.** Rhythm:_____ Rate:_____ P wave:_____

PR interval:_____ QRS complex:_____

Rhythm interpretation:_____

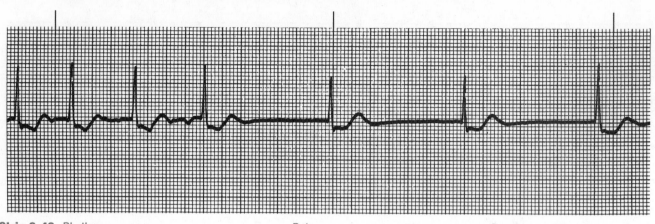

**Strip 8-43.** Rhythm: _____ Rate: _____ P wave: _____

PR interval: _____ QRS complex: _____

Rhythm interpretation: _____

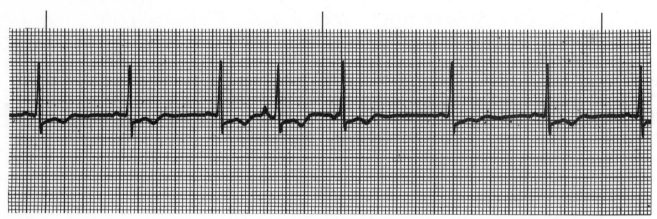

**Strip 8-44.** Rhythm: _____ Rate: _____ P wave: _____

PR interval: _____ QRS complex: _____

Rhythm interpretation: _____

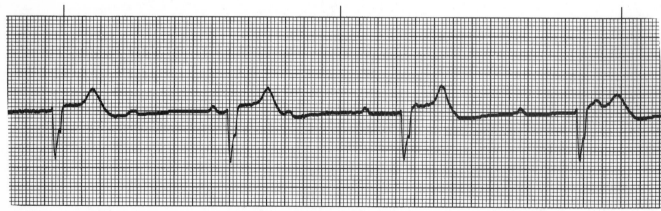

**Strip 8-45.** Rhythm: _____ Rate: _____ P wave: _____

PR interval: _____ QRS complex: _____

Rhythm interpretation: _____

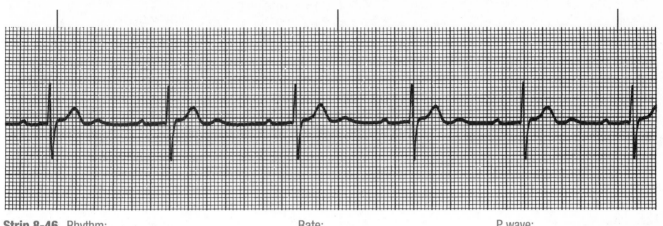

**Strip 8-46.** Rhythm: _____ Rate: _____ P wave: _____
PR interval: _____ QRS complex: _____
Rhythm interpretation: _____

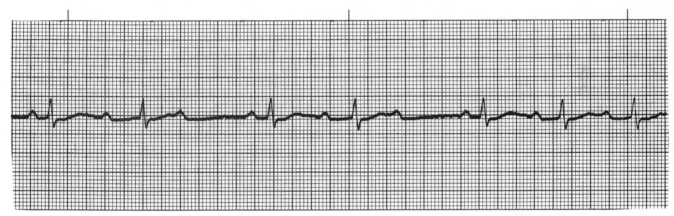

**Strip 8-47.** Rhythm: _____ Rate: _____ P wave: _____
PR interval: _____ QRS complex: _____
Rhythm interpretation: _____

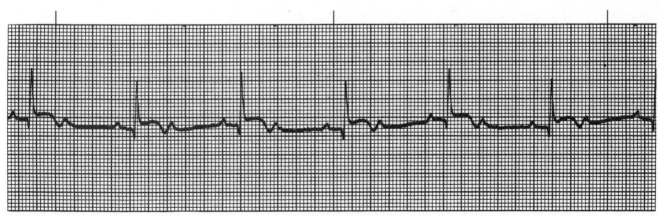

**Strip 8-48.** Rhythm: _____ Rate: _____ P wave: _____
PR interval: _____ QRS complex: _____
Rhythm interpretation: _____

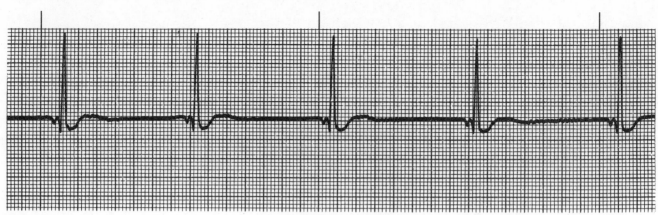

**Strip 8-49.** Rhythm: _____ Rate: _____ P wave: _____

PR interval: _____ QRS complex: _____

Rhythm interpretation: _____

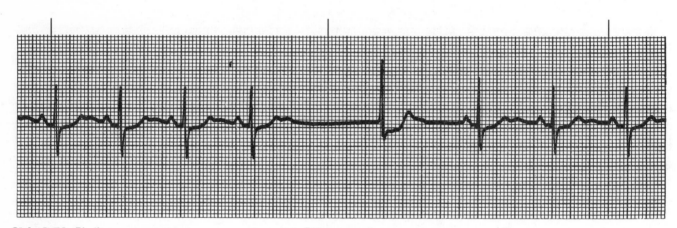

**Strip 8-50.** Rhythm: _____ Rate: _____ P wave: _____

PR interval: _____ QRS complex: _____

Rhythm interpretation: _____

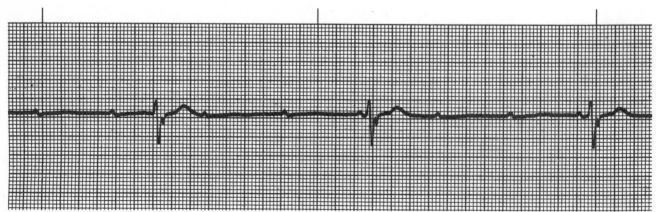

**Strip 8-51.** Rhythm: _____ Rate: _____ P wave: _____

PR interval: _____ QRS complex: _____

Rhythm interpretation: _____

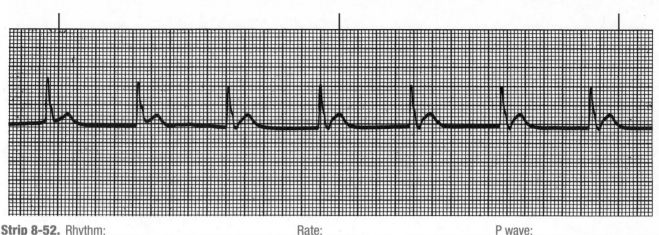

**Strip 8-52.** Rhythm: _____ Rate: _____ P wave: _____

PR interval: _____ QRS complex: _____

Rhythm interpretation: _____

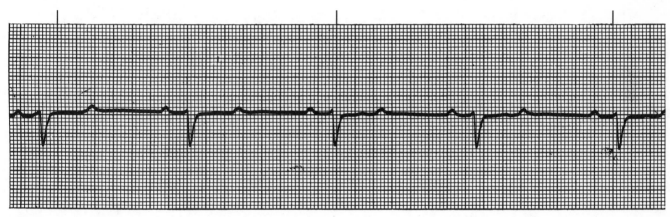

**Strip 8-53.** Rhythm: _____ Rate: _____ P wave: _____

PR interval: _____ QRS complex: _____

Rhythm interpretation: _____

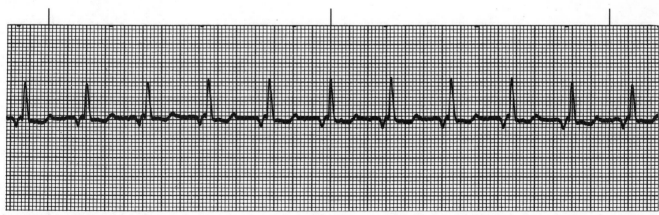

**Strip 8-54.** Rhythm: _____ Rate: _____ P wave: _____

PR interval: _____ QRS complex: _____

Rhythm interpretation: _____

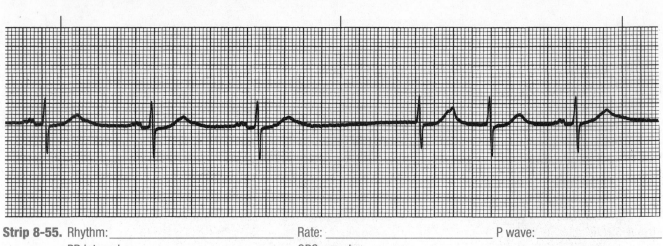

**Strip 8-55.** Rhythm:_____ Rate:_____ P wave:_____

PR interval:_____ QRS complex:_____

Rhythm interpretation:_____

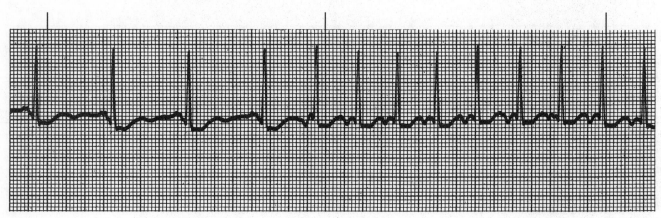

**Strip 8-56.** Rhythm:_____ Rate:_____ P wave:_____

PR interval:_____ QRS complex:_____

Rhythm interpretation:_____

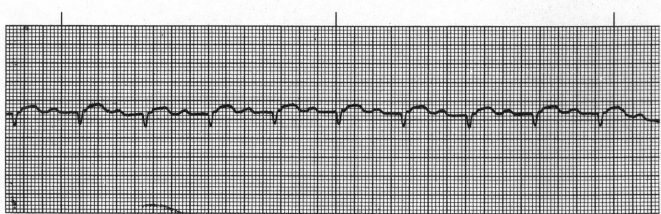

**Strip 8-57.** Rhythm:_____ Rate:_____ P wave:_____

PR interval:_____ QRS complex:_____

Rhythm interpretation:_____

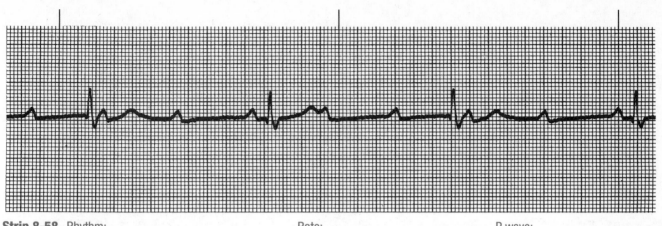

**Strip 8-58.** Rhythm: _____ Rate: _____ P wave: _____

PR interval: _____ QRS complex: _____

Rhythm interpretation: _____

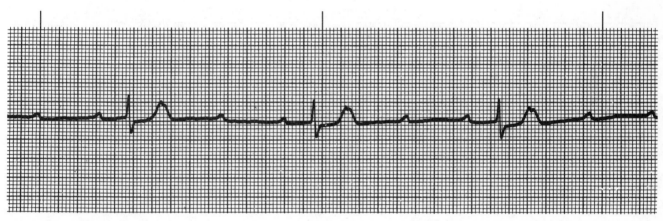

**Strip 8-59.** Rhythm: _____ Rate: _____ P wave: _____

PR interval: _____ QRS complex: _____

Rhythm interpretation: _____

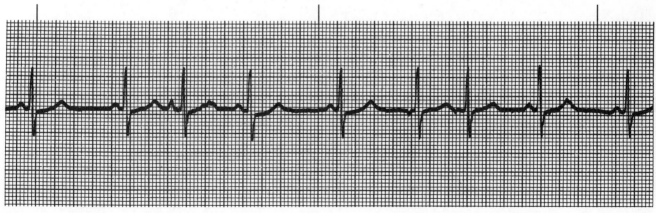

**Strip 8-60.** Rhythm: _____ Rate: _____ P wave: _____

PR interval: _____ QRS complex: _____

Rhythm interpretation: _____

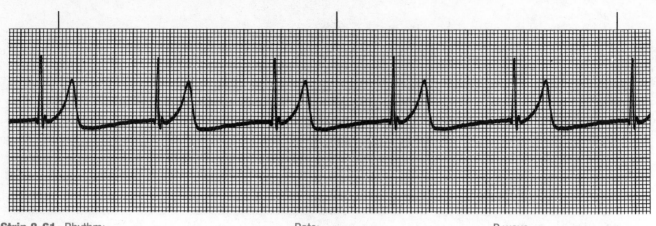

**Strip 8-61.** Rhythm: _____ Rate: _____ P wave: _____

PR interval: _____ QRS complex: _____

Rhythm interpretation: _____

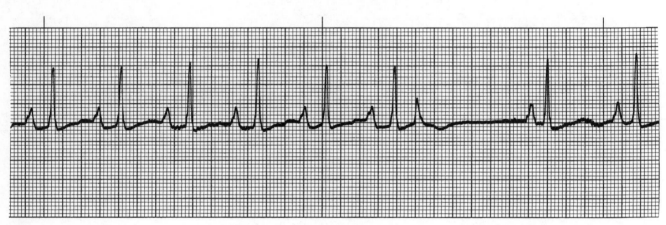

**Strip 8-62.** Rhythm: _____ Rate: _____ P wave: _____

PR interval: _____ QRS complex: _____

Rhythm interpretation: _____

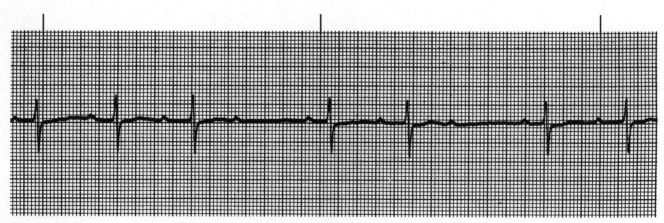

**Strip 8-63.** Rhythm: _____ Rate: _____ P wave: _____

PR interval: _____ QRS complex: _____

Rhythm interpretation: _____

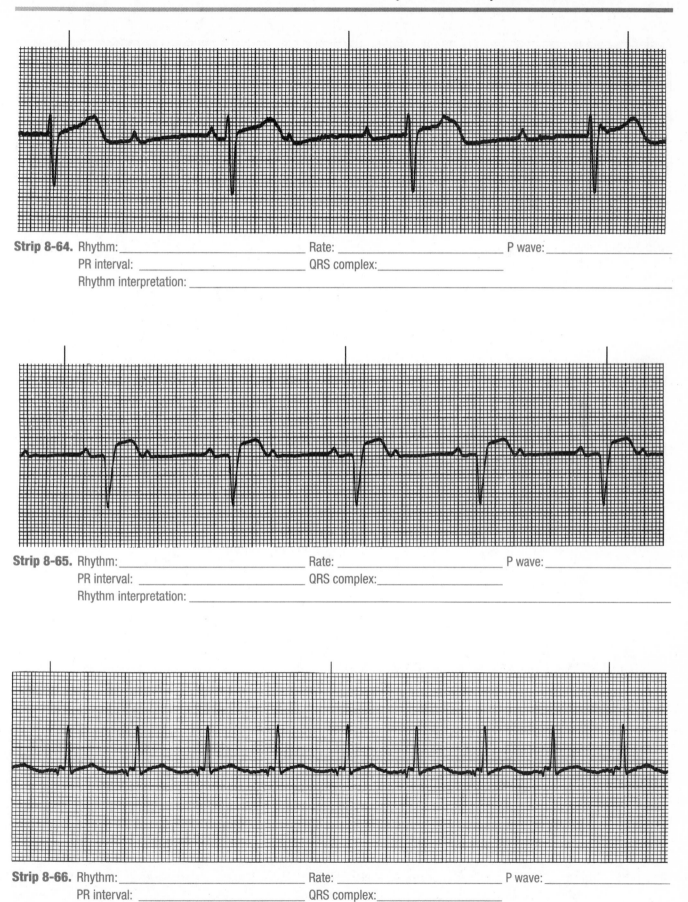

**Strip 8-64.** Rhythm:_____ Rate:_____ P wave:_____

PR interval: _____ QRS complex:_____

Rhythm interpretation: _____

**Strip 8-65.** Rhythm:_____ Rate:_____ P wave:_____

PR interval: _____ QRS complex:_____

Rhythm interpretation: _____

**Strip 8-66.** Rhythm:_____ Rate:_____ P wave:_____

PR interval: _____ QRS complex:_____

Rhythm interpretation: _____

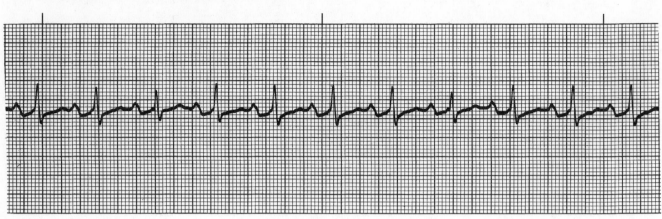

**Strip 8-67.** Rhythm:_____ Rate:_____ P wave:_____

PR interval:_____ QRS complex:_____

Rhythm interpretation:_____

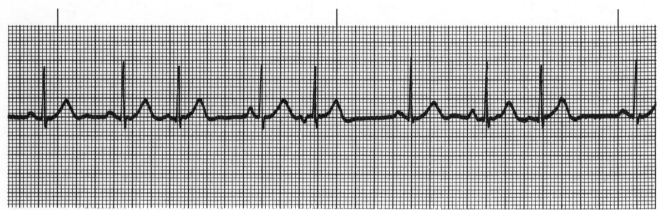

**Strip 8-68.** Rhythm:_____ Rate:_____ P wave:_____

PR interval:_____ QRS complex:_____

Rhythm interpretation:_____

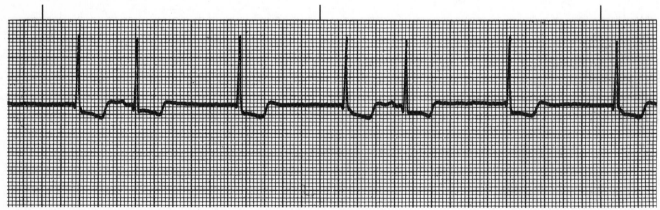

**Strip 8-69.** Rhythm:_____ Rate:_____ P wave:_____

PR interval:_____ QRS complex:_____

Rhythm interpretation:_____

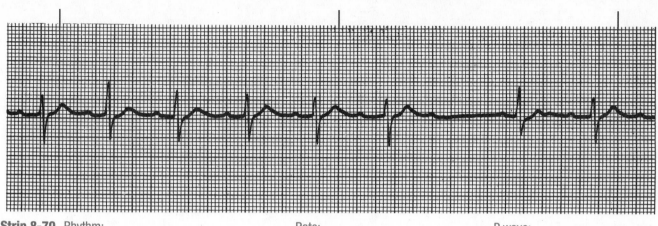

**Strip 8-70.** Rhythm: _____ Rate: _____ P wave: _____

PR interval: _____ QRS complex: _____

Rhythm interpretation: _____

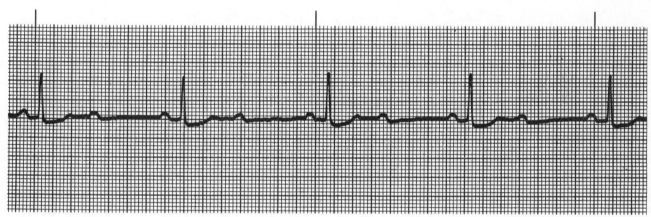

**Strip 8-71.** Rhythm: _____ Rate: _____ P wave: _____

PR interval: _____ QRS complex: _____

Rhythm interpretation: _____

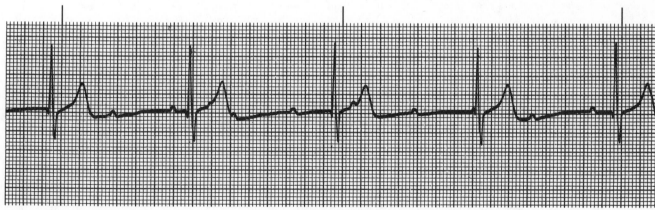

**Strip 8-72.** Rhythm: _____ Rate: _____ P wave: _____

PR interval: _____ QRS complex: _____

Rhythm interpretation: _____

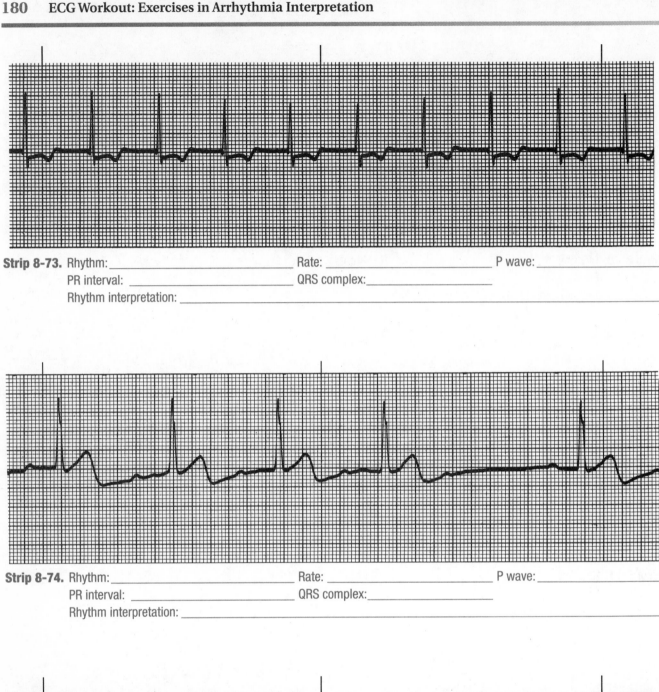

**Strip 8-73.** Rhythm: _____ Rate: _____ P wave: _____
PR interval: _____ QRS complex: _____
Rhythm interpretation: _____

**Strip 8-74.** Rhythm: _____ Rate: _____ P wave: _____
PR interval: _____ QRS complex: _____
Rhythm interpretation: _____

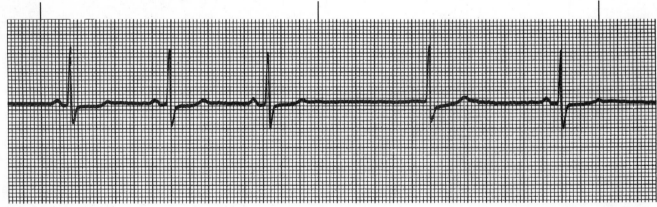

**Strip 8-75.** Rhythm: _____ Rate: _____ P wave: _____
PR interval: _____ QRS complex: _____
Rhythm interpretation: _____

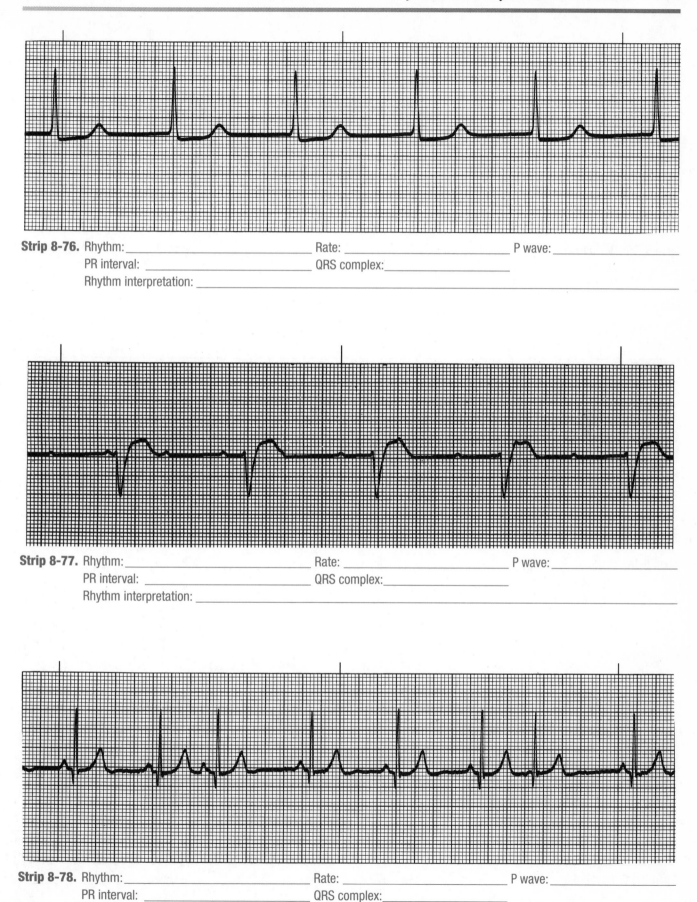

**Strip 8-76.** Rhythm:_____ Rate:_____ P wave:_____

PR interval:_____ QRS complex:_____

Rhythm interpretation:_____

**Strip 8-77.** Rhythm:_____ Rate:_____ P wave:_____

PR interval:_____ QRS complex:_____

Rhythm interpretation:_____

**Strip 8-78.** Rhythm:_____ Rate:_____ P wave:_____

PR interval:_____ QRS complex:_____

Rhythm interpretation:_____

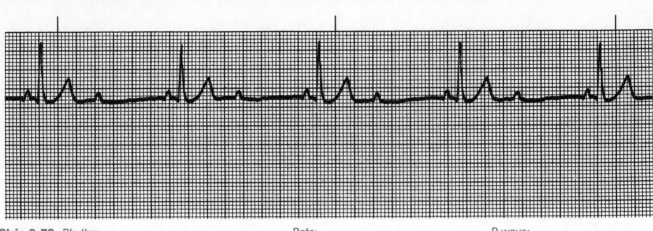

**Strip 8-79.** Rhythm:_____ Rate:_____ P wave:_____

PR interval:_____ QRS complex:_____

Rhythm interpretation:_____

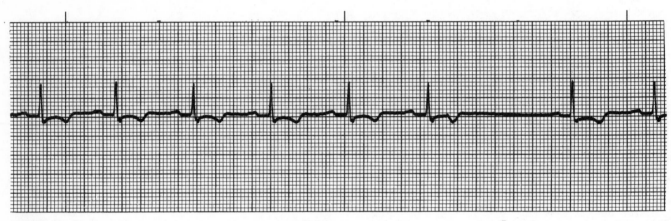

**Strip 8-80.** Rhythm:_____ Rate:_____ P wave:_____

PR interval:_____ QRS complex:_____

Rhythm interpretation:_____

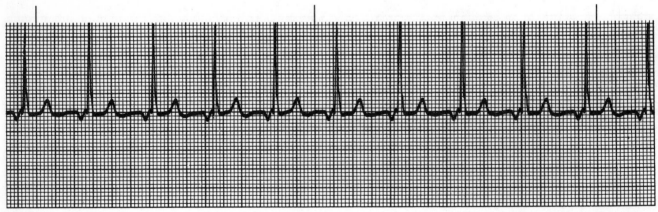

**Strip 8-81.** Rhythm:_____ Rate:_____ P wave:_____

PR interval:_____ QRS complex:_____

Rhythm interpretation:_____

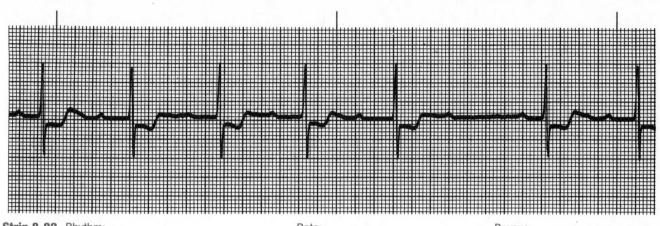

**Strip 8-82.** Rhythm:_____ Rate:_____ P wave:_____

PR interval:_____ QRS complex:_____

Rhythm interpretation:_____

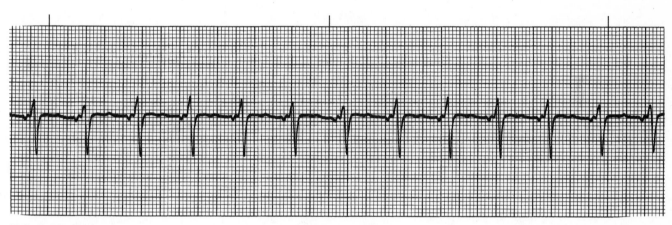

**Strip 8-83.** Rhythm:_____ Rate:_____ P wave:_____

PR interval:_____ QRS complex:_____

Rhythm interpretation:_____

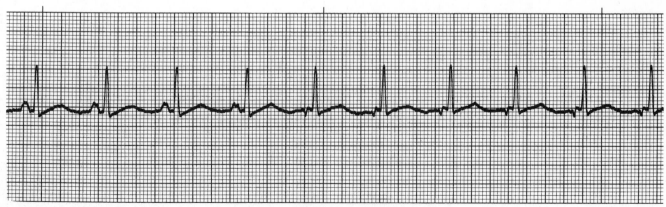

**Strip 8-84.** Rhythm:_____ Rate:_____ P wave:_____

PR interval:_____ QRS complex:_____

Rhythm interpretation:_____

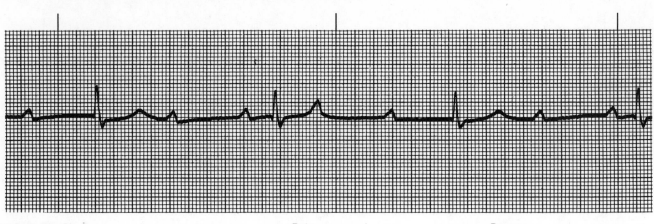

**Strip 8-85.** Rhythm:_____  Rate:_____  P wave:_____

PR interval: _____  QRS complex:_____

Rhythm interpretation: _____

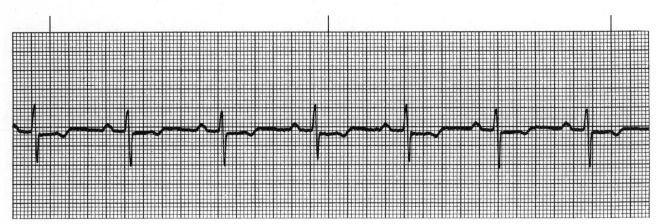

**Strip 8-86.** Rhythm:_____  Rate:_____  P wave:_____

PR interval: _____  QRS complex:_____

Rhythm interpretation: _____

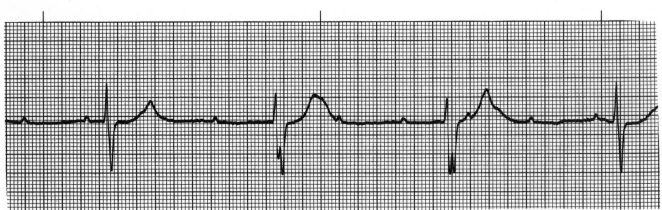

**Strip 8-87.** Rhythm:_____  Rate:_____  P wave:_____

PR interval: _____  QRS complex:_____

Rhythm interpretation: _____

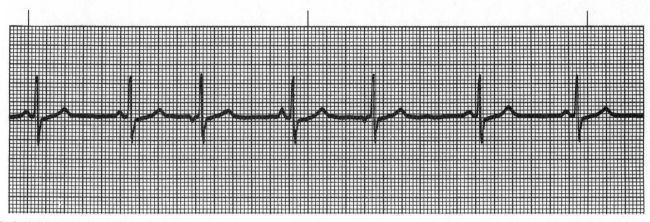

**Strip 8-88.** Rhythm:_____ Rate:_____ P wave:_____

PR interval:_____ QRS complex:_____

Rhythm interpretation:_____

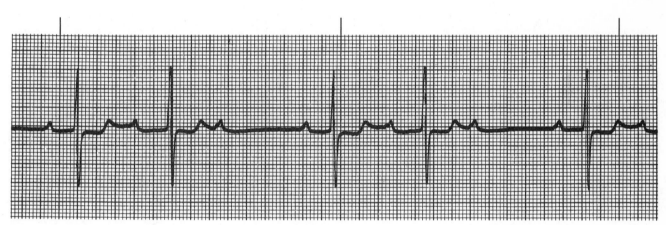

**Strip 8-89.** Rhythm:_____ Rate:_____ P wave:_____

PR interval:_____ QRS complex:_____

Rhythm interpretation:_____

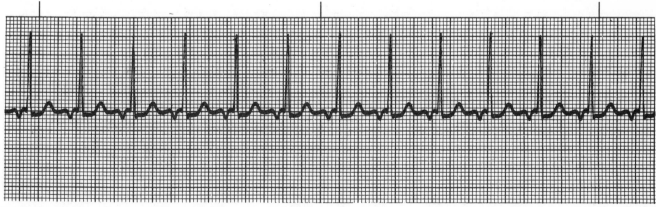

**Strip 8-90.** Rhythm:_____ Rate:_____ P wave:_____

PR interval:_____ QRS complex:_____

Rhythm interpretation:_____

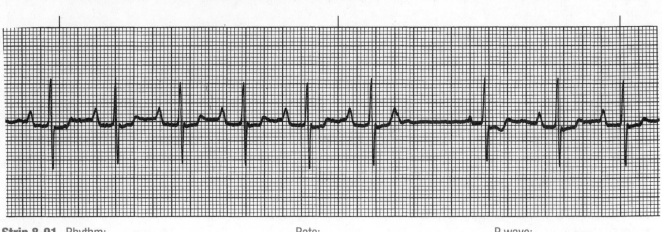

**Strip 8-91.** Rhythm: _____  Rate: _____  P wave: _____

PR interval: _____  QRS complex: _____

Rhythm interpretation: _____

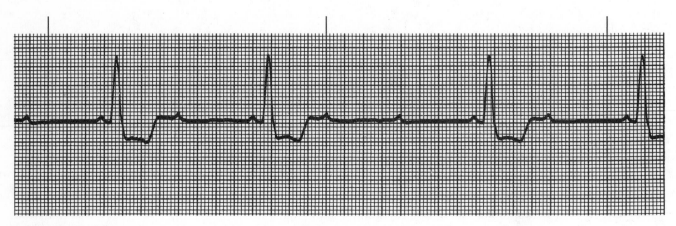

**Strip 8-92.** Rhythm: _____  Rate: _____  P wave: _____

PR interval: _____  QRS complex: _____

Rhythm interpretation: _____

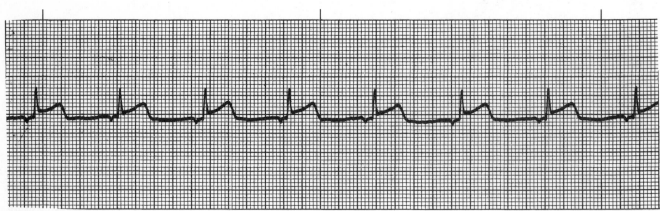

**Strip 8-93.** Rhythm: _____  Rate: _____  P wave: _____

PR interval: _____  QRS complex: _____

Rhythm interpretation: _____

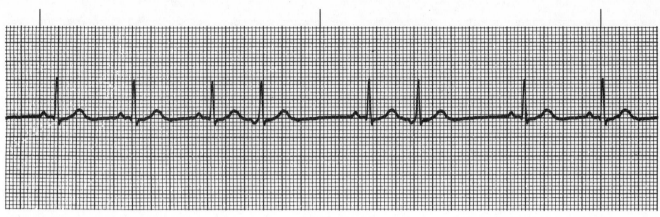

**Strip 8-94.** Rhythm:_____ Rate:_____ P wave:_____
PR interval: _____ QRS complex:_____
Rhythm interpretation: _____

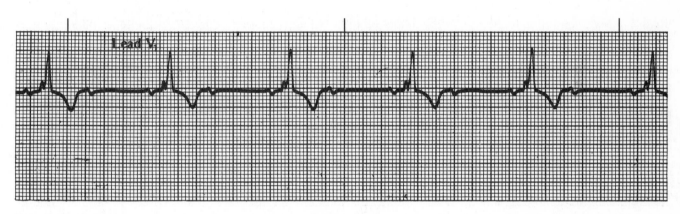

**Strip 8-95.** Rhythm:_____ Rate:_____ P wave:_____
PR interval: _____ QRS complex:_____
Rhythm interpretation: _____

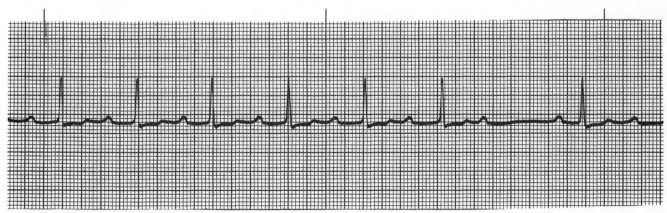

**Strip 8-96.** Rhythm:_____ Rate:_____ P wave:_____
PR interval: _____ QRS complex:_____
Rhythm interpretation: _____

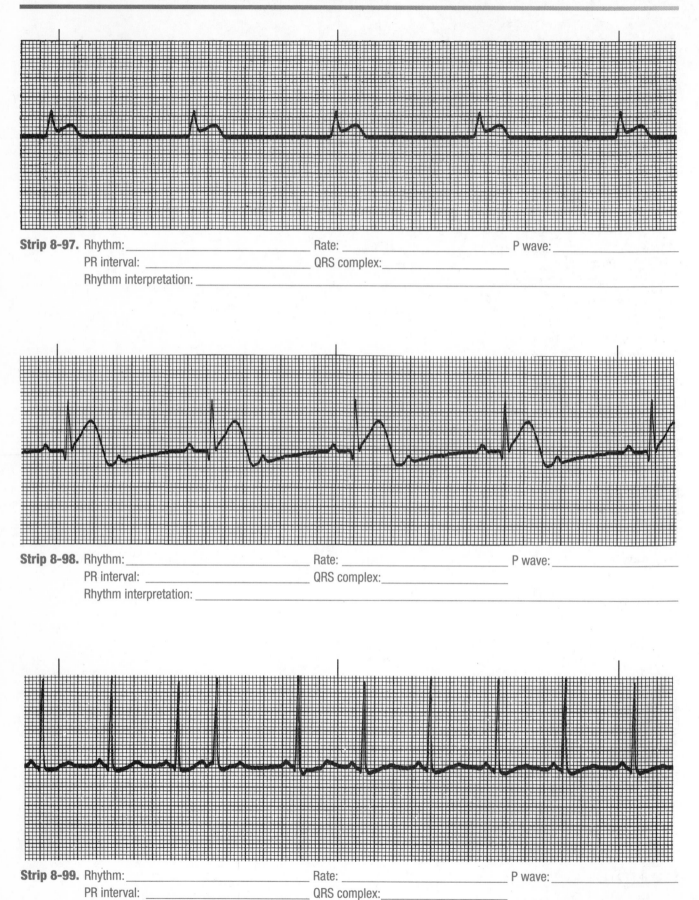

**Strip 8-97.** Rhythm: _____ Rate: _____ P wave: _____

PR interval: _____ QRS complex: _____

Rhythm interpretation: _____

**Strip 8-98.** Rhythm: _____ Rate: _____ P wave: _____

PR interval: _____ QRS complex: _____

Rhythm interpretation: _____

**Strip 8-99.** Rhythm: _____ Rate: _____ P wave: _____

PR interval: _____ QRS complex: _____

Rhythm interpretation: _____

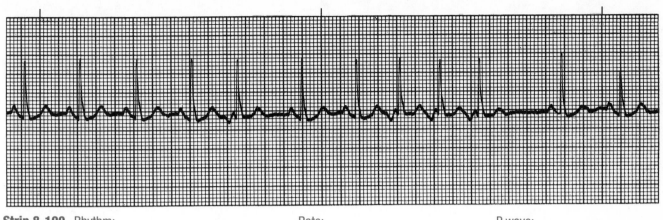

**Strip 8-100.** Rhythm:_____ Rate: _____ P wave: _____

PR interval: _____ QRS complex:_____

Rhythm interpretation: _____

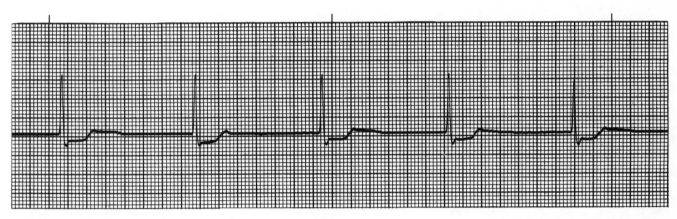

**Strip 8-101.** Rhythm:_____ Rate: _____ P wave: _____

PR interval: _____ QRS complex:_____

Rhythm interpretation: _____

# 9 Ventricular arrhythmias and bundle-branch block

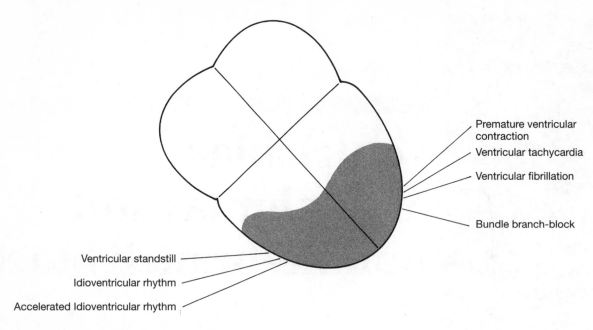

Premature ventricular contraction

Ventricular tachycardia

Ventricular fibrillation

Bundle branch-block

Ventricular standstill

Idioventricular rhythm

Accelerated Idioventricular rhythm

**Figure 9-1.** Ventricular arrhythmias and bundle-branch block.

## Overview

The three preceding chapters have focused on supraventricular arrhythmias. Normally, the electrical impulse produced by supraventricular rhythms follows the normal conduction pathway, resulting in simultaneous depolarization of the right and left ventricles. The resulting QRS complex is narrow (0.10 second or less in duration). Ventricular beats and rhythms (Figure 9-1) originate below the bundle of His in a pacemaker site in the ventricles. With ventricular

rhythms, the electrical impulse bypasses the normal conduction pathway and simultaneous depolarization of both ventricles doesn't occur. Instead, an electrical impulse originating from an ectopic site in one ventricle stimulates that ventricle first and then depolarizes the other ventricle. Depolarization of one ventricle before the other is called *sequential depolarization*. With sequential depolarization, conduction of the impulse is slower than normal and the resulting QRS complex is wide (0.12 second or longer in duration).

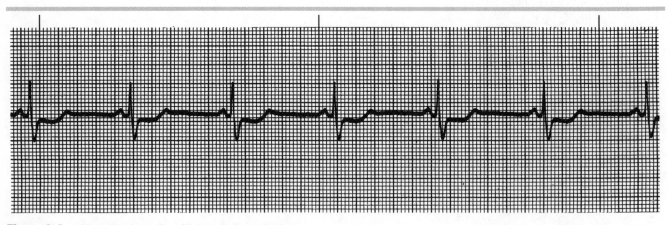

| **Figure 9-2.** | **Sinus bradycardia with bundle-branch block** |
|---|---|
| Rhythm: | Regular |
| Rate: | 54 beats/minute |
| P waves: | Sinus P waves are present. |
| PR interval: | 0.14 to 0.16 second |
| QRS complex: | 0.12 second |
| Comment: | ST segment depression is present. |

Ventricular arrhythmias include premature ventricular contractions (PVCs), ventricular tachycardia, ventricular fibrillation, idioventricular rhythm, accelerated idioventricular rhythm, and ventricular standstill. All of these rhythms are associated with a wide QRS complex (except ventricular fibrillation and ventricular standstill, which don't have QRS complexes). The electrophysiologic mechanism thought to be responsible for the ventricular rhythms is altered automaticity, triggered activity, or reentry. The electrical impulse in bundle-branch block originates in the sinoatrial (SA) node, not in ventricular tissue, but it's included in this rhythm group because of the location of the block in the ventricles, the sequential depolarization process, and the resulting wide QRS complex. Because the ventricles are the least efficient of the heart's pacemakers, most of these rhythms are—or have the potential to be—life-threatening and demand prompt recognition and treatment.

## Bundle-branch block

A bundle-branch block (Figures 9-2 through 9-4 and Box 9-1) refers to an obstruction in the transmission of the electrical impulse through one branch (either right or left) of the bundle of His. Normally, the electrical impulses travel through the right bundle branch and the left bundle branch and their fascicles at the same time, causing simultaneous depolarization of the right and left ventricles. Normal ventricular depolarization is completed within 0.10 second or

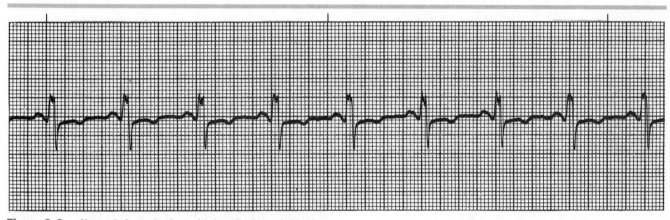

**Figure 9-3.** **Normal sinus rhythm with bundle-branch block**
**Rhythm:** Regular
**Rate:** 75 beats/minute
**P waves:** Sinus P waves are notched, which could indicate left atrial enlargement.
**PR interval:** 0.14 to 0.16 second
**QRS complex:** 0.12 second
**Comment:** A notched QRS complex is a common pattern with RBBB.

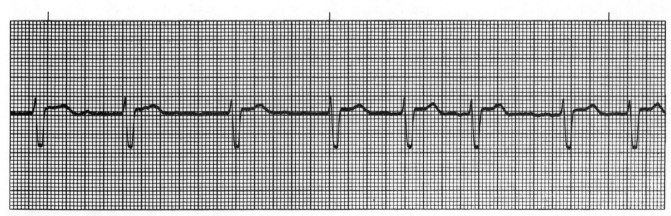

**Figure 9-4.** **Atrial fibrillation with bundle-branch block**
**Rhythm:** Irregular
**Rate:** 60 beats/minute
**P waves:** Wavy fibrillation waves
**PR interval:** Not measurable
**QRS complex:** 0.12 to 0.14 second

less. If a block occurs in one bundle branch, the ventricles are depolarized sequentially (one ventricle before the other). The impulse travels first down the unblocked branch and stimulates that ventricle, and then travels from cell to cell through the myocardium (instead of through the normal conduction pathway) to stimulate the other ventricle. Sequential depolarization results in slower conduction of the impulse, resulting in a wide QRS complex (0.12 second or more in duration). The presence of a bundle-branch block can be recognized by a single monitoring lead by the appearance of the wide, bizarre QRS complex. However, differentiating between right and left bundle-branch block requires a 12-lead electrocardiogram (ECG).

Right bundle-branch block (RBBB) may be present in individuals with organic heart disease, or it may occur in healthy people without any underlying heart disease. RBBB may be permanent or temporary. Sometimes, it appears only when the heart rate exceeds a certain critical value (rate-related bundle-branch block). Some causes of RBBB include coronary artery disease (the most common cause), hypertensive heart disease, cardiomyopathy, acute anteroseptal MI, acute pulmonary embolism, congenital RBBB, and chronic degeneration of the electrical conduction system.

### Box 9-1.
### Bundle-branch block: Identifying ECG features

| | |
|---|---|
| Rhythm: | Regular |
| Rate: | That of the underlying rhythm (usually sinus) |
| P waves: | Sinus |
| PR interval: | Normal (0.12 to 0.20 second) |
| QRS complex: | Wide (0.12 second or greater) |

Unlike RBBB, left bundle-branch block (LBBB) is usually a sign of organic heart disease. LBBB may also be permanent or temporary and may be rate related. Common causes of LBBB include hypertensive heart disease (the most common cause), coronary artery disease, cardiomyopathy, acute anteroseptal MI, and chronic degenerative disease of the electrical conduction system.

Specific treatment usually isn't indicated for a bundle-branch block if it's present alone. Temporary cardiac pacing may be indicated for the treatment of a bundle-branch block under the following conditions:

■ If a new RBBB or LBBB develops as a result of an acute MI.

■ If an RBBB is associated with a block in a fascicle of the left bundle branch (left anterior fascicle or left posterior fascicle).

■ If an RBBB or LBBB is complicated by AV block (first-degree, second-degree, or third-degree), especially if the patient has an acute MI.

## Premature ventricular contractions

A premature ventricular contraction (PVC) (Figures 9-5 through 9-13 and Box 9-2) is a premature, ectopic impulse that originates in either the right or left ventricle. Unlike premature beats in the atria and atrioventricular (AV) junction, which travel down the normal conduction pathway to the ventricles resulting in simultaneous depolarization of both ventricles, the electrical impulse arising from the ventricles doesn't enter the conduction pathway, but instead spreads through the ventricular muscle to depolarize the ventricles one ventricle at a time (*sequential depolarization*). As mentioned previously, sequential depolarization results in abnormal conduction of the impulse, resulting in a wide, bizarre QRS complex (0.12 second or greater in duration). PVCs have the following characteristics:

■ The QRS complex is premature.

■ A P wave isn't associated with the PVC. However, P waves associated with the underlying sinus rhythm can occasionally be seen before the PVC, or after the PVC in the ST segment or T wave (see Figure 9-8).

■ The QRS complex is wide (0.12 second or greater), distorted and bizarre, commonly notched, and appears different from the QRS complexes of the underlying rhythm.

■ The ST segment and T wave slope in the opposite direction from the main deflection of the QRS complex. Because depolarization is abnormal, repolarization is also abnormal.

■ The pause associated with the PVC is usually compensatory—that is, the measurement between the R wave before the PVC to the R wave after the PVC is equal to the sum of two R-R intervals of the underlying regular rhythm (Figure 9-5). The compensatory pause occurs because the SA node isn't depolarized by the ectopic ventricular beat, the discharge timing of the sinus node remains unchanged, and the basic underlying rhythm will resume on time after the PVC. Rarely, the PVC will depolarize the sinus node, resetting the discharge timing of the SA node and resulting in a noncompensatory pause (the measurement between the R wave before the PVC to the R wave after the PVC will be less than the sum of two R-R intervals of the underlying regular rhythm).

### Box 9-2.
### Premature ventricular contraction (PVC): Identifying ECG features

| | |
|---|---|
| Rhythm: | Underlying rhythm usually regular; irregular with PVC |
| Rate: | That of underlying rhythm (usually sinus) |
| P waves: | None associated with PVC; P waves associated with the underlying sinus rhythm can occasionally be seen just before the PVC or after the PVC in the ST segment or T wave; usually these P waves are hidden in the QRS complex |
| PR interval: | Not measurable |
| QRS complex: | Premature QRS complex; abnormal shape; wide (0.12 second or greater) |

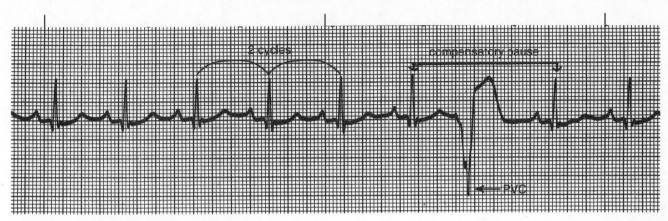

**Figure 9-5.** **Normal sinus rhythm with one PVC**
**Rhythm:** Basic rhythm regular; irregular with PVC
**Rate:** Basic rhythm rate 79 beats/minute
**P waves:** Sinus P waves with basic rhythm
**PR interval:** 0.16 to 0.20 second (basic rhythm)
**QRS complex:** 0.08 to 0.10 second (basic rhythm); 0.14 to 0.16 second (PVC)
**Comment:** The interval between the beat preceding the PVC and the beat following the PVC is equal to two cardiac cycles and represents a full compensatory pause.

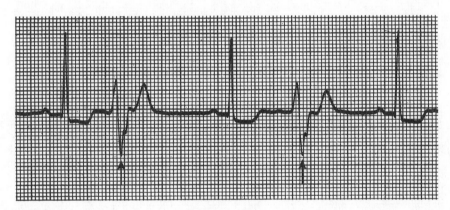

**Figure 9-6.** Bigeminal PVCs.

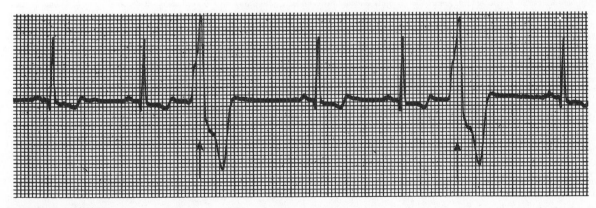

**Figure 9-7.** Trigeminal PVCs.

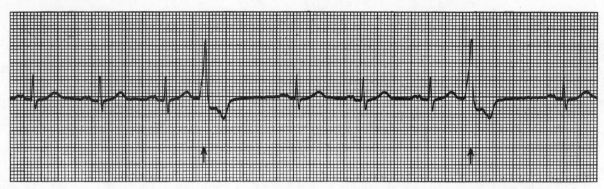

**Figure 9-8.** Quadrigeminal PVCs; the notched P wave associated with the underlying sinus rhythm can be seen after the PVCs in the ST segment.

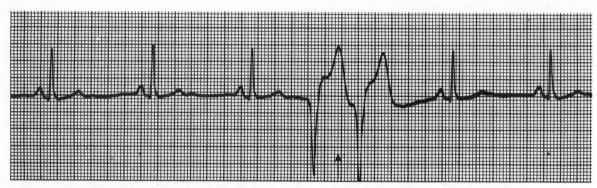

**Figure 9-9.** Paired PVCs.

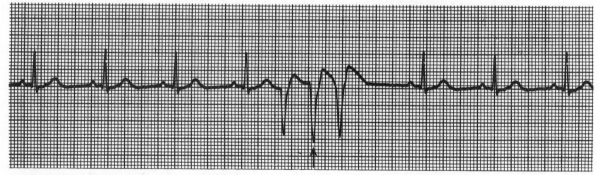

**Figure 9-10.** Run of PVCs (a burst of ventricular tachycardia).

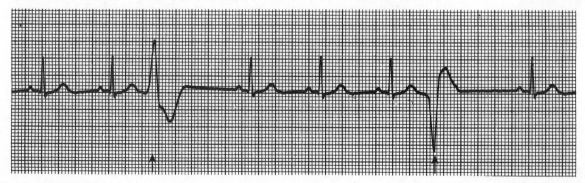

**Figure 9-11.** Multifocal PVCs.

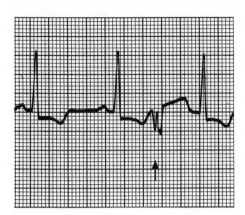

**Figure 9-12.** Interpolated PVC.

PVCs occur in addition to the patient's underlying rhythm and appear in various combinations. They may appear as a single beat, every other beat (bigeminal pattern, see Figure 9-6), every third beat (trigeminal pattern, see Figure 9-7), every fourth beat (quadrigeminal pattern, see Figure 9-8), in pairs (also called *couplets,* see Figure 9-9), or in runs (see Figure 9-10). A run of three or more consecutive PVCs constitutes a rhythm. The rate determines which rhythm is pres-

ent (that is, idioventricular rhythm, accelerated idioventricular rhythm, or ventricular tachycardia).

PVCs that are identical in size, shape, and direction arise from the same focus in the ventricles and are called *uniform* or *unifocal PVCs.* PVCs from different ectopic sites differ in size, shape, and direction and are called *multiform* or *multifocal PVCs* (see Figure 9-11). A PVC sandwiched between two normally conducted sinus beats, without greatly disturbing the regularity of the underlying rhythm, is called an *interpolated PVC* (see Figure 9-12). The compensatory pause, usually associated with the PVC, is absent.

The *R-on-T phenomenon* (see Figure 9-13) is a term used to indicate a PVC that has occurred during the vulnerable period of ventricular repolarization (on or near the peak of the T wave). During this period the myocardial fibers have repolarized enough to respond to a strong stimulus. Stimulation of the ventricle at this time may precipitate repetitive ventricular contractions, resulting in ventricular tachycardia or fibrillation.

Like premature atrial contractions, PVCs are common, even more so with age. They may occur in individuals with a healthy heart as well as in individuals with underlying heart disease. PVCs may be caused by enhanced automaticity of ventricular tissue, an increase in catecholamines and

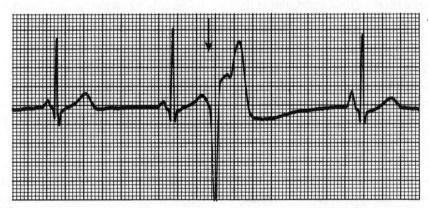

**Figure 9-13.** R-on-T PVC.

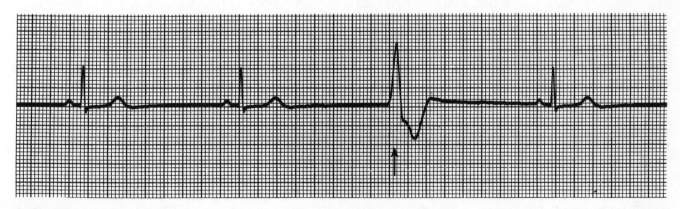

**Figure 9-14.** Ventricular escape beat.

sympathetic tone from emotional stress; ingestion of alcohol, caffeine, or tobacco; myocardial ischemia or acute myocardial infarction; cardiomyopathy; heart failure; hypoxia; digitalis toxicity; administration of drugs (such as epinephrine, norephinephrine, isoproterenol, or aminophylline); electrolyte imbalance (for example, hypokalemia or hypomagnesemia); and reperfusion after thrombolytic therapy or angioplasty. PVCs may also occur after heart surgery and after contact of the endocardium with invasive catheters (such as pacing leads or pulmonary artery catheters).

Treatment of PVCs should be guided by the clinical setting. Because occasional PVCs are a normal finding in healthy individuals, no treatment may be indicated. Initially, a search should be made for possible reversible causes (such as oxygen for hypoxia, replacement of electrolytes, a diuretic for heart failure, elimination of certain drugs). Treatment of PVCs depends on the cause, the patient's symptoms, and the clinical situation. Most patients with PVCs don't require treatment with an antiarrhythmic. However, treatment of significant PVCs (for example, frequent PVCs , multifocal PVCs, couplets, R-on-T PVCs, and PVCs occurring in nonsustained runs) is usually indicated, especially in the first 24 to 48 hours after an acute MI or cardiac surgery.

On some occasions a ventricular beat may occur late instead of early. These beats are called *ventricular escape beats* (see Figure 9-14). Escape beats are more likely to occur because of an increased vagal effect on the SA node rather than because of enhanced automaticity, as is commonly associated with the premature ventricular beat. Escape beats are common after a pause in the underlying rhythm. The morphologic characteristics of the late beat are the same as for the PVC. The ventricular escape beat is a protective mechanism, protecting the heart from slow rates and no treatment is required.

## Ventricular tachycardia

Ventricular tachycardia (VT) (Figures 9-15 through 9-19 and Box 9-3) is an arrhythmia originating in an ectopic focus in the ventricles, discharging impulses at a rate of 140 to 250 beats/minute. On the ECG the rhythm appears as a series of wide QRS complexes at a rapid rate. Impulses originating from ventricular tissue do not produce P waves. However, the sinus node continues to beat independently, and sinus P waves may occasionally be seen between the wide QRS complexes, but usually the sinus P waves are hidden in the QRS complexes. The QRS complexes are distorted and bizarre, many of them notched, with a duration of 0.12 second or greater. As a rule the QRS complexes are identical (monomorphic). When the QRS complexes differ, the VT is considered to be polymorphic. The QRS complexes are followed by large T waves, opposite in direction to the main deflection of the QRS complex. The rhythm is usually regular, but may be slightly irregular. VT may occasionally occur at rates greater than 250 beats/minute. At such extreme rates the QRS com-

plexes appear sawtooth in morphology, and the rhythm is commonly referred to as *ventricular flutter* (see Figure 9-16). The patient becomes hemodynamically compromised very quickly because there is virtually no cardiac output. VT of this type is commonly an immediate forerunner to ventricular fibrillation.

---

**Box 9-3.**

## Ventricular tachycardia: Identifying ECG features

| | |
|---|---|
| **Rhythm:** | Regular |
| **Rate:** | 140 to 250 beats/minute |
| **P waves:** | No P waves are associated with ventricular tachycardia. However, the SA node continues to beat independently and sinus P waves may occasionally be seen between the QRS complexes. Usually the P waves are hidden in the QRS. |
| **PR interval:** | Not measurable |
| **QRS complex:** | Wide (0.12 seconds or greater) |

---

VT usually occurs in patients with underlying heart disease. Common causes include myocardial ischemia, cardiomyopathy, mitral valve prolapse, heart failure, and digitalis toxicity. Other causes include electrolyte disturbances (especially hypokalemia and hypomagnesemia), mechanical stimulation of the endocardium by a pacing catheter or pulmonary artery catheter, and reperfusion after thrombolytic therapy or angioplasty. The most common cause of sustained monomorphic VT is coronary artery disease, usually with prior myocardial infarction. Certain medications (for example, antiarrhythmics, phenothiazines, and tricyclic antidepressants) may prolong the QT interval, causing the ventricles to be particularly vulnerable to polymorphic VT (torsades de pointes; see Figure 9-18).

VT is usually preceded by frequent and repetitive ventricular ectopy. VT may appear as a sustained rhythm (lasting longer than 30 seconds), or as a nonsustained rhythm (lasting less than 30 seconds) occurring in short bursts or paroxysms (see Figures 9-10 and 9-17). Three consecutive PVCs at a rate of 140 to 250 beats/minute is technically considered a burst of nonsustained VT. Nonsustained VT, unless frequent, usually doesn't cause hemodynamic compromise, but it can progress into sustained VT. Sustained VT is a life-threatening arrhythmia for two major reasons. First, the rapid ventricular rate and loss of atrial kick reduce cardiac output, leading to hypotension and decreased perfusion to vital organs. Second, the rhythm may degenerate into ventricular fibrillation.

Treatment of VT depends on how well the patient tolerates the rhythm. Patient tolerance is related to the ventricular rate and the underlying left ventricular function. As part of the initial assessment you should check for a pulse. If there is no pulse (pulseless VT), the rhythm must be treat-

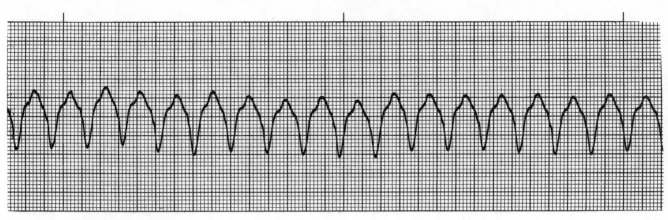

**Figure 9-15. Ventricular tachycardia**
Rhythm:      Regular
Rate:        150 beats/minute
P waves:     None identified
PR interval: Not measurable
QRS complex: 0.14 to 0.16 second

ed as ventricular fibrillation. If there is a pulse, protocols for VT with a pulse are followed and fall under stable and unstable categories.

## Stable monomorphic VT with a pulse

If there is a pulse and the patient's condition is stable (for example, adequate level of consciousness, warm skin, acceptable blood pressure [usually 90 mm Hg systolic or greater], no chest pain or dyspnea) the following guidelines are suggested:

■ Use any *one* of the following medications:

– Amiodarone is given as a 150 mg I.V. bolus over 10 minutes, followed by a 1 mg/minute infusion over 6 hours and then a 0.5 mg/minute infusion over 18 hours. Additional 150-mg I.V. bolus doses can be repeated for recurrent or resistant arrhythmias to a maximum dose of 2.2 g in 24 hours (maximum dose includes bolus and infusion doses). The major adverse effects from amiodarone are bradycardia and hypotension. Amiodarone can also induce torsades de pointes VT, although the drug has a lower incidence of proarrhythmic effects than other antiarrhythmics under similar circumstances.

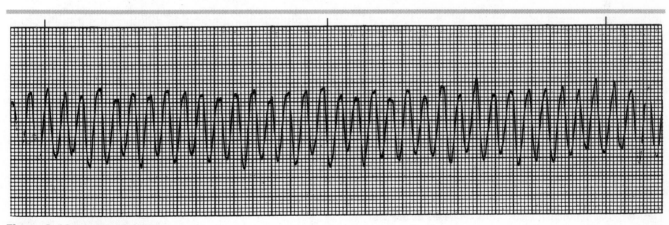

**Figure 9-16. Ventricular flutter**
Rhythm:      Regular
Rate:        375 beats/minute
P waves:     Not seen
PR interval: Not measurable
QRS complex: 0.12 to 0.14 second
Comment:     Ventricular flutter is a form of ventricular tachycardia. The ventricular rate is so fast the QRS complexes have a sawtooth appearance.

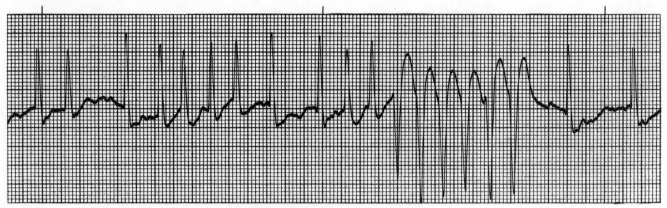

**Figure 9-17. Atrial fibrillation with a burst of ventricular tachycardia**

| | |
|---|---|
| **Rhythm:** | Basic rhythm irregular; ventricular tachycardia regular |
| **Rate:** | 160 beats/minute (basic rhythm); 250 beats/minute (VT) |
| **P waves:** | Fibrillation waves in basic rhythm; none with VT |
| **PR interval:** | Not measurable |
| **QRS complex:** | 0.08 to 0.10 second (basic rhythm); 0.12 second (VT) |

– Lidocaine is given as a 1 to 1.5 mg/kg I.V. bolus, followed by one-half the initial dose (0.5 to 0.75 mg/kg I.V. bolus) every 5 to 10 minutes to a maximum dose of 3 mg/kg. The maintenance infusion rate is 1 to 4 mg/minute. Reappearance of the arrhythmia during a continuous infusion of lidocaine should be treated with a small I.V. bolus dose (0.5 mg/kg) and an increase in the infusion rate. The half-life of lidocaine increases after 24 to 48 hours. Therefore, after 24 hours the dosage should be reduced or blood levels monitored. Signs of toxicity include slurred speech, altered consciousness, muscle twitching, seizures, and bradycardia.

■ If the rhythm is unresponsive to drug therapy, sedate the patient and perform electrical cardioversion beginning at 200 joules (or equivalent biphasic energy level), increasing joules (300, 360) with subsequent attempts.

If the patient has an ejection fraction of less than 40% or has heart failure, the recommended guidelines are:

■ Use *one* of the following medications:

– Amiodarone is given in the same dose as above.

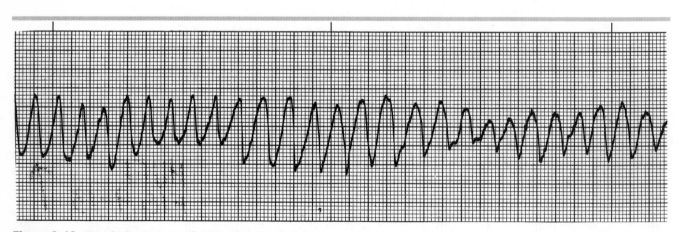

**Figure 9-18. Ventricular tachycardia (torsades de pointes)**

| | |
|---|---|
| **Rhythm:** | Regular |
| **Rate:** | 250 beats/minute |
| **P waves:** | None identified |
| **PR interval:** | Not measurable |
| **QRS complex:** | 0.12 to 0.22 second (some much wider than others) |
| **Comment:** | This type of ventricular tachycardia is called *torsades de pointes* (twists of points). The QRS changes from negative to positive polarity and appears to twist around the isoelectric line. It is associated with a prolonged QT interval and is refractory to antiarrhythmics. I.V. magnesium or overdrive pacing has been successful in the treatment of this rhythm. |

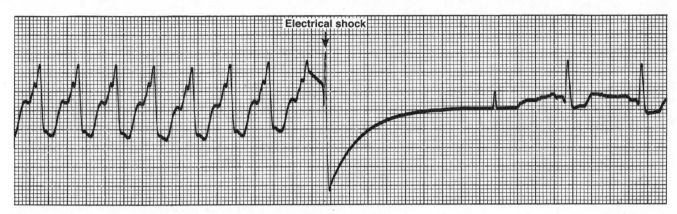

**Figure 9-19.** Electrical cardioversion of ventricular tachycardia to sinus rhythm.

– Lidocaine is given in a reduced dose of 0.5 to 0.75 mg/kg I.V. bolus, and this dose can be repeated every 5 to 10 minutes to a maximum dose of 3 mg/kg.

■ If the rhythm is unresponsive to drug therapy, sedate the patient and perform electrical cardioversion.

All antiarrhythmics have some degree of proarrhythmic effects. Sequential use of more than one antiarrhythmic compounds the adverse effects, particularly for bradycardia, hypotension, and torsades de pointes. Never use more than one agent unless absolutely necessary. When an appropriate dose of a single antiarrhythmic medication fails to terminate an arrhythmia, turn to electrical cardioversion rather than a second antiarrhythmic. Figure 9-19 shows electrical cardioversion of VT to a sinus rhythm.

## Unstable monomorphic VT with a pulse

If there is a pulse and the patient's condition is unstable (for example, decreased level of consciousness; cool, clammy skin; blood pressure less than 90 mm Hg systolic; complaints of chest pain or dyspnea; or in extreme situations, becomes unconscious and cyanotic and is having seizures), the following guidelines are suggested:

■ Sedate the patient (if conscious).

■ Convert the rhythm using cardioversion at 200 joules initially (or equivalent biphasic energy level) increasing the joules (300, 360) with subsequent attempts. Once electrical cardioversion has terminated the rhythm, an antiarrhythmic is usually started to prevent reoccurrence of the arrhythmia.

Treatment of chronic, recurrent VT usually includes therapy with an oral antiarrhythmic. Patients with refractory VT may require a nonpharmacologic approach. Further evaluation may include specialized electrophysiologic testing and endocardial mapping, with long-term options, including use of the implantable cardioverter defibrillator (ICD) or reentry circuit ablation. The ICD is a special, surgically implanted device developed to deliver an electric shock directly to the heart during a life-threatening tachycardia. Destruction (ab-

lation) of the reentry circuit involves delivering short pulses of radiofrequency current through an intracardiac catheter. It produces a small burn that effectively blocks the part of the circuit supporting the reentrant-type wave.

A special type of polymorphic VT is called *torsades de pointes* (see Figure 9-18), a French term meaning "twisting of the points." In this arrhythmia the direction of the QRS complexes seem to rotate, pointing downward for a series of beats and then twisting and pointing upward. The ventricular rate is extremely rapid (much faster than monomorphic VT) and the patient usually becomes hemodynamically compromised very quickly. VT of this type is commonly an immediate forerunner to ventricular fibrillation.

Torsades de pointes classically occurs in the setting of delayed ventricular repolarization, evidenced by prolongation of the QT interval or the presence of prominent U waves. A prolonged QT interval can be caused by an antiarrhythmic (such as procainamide or quinidine), a psychotropic drug (such as a phenothiazine or a tricyclic antidepressant), electrolyte imbalance (for example, hypokalemia, hypomagnesemia, or hypocalcemia), bradycardia, a liquid protein diet, or long QT syndrome.

Recognition of torsades de pointes is critical because the treatment plan differs greatly from the treatment of monomorphic VT. Drugs conventionally used in treating monomorphic VT can cause torsades de pointes and, if given, are usually ineffective and may make the rhythm worse. Treatment of torsades de pointes includes:

■ Removing or correcting causative factors (such as drug effects, electrolyte imbalances, or underlying bradycardia). The rhythm has a tendency to recur unless the precipitating factors are eliminated.

■ Magnesium may be administered as a loading dose of 1 to 2 g in 10 mL of dextrose 5% in water over 5 minutes, followed by a maintenance infusion of 0.5 to 1 g/hour. Rapid administration of magnesium may cause significant hypotension or asystole and should be avoided. Magnesium is unlikely to be effective in terminating polymorphic VT in patients with a normal QT interval, but amiodarone may be effective.

■ If the rhythm is felt to be precipitated by bradycardia, isoproterenol or ventricular pacing may be effective to accomplish "overdrive" suppression of the arrhythmia by increasing the underlying heart rate and thereby increasing ventricular repolarization time.

■ If the patient with polymorphic VT becomes unstable, provide high-energy (360 joules) unsynchronized shocks. The many QRS configurations and irregular rates present in polymorphic VT make it difficult or impossible to reliably synchronize to a QRS complex.

## Ventricular fibrillation

In ventricular fibrillation (Figures 9-20 and 9-21 and Box 9-4) a disorganized, chaotic, electrical focus in the ventricles takes over control of the heart. The ventricles don't beat in a coordinated fashion but, instead, quiver asynchronously and ineffectively, just as the atria respond in atrial fibrillation. The ECG tracing shows an undulating, wavy baseline composed of irregular waveforms that vary in amplitude and morphology. Ventricular fibrillation waves represent chaotic, incomplete, and haphazard depolarization of small groups of muscle fibers in the ventricles. Because organized depolarization of the atria and ventricles is absent, P waves and QRS complexes are also absent. If the fibrillatory waves are large the arrhythmia is described as *coarse ventricular fibrillation* (see Figure 9-20). If the fibrillatory waves are small the arrhythmia is described as *fine ventricular fibrillation* (see Figure 9-21). The distinction between the two may be significant because coarse ventricular fibrillation usually indicates a more recent onset and is more likely to be reversed by defibrillation alone. Fine ventricular fibrillation usually indicates that the arrhythmia has been present longer and may require drug therapy first, then defibrillation, before the arrhythmia can be reversed. Fine ventricular fibrillation will progress to ventricular asystole unless defibrillation restores the cardiac rhythm.

**Box 9-4.**
### Ventricular fibrillation: Identifying ECG features

| | |
|---|---|
| Rhythm: | None (P wave and QRS complex are absent) |
| Rate: | None (P wave and QRS complex are absent) |
| P waves: | Absent; wavy, irregular deflections seen, varying in size, shape, and height and representative of quivering of the ventricles instead of contraction; deflections may be small (described as *fine vetricular fibrillation*) or large (described as *coarse vetricular fibrillation*) |
| PR interval: | Not measurable |
| QRS complex: | Absent |

Ventricular fibrillation can occur in patients with heart disease of any type. It may be preceded by significant PVCs (for example, occurring in pairs, runs, multifocal, R-on-T type) or VT, but it can also occur spontaneously. It's the most common cause of sudden cardiac death in patients with an acute myocardial infarction. Other causes of ventricular fibrillation include myocardial ischemia, cardiomyopathy, mitral valve prolapse, cardiac trauma, hypoxia, cocaine toxicity, electrolyte imbalances, acidosis, and drug toxicity (especially digitalis and proarrhythmics). Ventricular fibrillation may also occur during anesthesia, cardiac catheterization procedures, pacemaker implantation, placement of a pulmonary artery catheter, or after accidental electrocution.

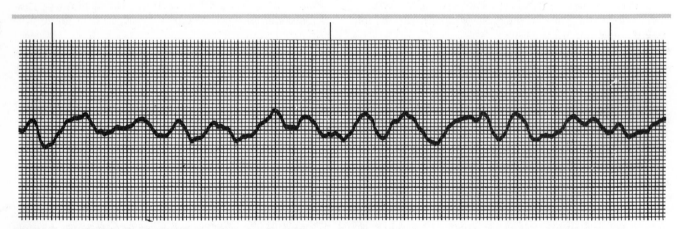

**Figure 9-20. Ventricular fibrillation (coarse wave forms)**

| | |
|---|---|
| Rhythm: | Chaotic |
| Rate: | 0 beats/minute (no QRS complexes are present) |
| P waves: | None; wave deflections are chaotic and vary in size, shape, and height |
| PR interval: | Not measurable |
| QRS complex: | Absent |

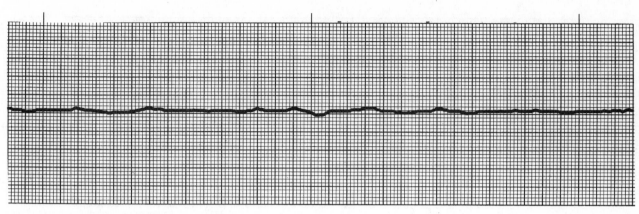

**Figure 9-21. Ventricular fibrillation (fine wave forms)**
Rhythm:         Chaotic
Rate:           0 beats/minute (no QRS complexes are present)
P waves:        Absent; wave deflections are chaotic and vary in size, shape, and height
PR interval:    Not measurable
QRS complex:    Absent

Once ventricular fibrillation occurs there is no cardiac output, peripheral pulses and blood pressure are absent, and the patient becomes unconscious immediately. Cyanosis and seizure activity may also be present. Death is imminent unless the arrhythmia is treated immediately. Treatment protocols include:

■ Check the pulse and rapidly assess the patient. If there is a pulse or the patient is conscious, ventricular fibrillation isn't the problem. ECG artifacts produced by loose or dry electrodes, patient movement, or muscle tremors may resemble ventricular fibrillation.

■ If there is no pulse and the patient is unconscious, defibrillate at 360 joules (or equivalent biphasic) × 1. If the arrest is unwitnessed, perform CPR for 5 cycles before the initial shock.

■ If unsuccessful start cardiopulmonary resuscitation (CPR), establish an I.V. line, and intubate the patient.

■ Administer epinephrine 1 mg I.V. push and repeat every 3 to 5 minutes. Vasopressin 40 units I.V. push may be given × 1 dose to replace first or second dose epinephrine.

■ Continue CPR for 5 cycles to circulate drug; defibrillate at 360 joules × 1.

■ Consider ONE of the following antiarrhythmics:
  – Amiodarone 300 mg I.V. push (cardiac arrest dose); if ventricular fibrillation is refractory or recurs, consider an additional dose of 150 mg I.V. push; if drug therapy is successful, a maintenance infusion of amiodarone can be started at 1 mg/minute for 6 hours followed by 0.5 mg/minute for 18 hours (maximum cumulative dose: 2.2 g in 24 hours).
  – Lidocaine 1 to 1.5 mg/kg I.V. push followed by one-half the initial dose (0.5 to 0.75 mg/kg I.V. push) every 5 to 10 minutes to a maximum dose of 3 mg/kg. If drug therapy is successful, a maintenance infusion of lidocaine can be started at 1 to 4 mg/minute.

■ Continue drug therapy, CPR, and defibrillation attempts (drug-CPR-shock pattern) until rhythm resolves or a decision is made to stop resuscitative efforts.

## Idioventricular rhythm (ventricular escape rhythm)

Idioventricular rhythm (IVR) (Figure 9-22 and Box 9-5) is an arrhythmia originating in a secondary pacemaker site in the ventricles, with a heart rate between 30 and 40 beats/minute (sometimes less). Because the impulse focus is in the ventricles, the ECG tracing is characterized by an absence of P waves and the presence of wide QRS complexes occurring at a regular rate.

**Box 9-5.**
### Idioventricular rhythm: Identifying ECG features

Rhythm:         Regular
Rate:           30 to 40 beats/minute (sometimes less)
P waves:        Absent
PR interval:    Not measurable
QRS complex:    Wide (0.12 second or greater)

Idioventricular rhythm is considered an escape rhythm. It occurs when the rate of impulse formation of the dominant pacemaker (usually the sinus node) and the backup pacemaker in the AV node becomes less than the pacemaker in the ventricles or when the electrical impulse from the SA node, atria, or AV node fails to reach the ventricles. When an electrical impulse fails to arrive in the ventricles, pacemaker cells in the ventricles take over pacemaker function

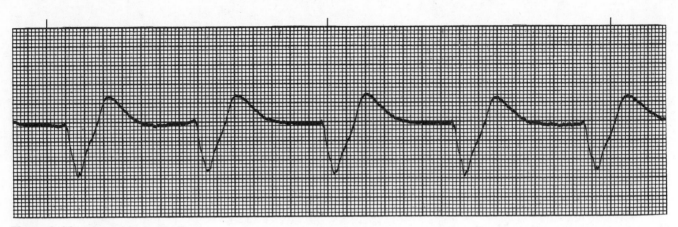

**Figure 9-22.  Idioventricular rhythm**
**Rhythm:**        Regular
**Rate:**          44 beats/minute
**P waves:**       Absent
**PR interval:**   Not measurable
**QRS complex:** 0.32 second

at their inherent firing rate of 40 beats/minute or less. The result may be an escape beat (see Figure 9-14) or a ventricular escape rhythm.

Ventricular escape rhythm may be temporary or continuous. Temporary idioventricular rhythm is seen as three or more ventricular beats lasting only a few seconds or minutes, is usually related to increased vagal effect on the higher pacing centers, and is insignificant. Continuous idioventricular rhythm associated with third-degree heart block can generally be treated with pacemaker therapy and has a better prognosis than idioventricular rhythm not associated with AV block. Continuous idioventricular rhythm not associated with AV block is seen in advanced heart disease and is commonly the cardiac arrhythmia present just be-

fore the final arrhythmia, ventricular standstill (asystole). Continuous idioventricular rhythm is generally symptomatic because of the marked reduction in cardiac output from the slow rate and loss of the atrial kick. If the rate of IVR falls below 20 beats/minute and the QRS complexes deteriorate into irregular, wide, indistinguishable waveforms, the rhythm is commonly referred to as an *agonal rhythm* or "dying heart."

The goal of treatment isn't to eradicate the rhythm with suppressive agents, but to stimulate a rhythm from a higher pacemaker site if possible. Treatment may include:
■ Administer atropine 0.5 to 1.0 mg I.V. push; may repeat every 3 to 5 minutes until the heart rate increases or a total dose of 3 mg is given.

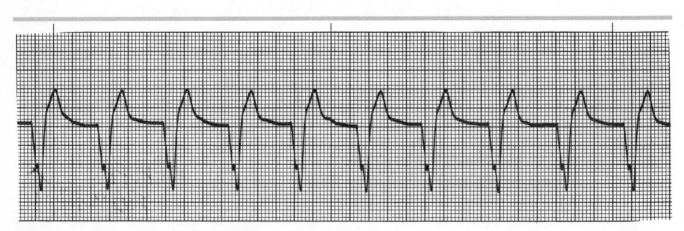

**Figure 9-23.  Accelerated idioventricular rhythm**
**Rhythm:**        Regular
**Rate:**          84 beats/minute
**P waves:**       None identified
**PR interval:**   Not measurable
**QRS complex:** 0.16 second

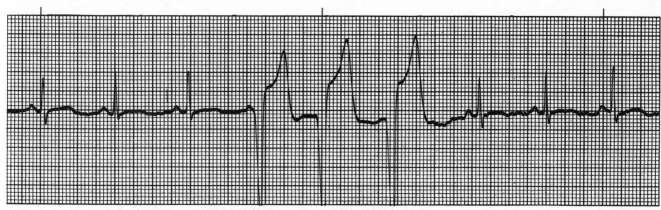

**Figure 9-24.** **Normal sinus rhythm with episode of accelerated idioventricular rhythm**
**Rhythm:**        Basic rhythm regular; AIVR basically regular (off by 2 squares)
**Rate:**            79 beats/minute basic rhythm; around 80 beats/minute AIVR rate
**P waves:**        Sinus P waves with basic rhythm; none with AIVR
**PR interval:**    0.12 to 0.16 second
**QRS complex:**   0.06 to 0.08 second (basic rhythm); 0.12 seconds (AIVR)

■ Initiate transcutaneous pacing.
■ If the patient is hypotensive, start a dopamine infusion at 5 to 20 mcg/minute or, if symptoms are severe, go directly to an epinephrine infusion at 2 to 10 mcg/minute.
■ Consider inserting a temporary transvenous pacemaker; chronic idioventricular rhythm associated with third-degree AV block requires insertion of a permanent pacemaker.

## Accelerated idioventricular rhythm

Accelerated idioventricular rhythm (AIVR) (Figures 9-23 and 9-24 and Box 9-6) is an arrhythmia originating in an ectopic pacemaker site in the ventricles with a rate between 50 and 100 beats/minute. The term *accelerated* denotes a rhythm that exceeds the inherent idioventricular escape rate of 30 to 40 beats/minute but isn't fast enough to be VT. Accelerated idioventricular rhythm has the same ECG characteristics as idioventricular rhythm and is differentiated by the heart rate.

Accelerated idioventricular rhythm is common after an inferior MI and is commonly a reperfusion rhythm as a result of thrombolytic therapy, angioplasty, or spontaneous reperfusion. AIVR may also result from digitalis toxicity. Brief episodes of AIVR commonly alternate with periods of normal sinus rhythm (see Figure 9-24).

Accelerated idioventricular rhythm is a temporary arrhythmia that is usually well tolerated and produces no hemodynamic effects. The ventricular rate is within normal limits and usually adequate to maintain cardiac output. Suppressive therapy isn't recommended because abolishing the ventricular rhythm may leave an even less desirable heart rate. Treatment usually isn't required.

## Ventricular standstill (ventricular asystole)

Ventricular standstill, or *asystole* (Figures 9-25 and 9-26 and Box 9-7), is the absence of all electrical activity in the ventricles. The ECG tracing shows either P waves without QRS complexes or a straight line. If P waves are present then some type of advanced AV block (Mobitz II or third-degree) probably preceded the arrhythmia. Ventricular standstill with a straight line is usually the terminal arrhythmia after VT, ventricular fibrillation, or idioventricular rhythm. Ventricular standstill may also occur because of acidosis, hypoxia, hyperkalemia, hypothermia, or drug overdose. Prognosis is extremely poor despite resuscitative efforts (usually as low as 1 to 2 people out of 100 cardiac arrests). The only hope for resuscitation of a person in asystole is to identify and treat a reversible cause.

**Box 9-6.**
### Accelerated idioventricular rhythm: Identifying ECG features

| | |
|---|---|
| **Rhythm:** | Regular |
| **Rate:** | 50 to 100 beats/minute |
| **P waves:** | Absent |
| **PR interval:** | Not measurable |
| **QRS complex:** | Wide (0.12 second or greater) |

**Box 9-7.**
### Ventricular standstill: Identifying ECG features

| | |
|---|---|
| **Rhythm:** | Atrial: If P waves present, will have atrial rhythm Ventricular: None |
| **Rate:** | Atrial: If P waves present, will have atrial rate Ventricular: None |
| **P waves:** | ECG tracings will show either P waves without a QRS complex or a straight line |
| **PR interval:** | Not measurable |
| **QRS complex:** | Absent |

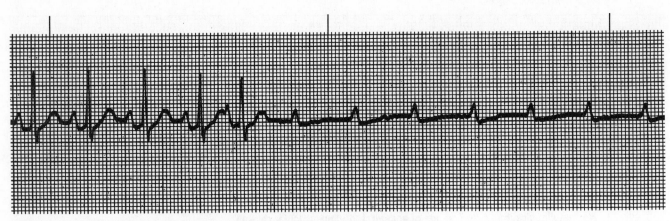

**Figure 9-25. Normal sinus rhythm with one PAC changing to ventricular standstill**

Rhythm:      Basic rhythm regular
Rate:        Basic rhythm 100 beats/minute
P waves:     Sinus P waves are present
PR interval: 0.16 to 0.18 second (basic rhythm)
QRS complex: 0.06 second (basic rhythm)

Once ventricular standstill occurs there is no cardiac output, peripheral pulses and blood pressure are absent, and the patient becomes unconscious immediately. Cyanosis and seizure activity may also be present. Death is imminent unless the arrhythmia is treated immediately. Without ECG monitoring ventricular standstill cannot be distinguished from ventricular fibrillation at the bedside. Treatment protocols include:

■ Check pulse and rapidly assess the patient. If there is a pulse or the patient is conscious, ventricular standstill isn't the problem.

■ Check monitor lead system—a loose electrode pad or lead wire will show a straight line. Check monitor rhythm

in two leads if possible—fine waveform ventricular fibrillation may mimic ventricular standstill.

■ Start CPR, establish an I.V. line, and intubate the patient.

■ Apply a transcutaneous pacemaker. To be effective, this must be performed early and combined with drug therapy.

■ Give epinephrine 1 mg I.V. and continue CPR to circulate the drug; the drug may be repeated every 3 to 5 minutes.

■ Give atropine 1 mg I.V. and continue CPR to circulate the drug; the drug may be repeated every 3 to 5 minutes until a total dose of 3 mg is given.

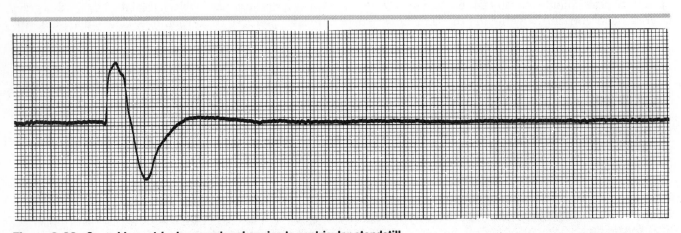

**Figure 9-26. One wide ventricular complex changing to ventricular standstill**

Rhythm:      0
Rate:        0
P waves:     None identified
PR interval: Not measurable
QRS complex: 0.28 second or wider

**Table 9-1.**
## Ventricular arrhythmias and bundle-branch block: Summary of identifying ECG features

| Name | Rhythm | Rate (beats/minute) | P waves (lead II) | PR interval | QRS complex |
|---|---|---|---|---|---|
| Bundle-branch block | Regular | That of underlying rhythm (usually sinus) | Sinus origin | Normal (0.12 to 0.20 second) | Wide (0.12 second or greater) |
| Premature ventricular contraction (PVC) | Basic rhythm usually regular; irregular with PVC | That of underlying rhythm (usually sinus) | None associated with PVC; P waves associated with underlying sinus rhythm can sometimes be seen just before PVC or after PVC in ST segment or T wave, but these waves are usually hidden within PVC | Not measurable | Premature QRS complex; abnormal shape; wide (0.12 second or greater) |
| Ventricular tachycardia (VT) | Regular | 140 to 250 | None associated with VT, but the sinoatrial node continues to beat independently and sinus P waves may occasionally be seen between the QRS complexes (usually these P waves are hidden in the QRS complex) | Not measurable | Wide (0.12 second or greater) |
| Ventricular fibrillation | None (P wave and QRS complex are absent) | None (P wave and QRS complex are absent) | Absent; wavy, irregular deflections seen in various sizes, shapes, and heights, representative of ventricular quivering instead of contraction; deflections may be small (described as *fine ventricular fibrillation*) or large (described as *coarse ventricular fibrillation*) | Not measurable | Absent |
| Idioventricular rhythm (IVR) | Regular | 30 to 40 (sometimes less) | Absent | Not measurable | Wide (0.12 second or greater) |
| Accelerated IVR | Regular | 50 to 100 | Absent | Not measurable | Wide (0.12 second or greater) |
| Ventricular standstill (ventricular asystole) | Atrial: if P waves present, will have atrial rhythm Ventricular: None | Atrial: if P waves present, will have atrial rate Ventricular: None | Tracing will show either P waves without a QRS complex or a straight line | Not measurable | Absent |

■ Continue administering epinephrine, atropine, and CPR until the rhythm is resolved or a decision is made to discontinue resuscitative efforts.

With asystole refractory to treatment, the patient is making the transition from life to death. Medical personnel should try to make that transition as sensitive and dignified as possible.

A summary of the identifying ECG features of ventricular arrhythmias and bundle-branch block can be found in Table 9-1.

# Rhythm strip practice: Ventricular arrhythmias and bundle-branch block

For each of the following rhythm strips:

- determine the rhythm regularity and the ventricular rate (also the atrial rate if it differs from the ventricular rate)
- identify and examine the P waves
- measure the duration of the PR interval and QRS complex

- interpret the rhythm.

All rhythm strips are lead II unless otherwise noted. Check your answers with the answer key in the appendix.

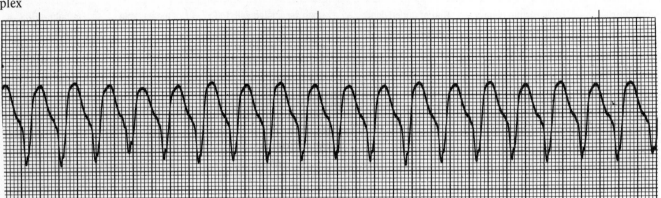

**Strip 9-1.** Rhythm: _____ Rate: _____ P wave: _____

PR interval: _____ QRS complex: _____

Rhythm interpretation: _____

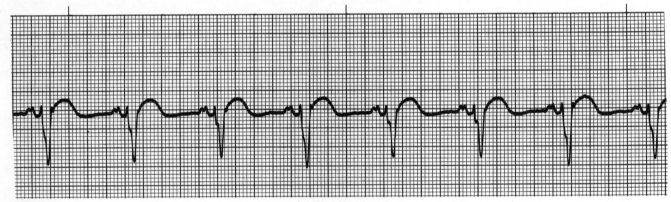

**Strip 9-2.** Rhythm: _____ Rate: _____ P wave: _____

PR interval: _____ QRS complex: _____

Rhythm interpretation: _____

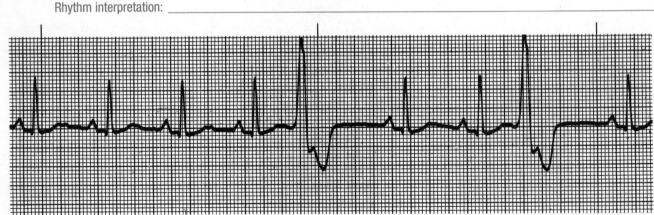

**Strip 9-3.** Rhythm: _____ Rate: _____ P wave: _____

PR interval: _____ QRS complex: _____

Rhythm interpretation: _____

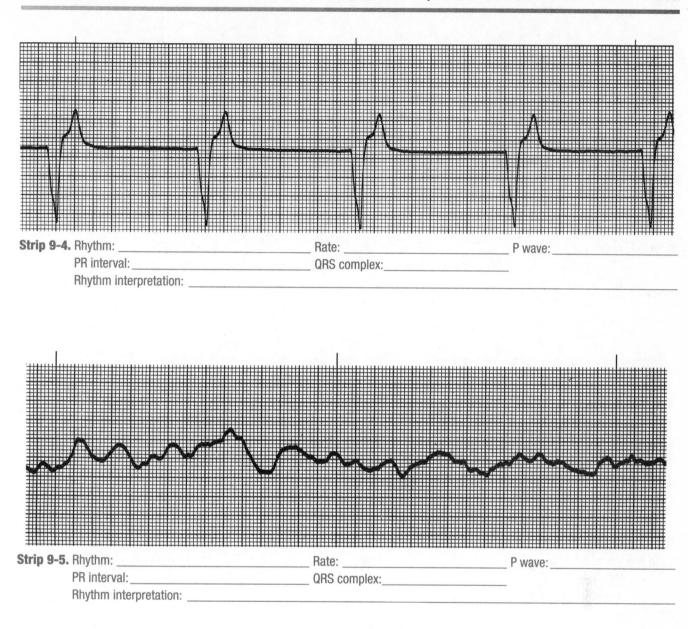

**Strip 9-4.** Rhythm: _____ Rate: _____ P wave: _____
PR interval: _____ QRS complex: _____
Rhythm interpretation: _____

**Strip 9-5.** Rhythm: _____ Rate: _____ P wave: _____
PR interval: _____ QRS complex: _____
Rhythm interpretation: _____

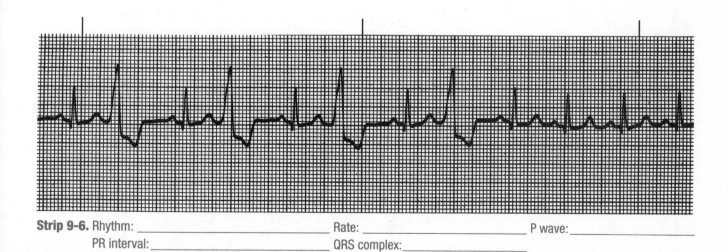

**Strip 9-6.** Rhythm: _____ Rate: _____ P wave: _____
PR interval: _____ QRS complex: _____
Rhythm interpretation: _____

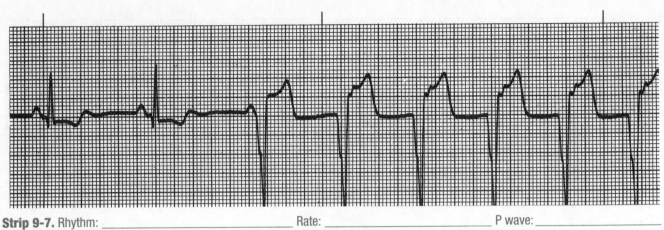

**Strip 9-7.** Rhythm: _____ Rate: _____ P wave: _____

PR interval: _____ QRS complex: _____

Rhythm interpretation: _____

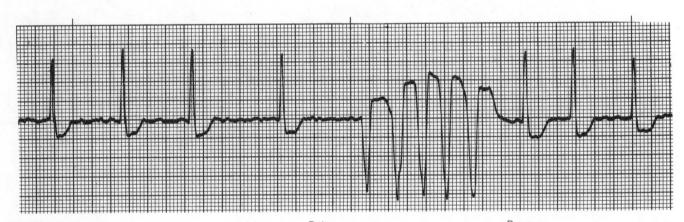

**Strip 9-8.** Rhythm: _____ Rate: _____ P wave: _____

PR interval: _____ QRS complex: _____

Rhythm interpretation: _____

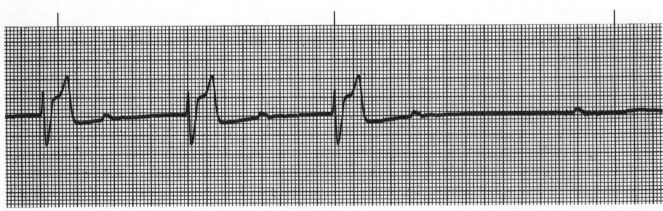

**Strip 9-9.** Rhythm: _____ Rate: _____ P wave: _____

PR interval: _____ QRS complex: _____

Rhythm interpretation: _____

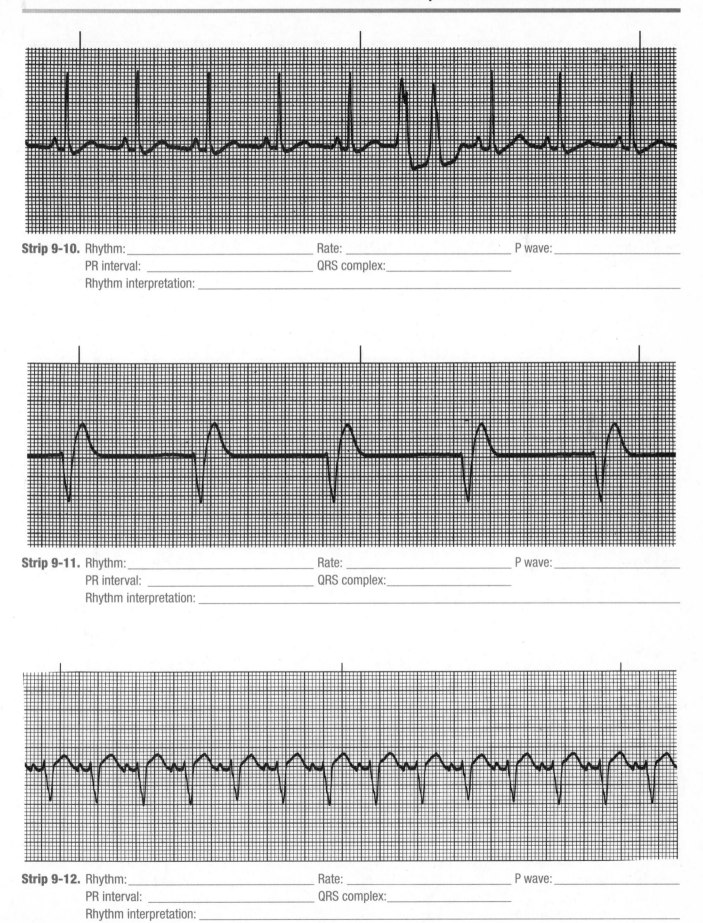

**Strip 9-10.** Rhythm: _____ Rate: _____ P wave: _____

PR interval: _____ QRS complex: _____

Rhythm interpretation: _____

**Strip 9-11.** Rhythm: _____ Rate: _____ P wave: _____

PR interval: _____ QRS complex: _____

Rhythm interpretation: _____

**Strip 9-12.** Rhythm: _____ Rate: _____ P wave: _____

PR interval: _____ QRS complex: _____

Rhythm interpretation: _____

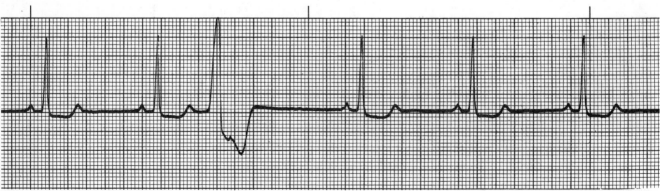

**Strip 9-13.** Rhythm: _____ Rate: _____ P wave: _____

PR interval: _____ QRS complex: _____

Rhythm interpretation: _____

**Strip 9-14.** Rhythm: _____ Rate: _____ P wave: _____

PR interval: _____ QRS complex: _____

Rhythm interpretation: _____

**Strip 9-15.** Rhythm: _____ Rate: _____ P wave: _____

PR interval: _____ QRS complex: _____

Rhythm interpretation: _____

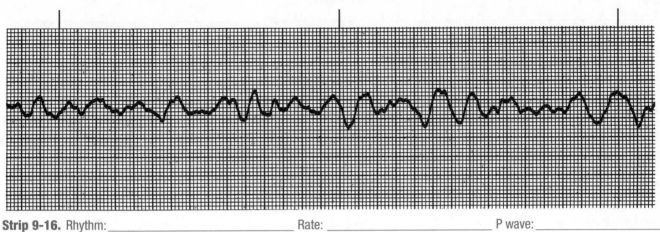

**Strip 9-16.** Rhythm:_____ Rate:_____ P wave:_____

PR interval:_____ QRS complex:_____

Rhythm interpretation:_____

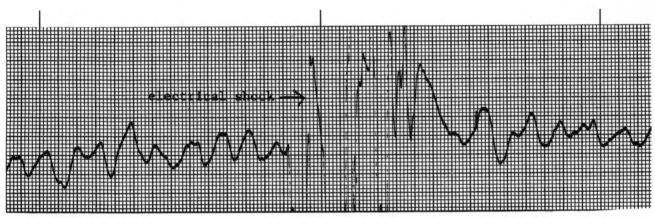

**Strip 9-17.** Rhythm:_____ Rate:_____ P wave:_____

PR interval:_____ QRS complex:_____

Rhythm interpretation:_____

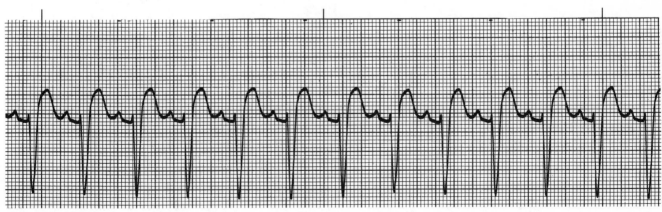

**Strip 9-18.** Rhythm:_____ Rate:_____ P wave:_____

PR interval:_____ QRS complex:_____

Rhythm interpretation:_____

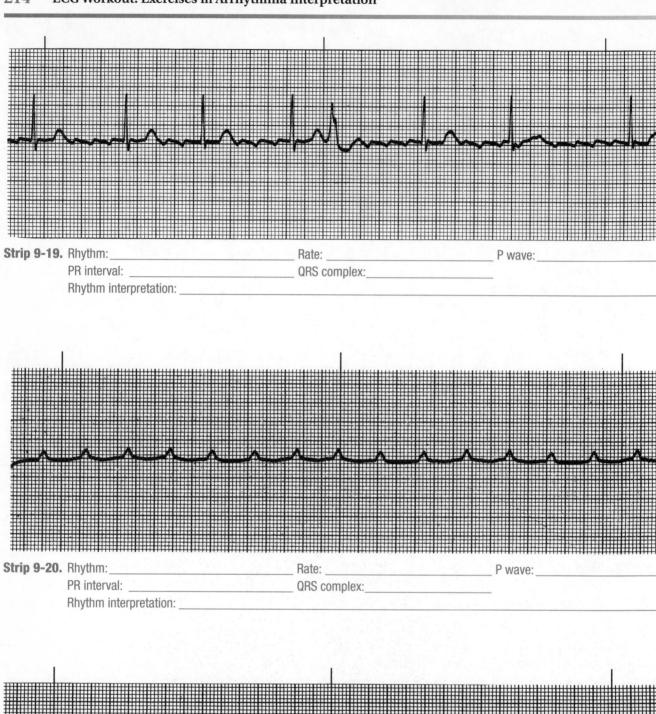

**Strip 9-19.** Rhythm:_____ Rate:_____ P wave:_____

PR interval: _____ QRS complex:_____

Rhythm interpretation: _____

**Strip 9-20.** Rhythm:_____ Rate:_____ P wave:_____

PR interval: _____ QRS complex:_____

Rhythm interpretation: _____

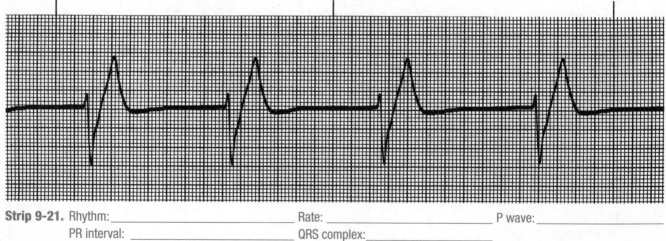

**Strip 9-21.** Rhythm:_____ Rate:_____ P wave:_____

PR interval: _____ QRS complex:_____

Rhythm interpretation: _____

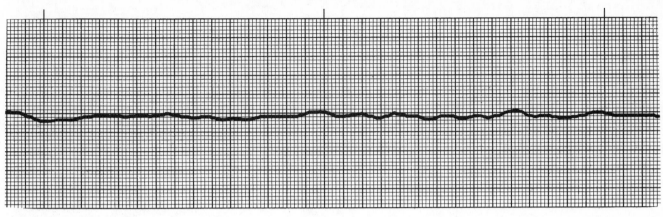

**Strip 9-22.** Rhythm:_____ Rate:_____ P wave:_____

PR interval:_____ QRS complex:_____

Rhythm interpretation:_____

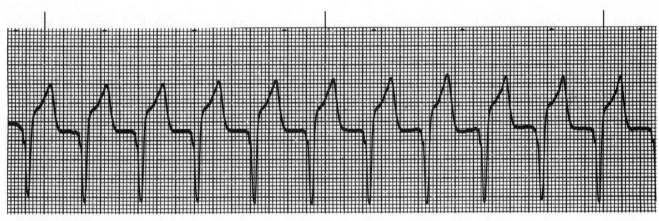

**Strip 9-23.** Rhythm:_____ Rate:_____ P wave:_____

PR interval:_____ QRS complex:_____

Rhythm interpretation:_____

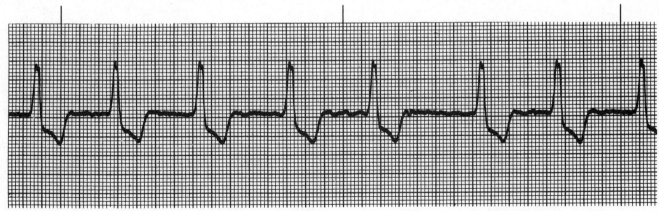

**Strip 9-24.** Rhythm:_____ Rate:_____ P wave:_____

PR interval:_____ QRS complex:_____

Rhythm interpretation:_____

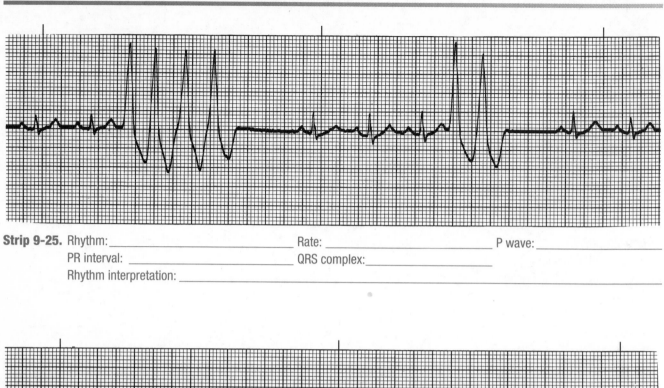

**Strip 9-25.** Rhythm:_____ Rate:_____ P wave:_____

PR interval:_____ QRS complex:_____

Rhythm interpretation:_____

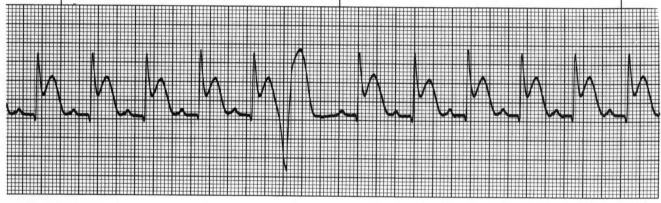

**Strip 9-26.** Rhythm:_____ Rate:_____ P wave:_____

PR interval:_____ QRS complex:_____

Rhythm interpretation:_____

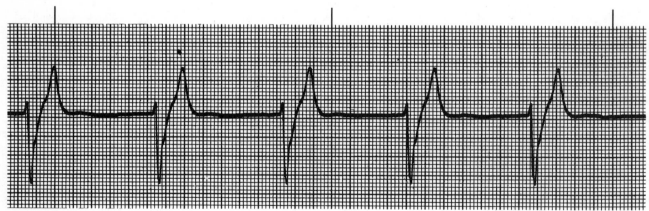

**Strip 9-27.** Rhythm:_____ Rate:_____ P wave:_____

PR interval:_____ QRS complex:_____

Rhythm interpretation:_____

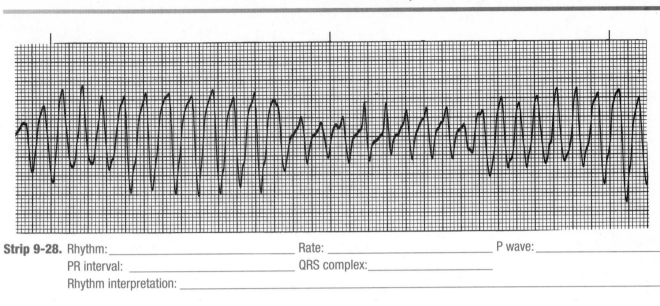

**Strip 9-28.** Rhythm: _____ Rate: _____ P wave: _____
PR interval: _____ QRS complex: _____
Rhythm interpretation: _____

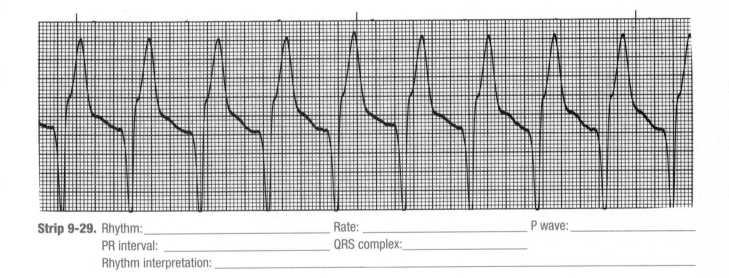

**Strip 9-29.** Rhythm: _____ Rate: _____ P wave: _____
PR interval: _____ QRS complex: _____
Rhythm interpretation: _____

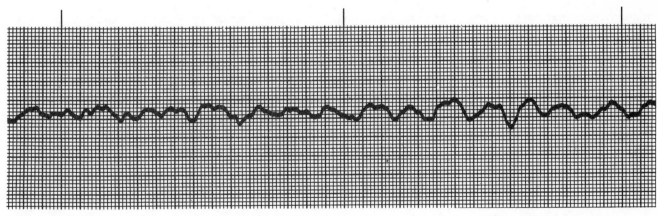

**Strip 9-30.** Rhythm: _____ Rate: _____ P wave: _____
PR interval: _____ QRS complex: _____
Rhythm interpretation: _____

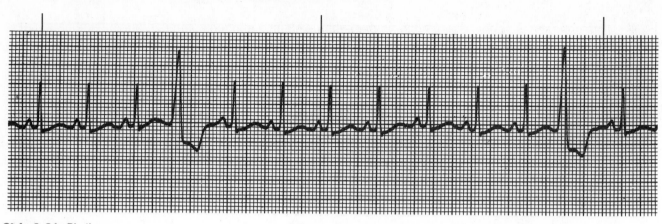

**Strip 9-31.** Rhythm:_____ Rate:_____ P wave:_____
PR interval:_____ QRS complex:_____
Rhythm interpretation:_____

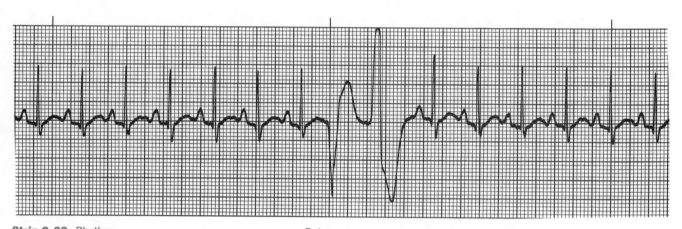

**Strip 9-32.** Rhythm:_____ Rate:_____ P wave:_____
PR interval:_____ QRS complex:_____
Rhythm interpretation:_____

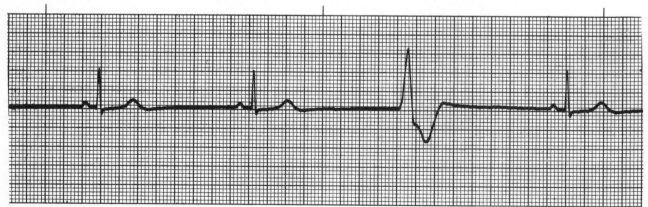

**Strip 9-33.** Rhythm:_____ Rate:_____ P wave:_____
PR interval:_____ QRS complex:_____
Rhythm interpretation:_____

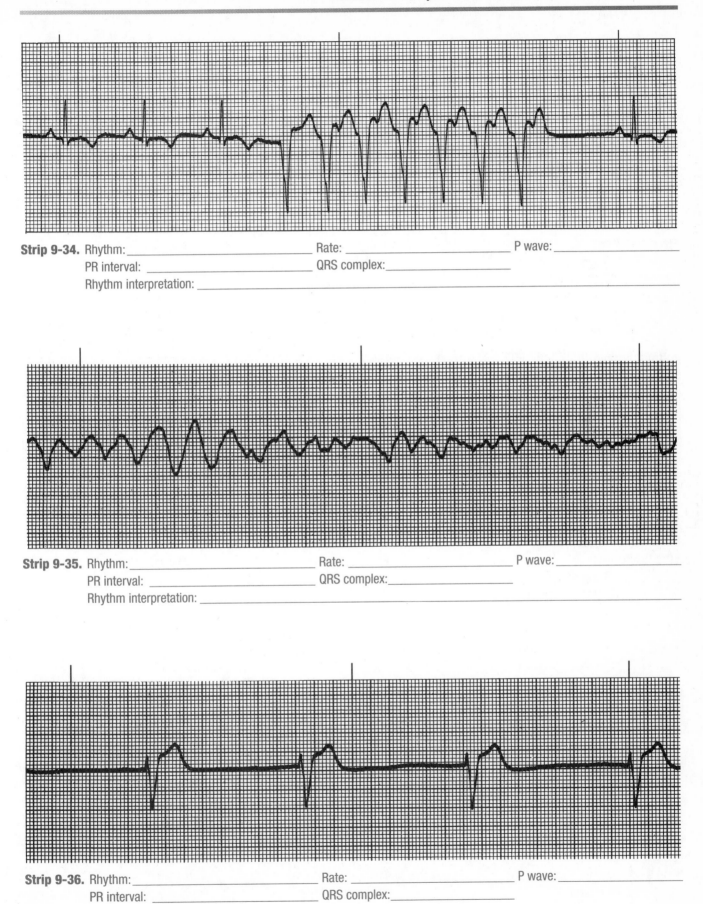

**Strip 9-34.** Rhythm:_____ Rate: _____ P wave: _____

PR interval: _____ QRS complex:_____

Rhythm interpretation: _____

**Strip 9-35.** Rhythm:_____ Rate: _____ P wave: _____

PR interval: _____ QRS complex:_____

Rhythm interpretation: _____

**Strip 9-36.** Rhythm:_____ Rate: _____ P wave: _____

PR interval: _____ QRS complex:_____

Rhythm interpretation: _____

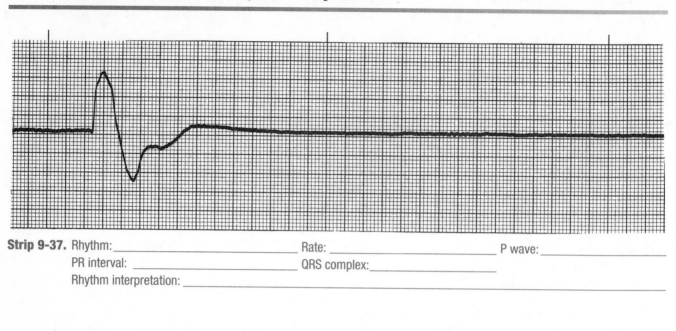

**Strip 9-37.** Rhythm:_____ Rate: _____ P wave: _____
PR interval: _____ QRS complex:_____
Rhythm interpretation: _____

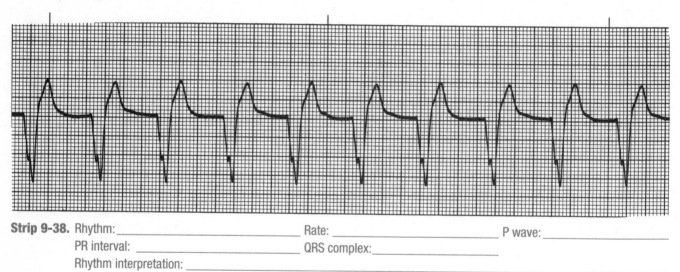

**Strip 9-38.** Rhythm:_____ Rate: _____ P wave: _____
PR interval: _____ QRS complex:_____
Rhythm interpretation: _____

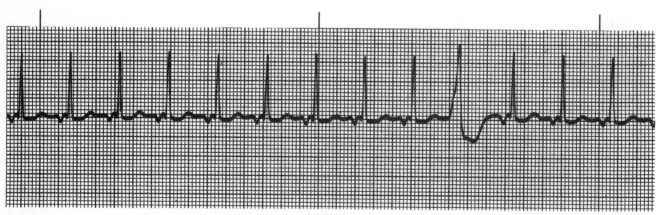

**Strip 9-39.** Rhythm:_____ Rate: _____ P wave: _____
PR interval: _____ QRS complex:_____
Rhythm interpretation: _____

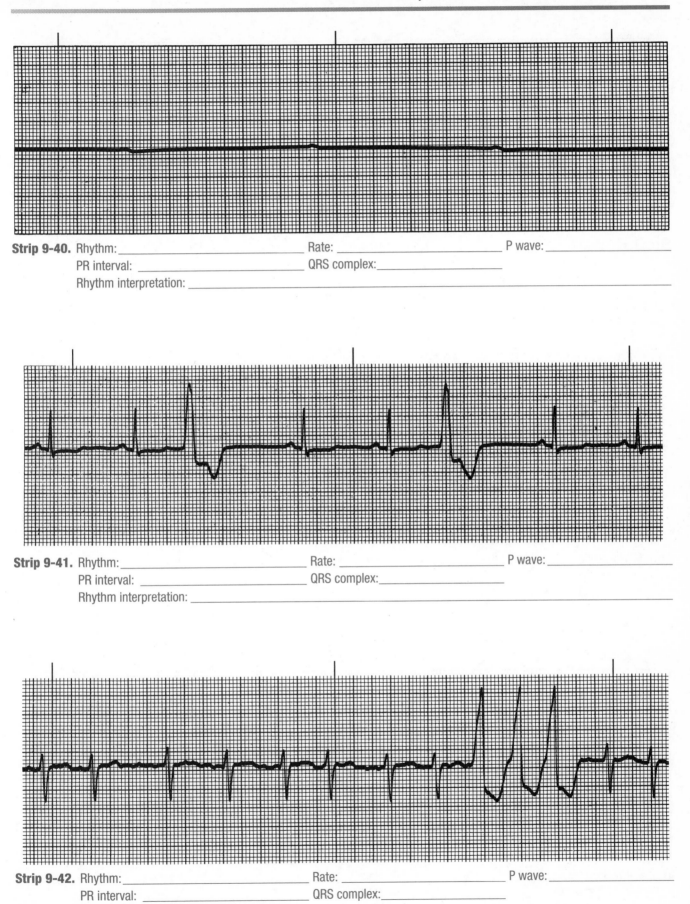

**Strip 9-40.** Rhythm: _____ Rate: _____ P wave: _____
PR interval: _____ QRS complex: _____
Rhythm interpretation: _____

**Strip 9-41.** Rhythm: _____ Rate: _____ P wave: _____
PR interval: _____ QRS complex: _____
Rhythm interpretation: _____

**Strip 9-42.** Rhythm: _____ Rate: _____ P wave: _____
PR interval: _____ QRS complex: _____
Rhythm interpretation: _____

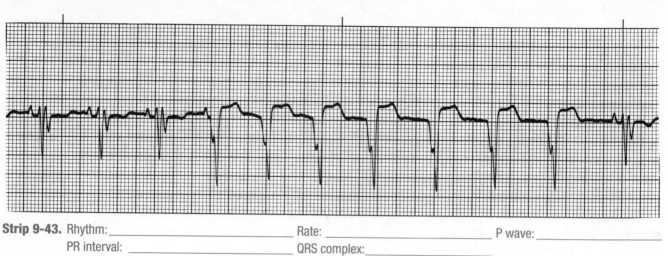

**Strip 9-43.** Rhythm:_____ Rate:_____ P wave:_____

PR interval: _____ QRS complex:_____

Rhythm interpretation: _____

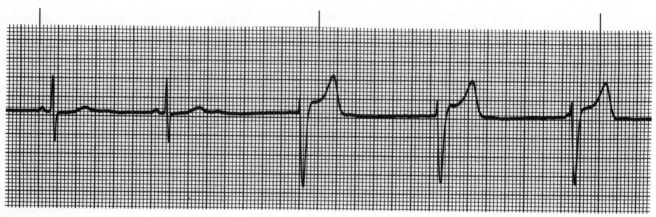

**Strip 9-44.** Rhythm:_____ Rate:_____ P wave:_____

PR interval: _____ QRS complex:_____

Rhythm interpretation: _____

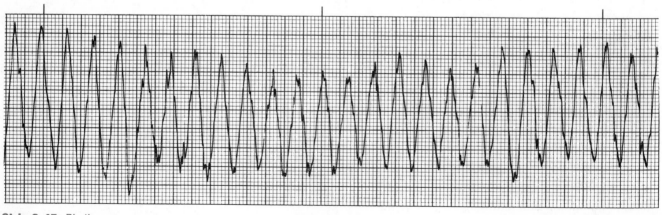

**Strip 9-45.** Rhythm:_____ Rate:_____ P wave:_____

PR interval: _____ QRS complex:_____

Rhythm interpretation: _____

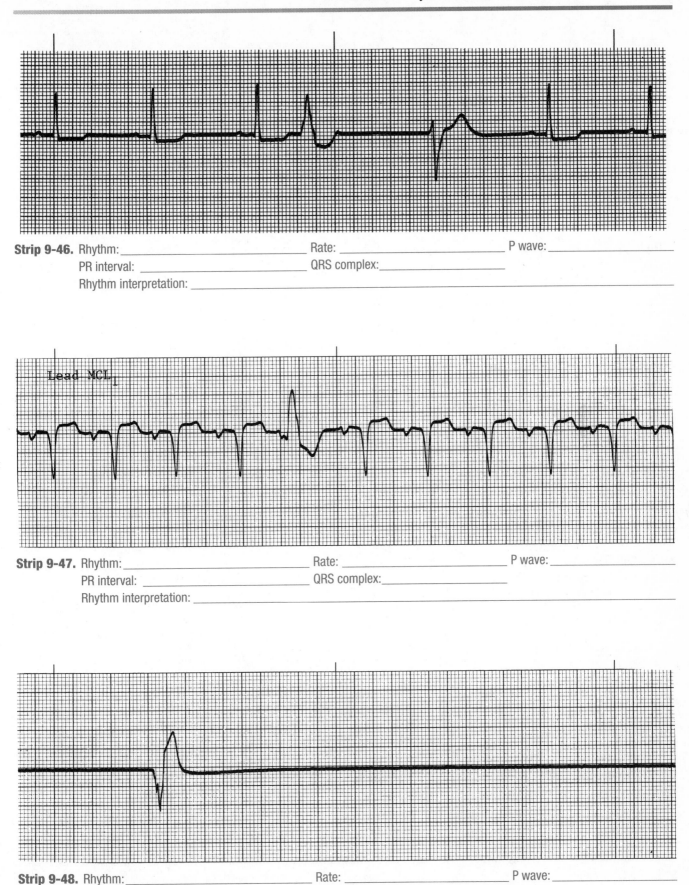

**Strip 9-46.** Rhythm: _____ Rate: _____ P wave: _____
PR interval: _____ QRS complex: _____
Rhythm interpretation: _____

Lead MCL₁

**Strip 9-47.** Rhythm: _____ Rate: _____ P wave: _____
PR interval: _____ QRS complex: _____
Rhythm interpretation: _____

**Strip 9-48.** Rhythm: _____ Rate: _____ P wave: _____
PR interval: _____ QRS complex: _____
Rhythm interpretation: _____

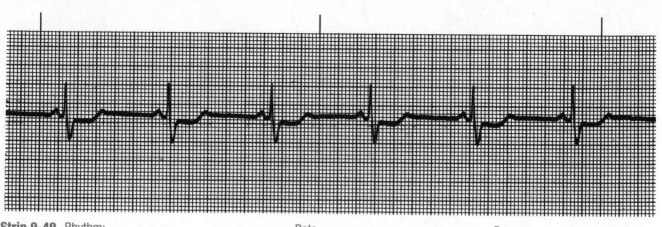

**Strip 9-49.** Rhythm:_____ Rate:_____ P wave:_____
PR interval:_____ QRS complex:_____
Rhythm interpretation:_____

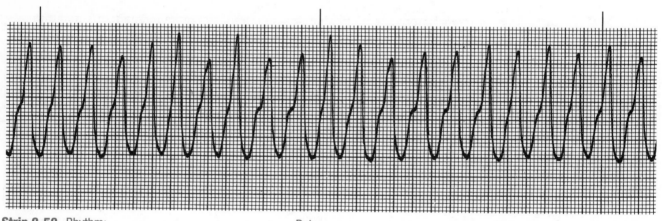

**Strip 9-50.** Rhythm:_____ Rate:_____ P wave:_____
PR interval:_____ QRS complex:_____
Rhythm interpretation:_____

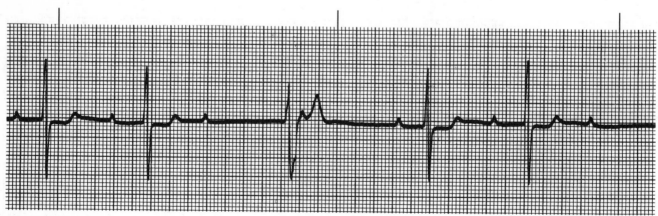

**Strip 9-51.** Rhythm:_____ Rate:_____ P wave:_____
PR interval:_____ QRS complex:_____
Rhythm interpretation:_____

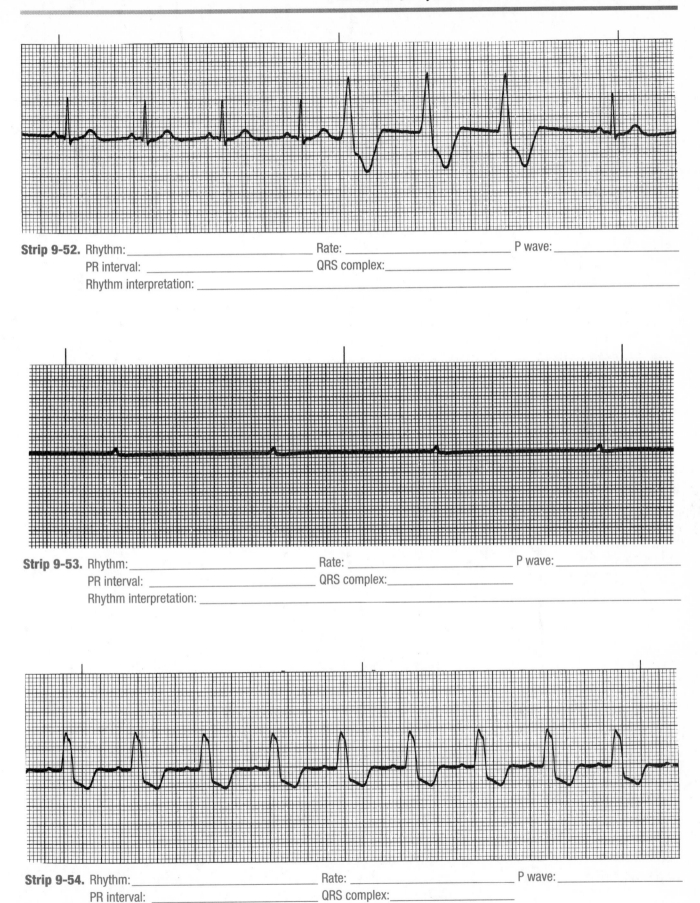

**Strip 9-52.** Rhythm: _____ Rate: _____ P wave: _____

PR interval: _____ QRS complex: _____

Rhythm interpretation: _____

**Strip 9-53.** Rhythm: _____ Rate: _____ P wave: _____

PR interval: _____ QRS complex: _____

Rhythm interpretation: _____

**Strip 9-54.** Rhythm: _____ Rate: _____ P wave: _____

PR interval: _____ QRS complex: _____

Rhythm interpretation: _____

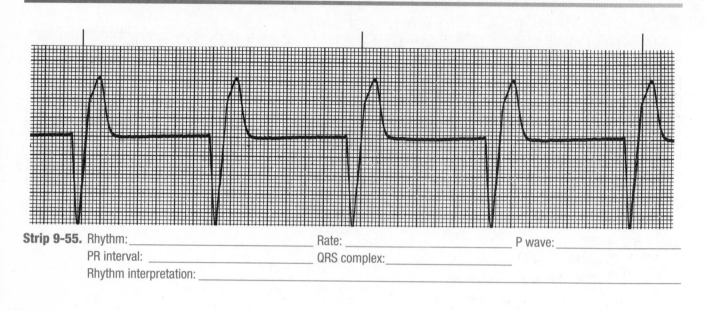

**Strip 9-55.** Rhythm:_____ Rate: _____ P wave:_____

PR interval: _____ QRS complex:_____

Rhythm interpretation: _____

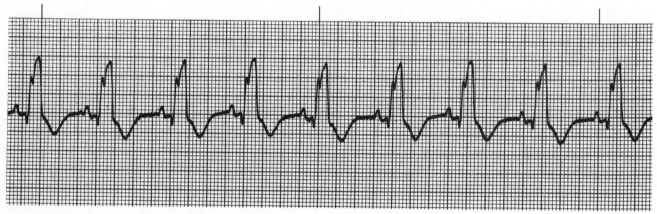

**Strip 9-56.** Rhythm:_____ Rate: _____ P wave:_____

PR interval: _____ QRS complex:_____

Rhythm interpretation: _____

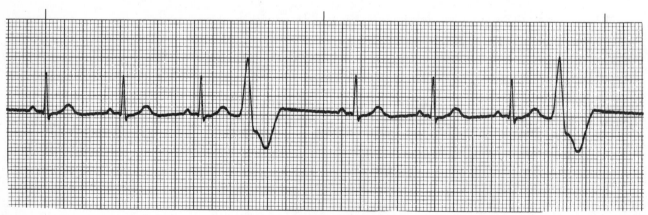

**Strip 9-57.** Rhythm:_____ Rate: _____ P wave:_____

PR interval: _____ QRS complex:_____

Rhythm interpretation: _____

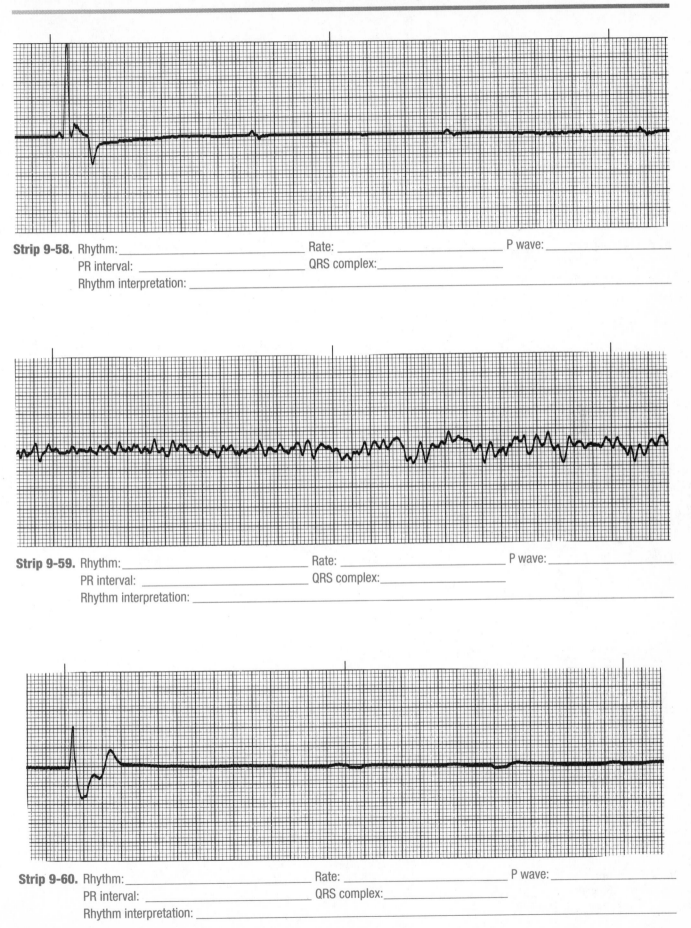

**Strip 9-58.** Rhythm: _____ Rate: _____ P wave: _____

PR interval: _____ QRS complex: _____

Rhythm interpretation: _____

**Strip 9-59.** Rhythm: _____ Rate: _____ P wave: _____

PR interval: _____ QRS complex: _____

Rhythm interpretation: _____

**Strip 9-60.** Rhythm: _____ Rate: _____ P wave: _____

PR interval: _____ QRS complex: _____

Rhythm interpretation: _____

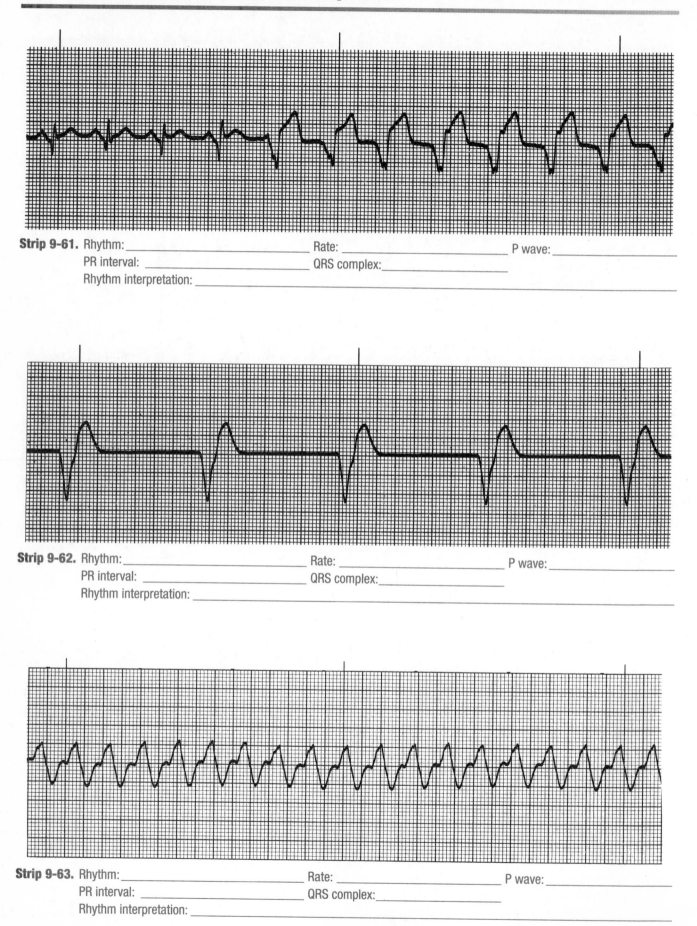

**Strip 9-61.** Rhythm:_____ Rate:_____ P wave:_____

PR interval:_____ QRS complex:_____

Rhythm interpretation:_____

**Strip 9-62.** Rhythm:_____ Rate:_____ P wave:_____

PR interval:_____ QRS complex:_____

Rhythm interpretation:_____

**Strip 9-63.** Rhythm:_____ Rate:_____ P wave:_____

PR interval:_____ QRS complex:_____

Rhythm interpretation:_____

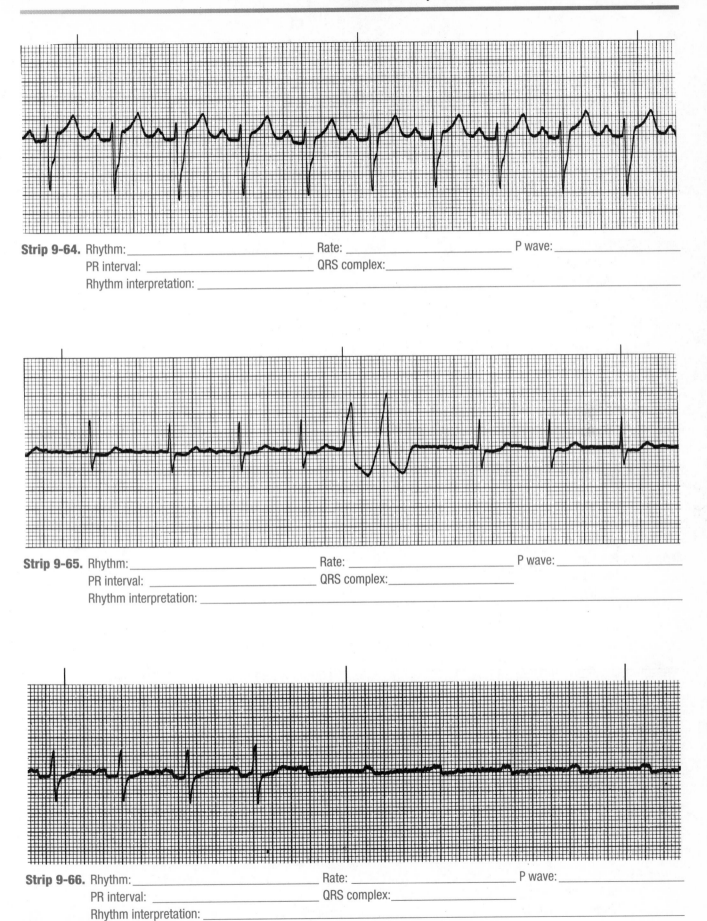

**Strip 9-64.** Rhythm: _____ Rate: _____ P wave: _____

PR interval: _____ QRS complex: _____

Rhythm interpretation: _____

**Strip 9-65.** Rhythm: _____ Rate: _____ P wave: _____

PR interval: _____ QRS complex: _____

Rhythm interpretation: _____

**Strip 9-66.** Rhythm: _____ Rate: _____ P wave: _____

PR interval: _____ QRS complex: _____

Rhythm interpretation: _____

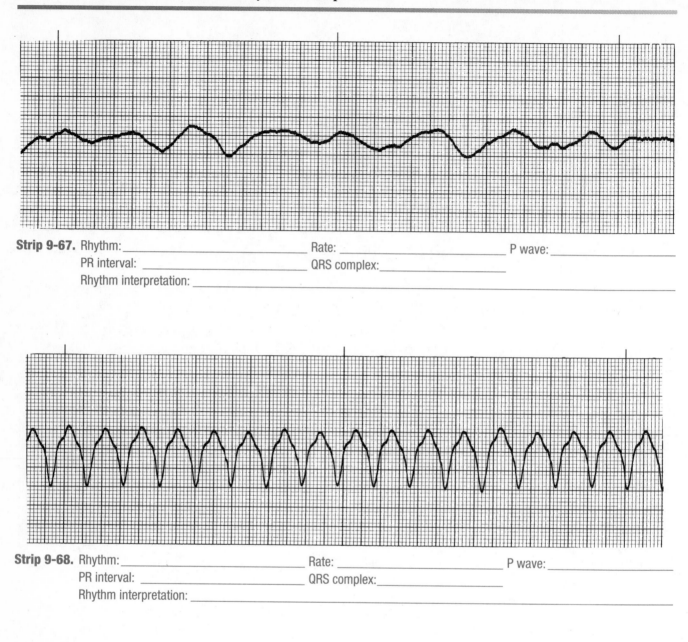

**Strip 9-67.** Rhythm:_____ Rate:_____ P wave:_____

PR interval:_____ QRS complex:_____

Rhythm interpretation:_____

**Strip 9-68.** Rhythm:_____ Rate:_____ P wave:_____

PR interval:_____ QRS complex:_____

Rhythm interpretation:_____

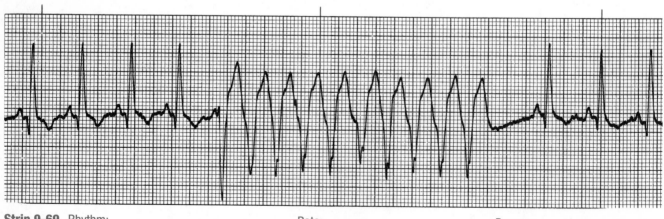

**Strip 9-69.** Rhythm:_____ Rate:_____ P wave:_____

PR interval:_____ QRS complex:_____

Rhythm interpretation:_____

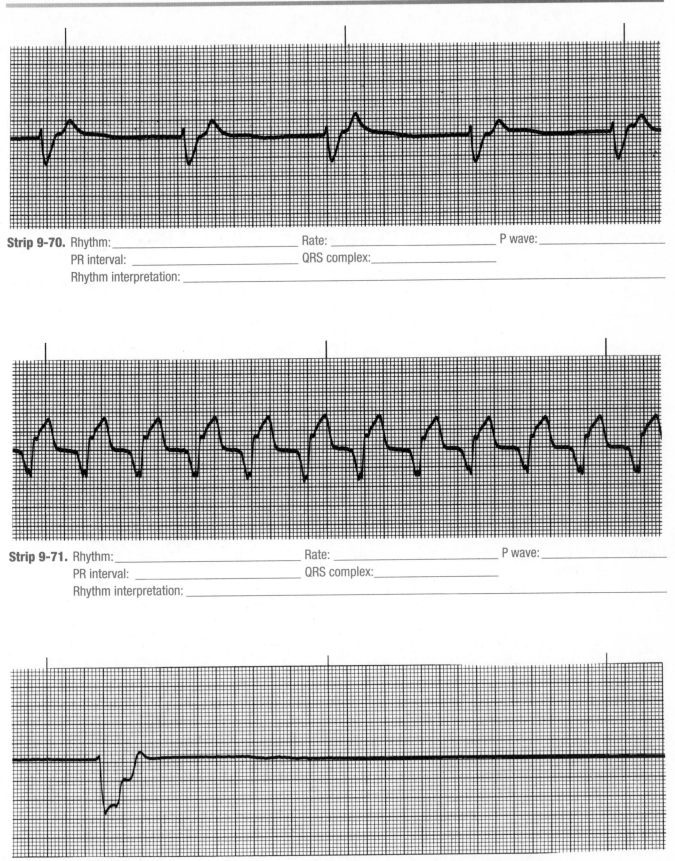

**Strip 9-70.** Rhythm: _____ Rate: _____ P wave: _____
PR interval: _____ QRS complex: _____
Rhythm interpretation: _____

**Strip 9-71.** Rhythm: _____ Rate: _____ P wave: _____
PR interval: _____ QRS complex: _____
Rhythm interpretation: _____

**Strip 9-72.** Rhythm: _____ Rate: _____ P wave: _____
PR interval: _____ QRS complex: _____
Rhythm interpretation: _____

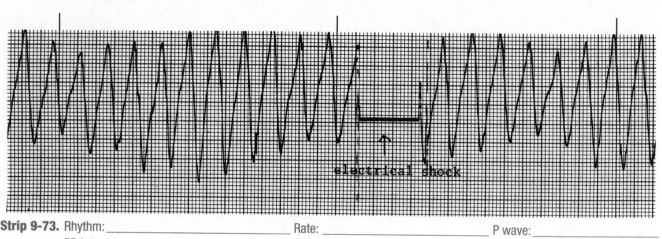

electrical shock

**Strip 9-73.** Rhythm:_____ Rate:_____ P wave:_____

PR interval:_____ QRS complex:_____

Rhythm interpretation:_____

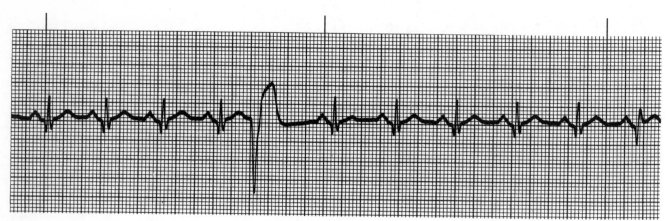

**Strip 9-74.** Rhythm:_____ Rate:_____ P wave:_____

PR interval:_____ QRS complex:_____

Rhythm interpretation:_____

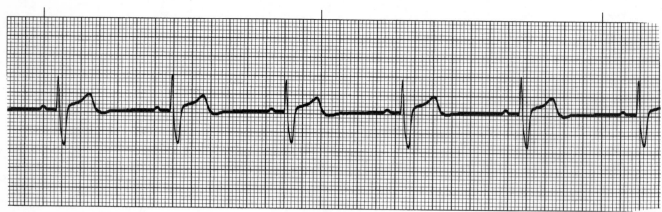

**Strip 9-75.** Rhythm:_____ Rate:_____ P wave:_____

PR interval:_____ QRS complex:_____

Rhythm interpretation:_____

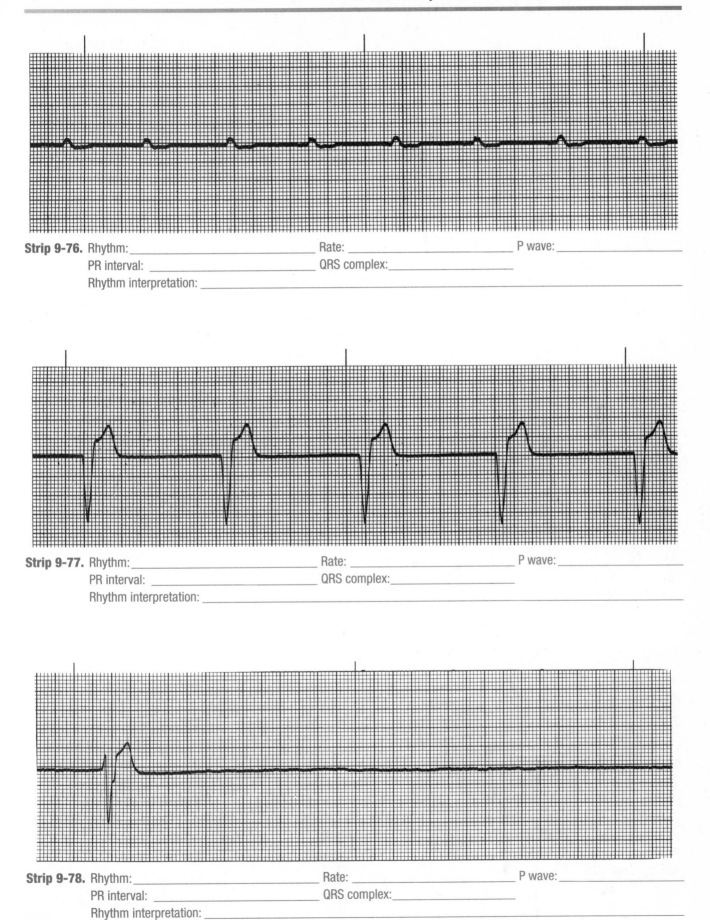

**Strip 9-76.** Rhythm:_____ Rate:_____ P wave:_____

PR interval:_____ QRS complex:_____

Rhythm interpretation:_____

**Strip 9-77.** Rhythm:_____ Rate:_____ P wave:_____

PR interval:_____ QRS complex:_____

Rhythm interpretation:_____

**Strip 9-78.** Rhythm:_____ Rate:_____ P wave:_____

PR interval:_____ QRS complex:_____

Rhythm interpretation:_____

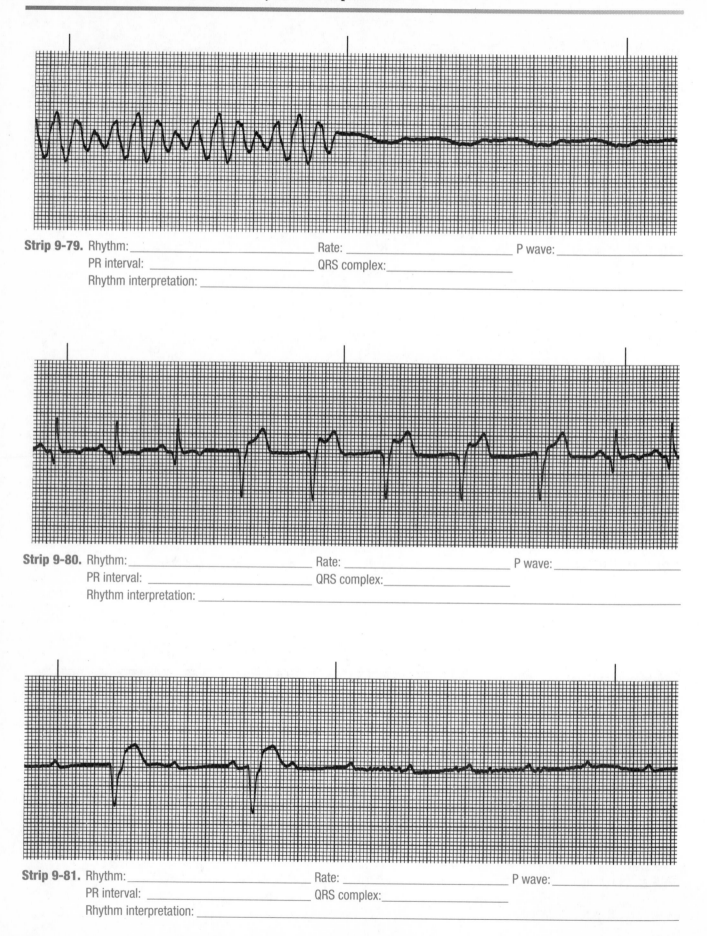

**Strip 9-79.** Rhythm:_____ Rate:_____ P wave:_____

PR interval: _____ QRS complex:_____

Rhythm interpretation: _____

**Strip 9-80.** Rhythm:_____ Rate:_____ P wave:_____

PR interval: _____ QRS complex:_____

Rhythm interpretation: _____

**Strip 9-81.** Rhythm:_____ Rate:_____ P wave:_____

PR interval: _____ QRS complex:_____

Rhythm interpretation: _____

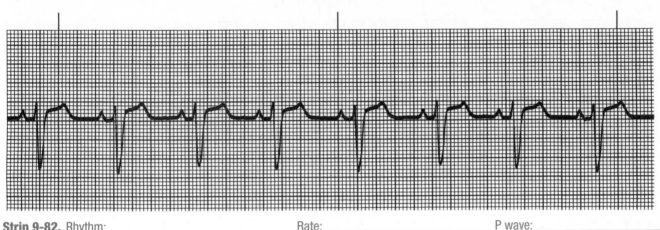

**Strip 9-82.** Rhythm: _____ Rate: _____ P wave: _____
PR interval: _____ QRS complex: _____
Rhythm interpretation: _____

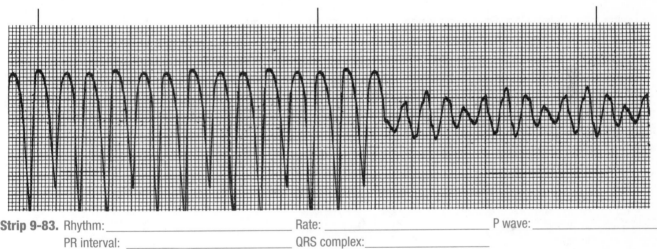

**Strip 9-83.** Rhythm: _____ Rate: _____ P wave: _____
PR interval: _____ QRS complex: _____
Rhythm interpretation: _____

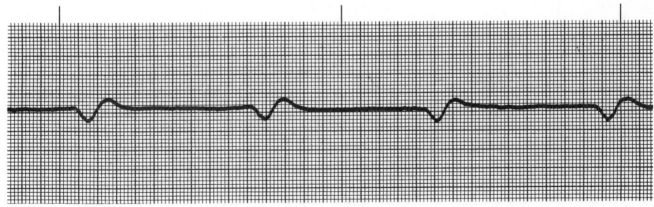

**Strip 9-84.** Rhythm: _____ Rate: _____ P wave: _____
PR interval: _____ QRS complex: _____
Rhythm interpretation: _____

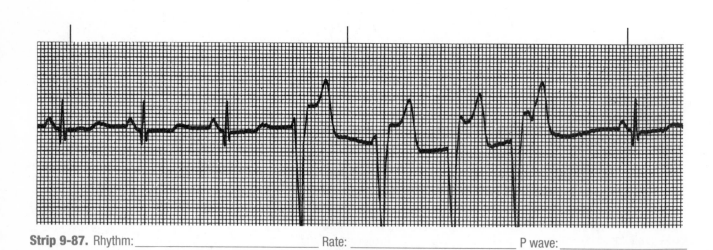

**Strip 9-85.** Rhythm: _____ Rate: _____ P wave: _____

PR interval: _____ QRS complex: _____

Rhythm interpretation: _____

**Strip 9-86.** Rhythm: _____ Rate: _____ P wave: _____

PR interval: _____ QRS complex: _____

Rhythm interpretation: _____

**Strip 9-87.** Rhythm: _____ Rate: _____ P wave: _____

PR interval: _____ QRS complex: _____

Rhythm interpretation: _____

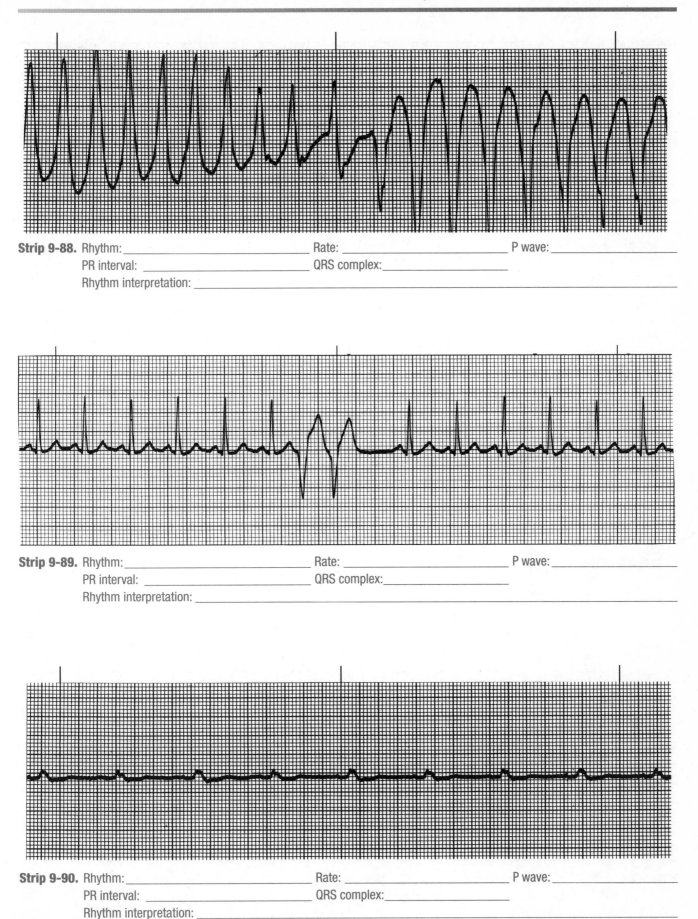

**Strip 9-88.** Rhythm:_____ Rate:_____ P wave:_____
PR interval:_____ QRS complex:_____
Rhythm interpretation:_____

**Strip 9-89.** Rhythm:_____ Rate:_____ P wave:_____
PR interval:_____ QRS complex:_____
Rhythm interpretation:_____

**Strip 9-90.** Rhythm:_____ Rate:_____ P wave:_____
PR interval:_____ QRS complex:_____
Rhythm interpretation:_____

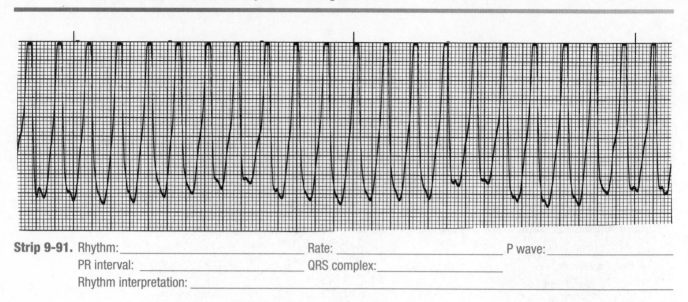

**Strip 9-91.** Rhythm: _____ Rate: _____ P wave: _____

PR interval: _____ QRS complex: _____

Rhythm interpretation: _____

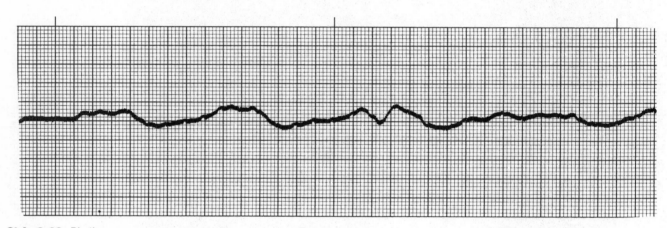

**Strip 9-92.** Rhythm: _____ Rate: _____ P wave: _____

PR interval: _____ QRS complex: _____

Rhythm interpretation: _____

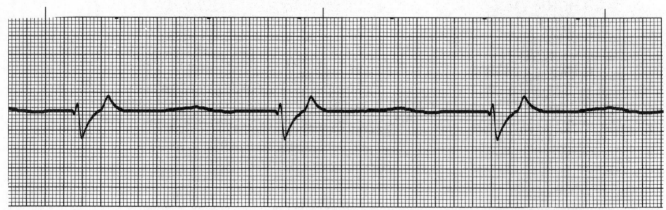

**Strip 9-93.** Rhythm: _____ Rate: _____ P wave: _____

PR interval: _____ QRS complex: _____

Rhythm interpretation: _____

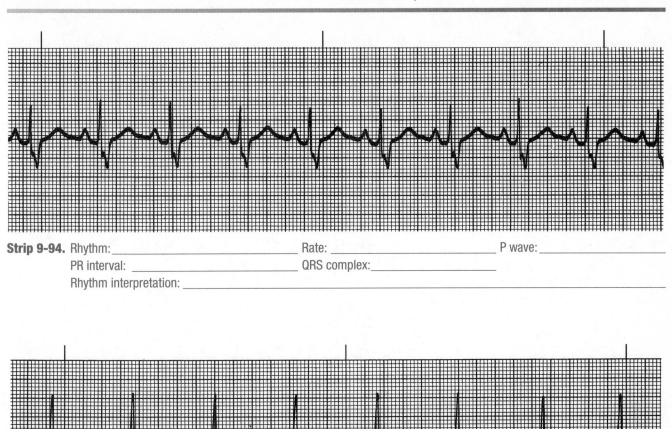

**Strip 9-94.** Rhythm:_____ Rate:_____ P wave:_____

PR interval:_____ QRS complex:_____

Rhythm interpretation:_____

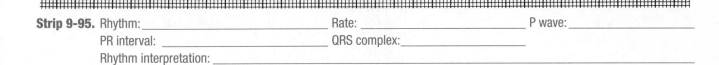

**Strip 9-95.** Rhythm:_____ Rate:_____ P wave:_____

PR interval:_____ QRS complex:_____

Rhythm interpretation:_____

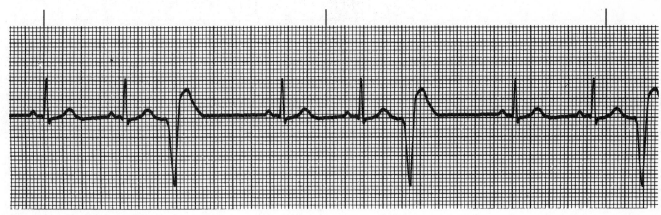

**Strip 9-96.** Rhythm:_____ Rate:_____ P wave:_____

PR interval:_____ QRS complex:_____

Rhythm interpretation:_____

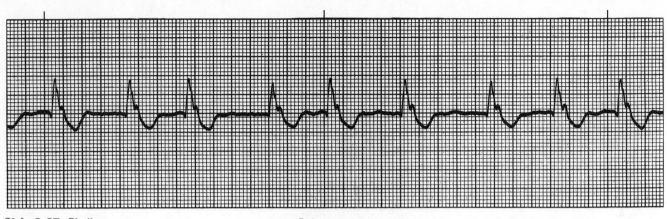

**Strip 9-97.** Rhythm: _____ Rate: _____ P wave: _____
PR interval: _____ QRS complex: _____
Rhythm interpretation: _____

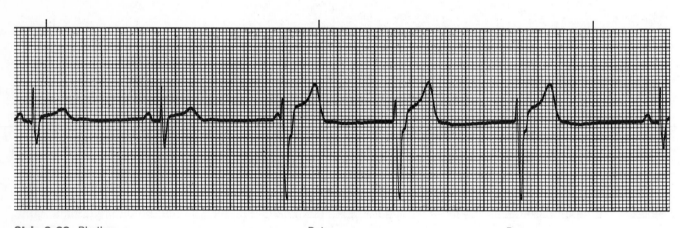

**Strip 9-98.** Rhythm: _____ Rate: _____ P wave: _____
PR interval: _____ QRS complex: _____
Rhythm interpretation: _____

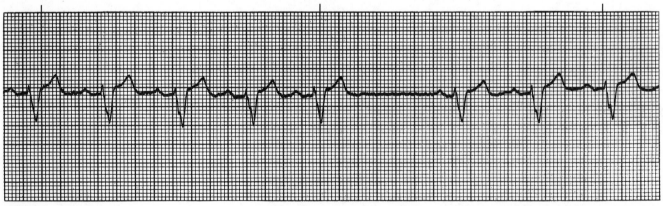

**Strip 9-99.** Rhythm: _____ Rate: _____ P wave: _____
PR interval: _____ QRS complex: _____
Rhythm interpretation: _____

**Strip 9-100.** Rhythm:_____ Rate: _____ P wave: _____

PR interval: _____ QRS complex:_____

Rhythm interpretation: _____

# 10  Pacemakers

## Overview

A pacemaker is a battery-powered device that delivers an electrical stimulus to the myocardium resulting in contraction. Pacemakers can be temporary or permanent and are used primarily when the patient's own heart rate is excessively slow, as in symptomatic sinus bradycardia, sinus arrest, sinus exit block, sick sinus syndrome (a degenerative process of the sinus node that produces alternating periods of bradycardia and tachycardia), slow atrial fibrillation; or when there is a potential for ventricular standstill to occur, as in second-degree atrioventricular (AV) block Mobitz II or third-degree AV block. Prophylactic temporary pacing is commonly done if a new bundle-branch block results from an acute myocardial infarction (MI); if a right bundle-branch block is associated with a block in one fascicle of the left bundle branch, or if a right or left bundle branch block is complicated by AV block, especially if the patient has an acute MI.

A pacemaker functions in one of two ways: as a fixed-rate pacemaker or as a demand pacemaker. Fixed-rate pacemakers initiate impulses at a set rate, regardless of the patient's intrinsic rate. The fixed-rate pacemaker competes with the patient's own heart rhythm and is potentially dangerous because the pacing stimulus may fall during the vulnerable period of the cardiac cycle and induce serious ventricular arrhythmias. This type of pacemaker is used primarily when the patient has no intrinsic heart rate, such as during cardiac arrest. Demand pacemakers are designed with a sensing mechanism that inhibits discharge when the patient's heart rate is adequate and a pacing mechanism that triggers the pacemaker to fire when no intrinsic activity occurs within a predetermined period. Different types of demand pacemakers are available:

- Single-chamber pacemakers sense and pace either the atrium or the ventricle.
- Dual-chamber pacemakers sense and pace both the atrium and the ventricle.

An advantage of the dual-chamber pacemakers is their ability to stimulate the atria and ventricles in sequence, thereby preserving normal AV synchrony and the atrial kick that contributes 20% to 30% of cardiac output.

All pacemakers have some components in common — the pulse generator and the pacing catheter. The pulse generator houses the battery that creates the electrical signal and contains the various controls or settings for pacemaker function (electrical output or milliamperes [mA], sensitivity or millivolts [mV], heart rate setting, mode of pacing, specialized settings, and so forth). The pacing catheter (commonly called the *lead* or *electrode*) serves as a transmission line between the pulse generator and the endocardium. Electrical impulses are conducted from the pulse generator to the endocardium while information about intrinsic electrical activity is relayed from the catheter tip back to the generator for processing.

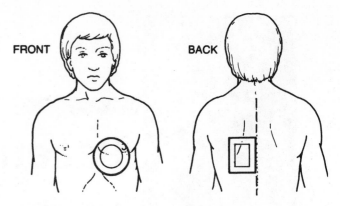

**Figure 10-1.** External pacing pad placement.

## Temporary pacemakers

Temporary pacing can be accomplished with transvenous, epicardial, or transcutaneous (external) methods. With the external pacemaker system, large pacing pads are placed on the anterior and posterior chest (see Figure 10-1). Placement of the pacing pads affects the current required to obtain ventricular capture. The placement that offers the most direct current pathway to the heart usually produces the lowest threshold. The pacing pads are attached to a pacing cable, which is then connected to a defibrillator/monitor. Electrocardiogram (ECG) leads are also attached to the patient. A pacing rate is set, and the mA dial turned up until consistent capture is seen. The myocardium is stimulated indirectly by electric currents transmitted through the chest wall. There are also systems available that have the capability to monitor, externally pace, and defibrillate the patient through one set of chest pads.

External pacemakers are noninvasive, quick and easy to apply, and designed to function in the demand mode. Successful transcutaneous pacing requires a higher current output (mA) than conventional transvenous pacing. Delivery of this stronger current may cause chest wall pain and skin burns (although the larger pacing pad minimizes the risk of burns). Transcutaneous pacing is effective as a treatment when meaningful contractile activity is present (for example, in the hemodynamically significant bradycardias, such as symptomatic sinus bradycardia, second-degree AV block Mobitz II, and third-degree AV block). External pacing usually isn't effective for treatment of ventricular standstill or pulseless electrical activity (PEA) that occurs in the setting of cardiac arrest. This is because the primary problem in these situations is the inability of the myocardium to contract when appropriately stimulated. External pacemakers are used as a temporary measure in emergency situations where transvenous access isn't readily available. Transvenous pacing is still the treatment of choice for patients requiring a temporary but longer period of pacemaker support.

With the temporary transvenous pacemaker (see Figure 10-2), the pacing electrode is inserted by transvenous route

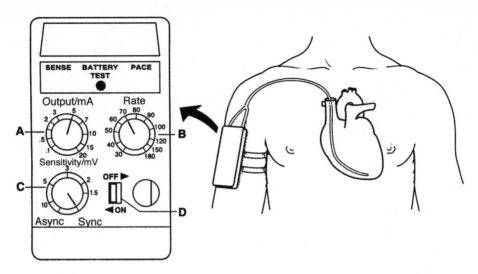

**Figure 10-2.** Temporary pacemaker.

A. Output or mA dial
   1. Controls the amount of electrical energy delivered to the endocardium.
B. Rate dial
   1. Determines the rate in beats per minute at which the stimulus is to be delivered.
C. Sensitivity or mV dial
   1. Controls the ability of the generator to sense intrinsic activity.
   2. In maximum clockwise position, this provides demand (synchronous) pacing.
   3. In maximum counterclockwise position, this provides fixed rate (asynchronous) pacing.
D. On/off control
   1. Activates/inactivates the pulse generator.

(internal jugular, subclavian, antecubital, or femoral vein) into the apex of the right ventricle for ventricular pacing, the right atrium for atrial pacing, or both chambers for dual-chamber pacing. The electrode is then connected via a bridging cable to an external pulse generator. The endocardium is stimulated directly by electric currents transmitted from the pulse generator. Controls on the face of the pulse generator allow operator manipulation of pacing parameters. Removable batteries are contained within the generator housing. Although temporary transvenous atrial or dual-chamber pacing can be done, it's difficult to place temporary atrial wires and it isn't as reliable as single-chamber ventricular pacing.

Like transcutaneous pacing, the temporary transvenous pacemaker is also used to treat the hemodynamically significant bradycardias and usually isn't effective when meaningful contractile activity is absent (ventricular standstill and PEA). For significant unresolved rhythm or conduction disorders, permanent pacing is required.

Epicardial pacing electrodes (epicardial wires) are placed on the atria or ventricles during cardiac surgery. The electrode end of the wire is looped through or loosely sutured to the epicardial surface of the atria or ventricles and the other end is pulled through the chest wall, sutured to the skin, attached to a bridging cable, and connected to an external pulse generator. A ground wire is commonly attached to the chest wall and pulled through with the other pacing wires. The number of wires present varies with the surgeon—there may be one or two atrial wires, one or two ventricular wires, one or two ground wires, or no ground wire. Atrial wires usually exit to the right of the sternum, and ventricular wires exit to the left. Epicardial pacing is used after cardiac surgery to treat hemodynamically significant bradycardias, and can also be used to treat tachyarrhythmias using overdrive pacing techniques.

## Permanent pacemakers

Implantation of a permanent pacemaker (see Figure 10-3) doesn't automatically follow temporary pacing. The procedure is performed only after careful analysis of each patient's clinical situation. Permanent pacemakers are usually implanted using I.V. conscious sedation and local anesthesia in the cardiac catheterization laboratory. The pulse generator is placed in a subcutaneous pocket in either the right or the left pectoral area. The patient's occupation, hobbies, and dominant side determine whether the pacemaker is implanted on the right or the left side. Usually the nondominant side is chosen to minimize interference with the patient's activities of daily living. The pacing lead is inserted through the cephalic vein or the subclavian vein into the right ventricular apex. For dual-chamber pacing a second lead is placed in the right atrial appendage. Permanent pulse generators are powered by lithium batteries. Their life span

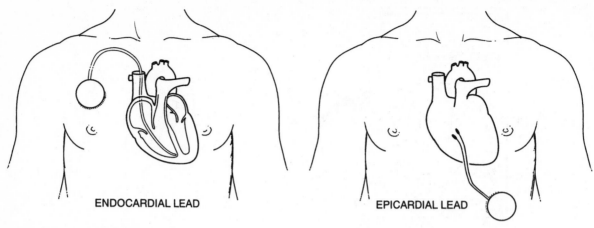

**Figure 10-3.** Permanent pacemaker.

is about 10 years, but this will depend on how the pacemaker is programmed and how often it paces. Many of the permanent pacemakers used today are multiprogramable. Some are capable of increasing the pacing rate in response to the body's need for increased cardiac output (rate-responsive capabilities), whereas others are programmed with antitachycardia features designed to terminate superventricular and ventricular tachyarrhythmias using pacing techniques or shock. In situations where endocardial pacing can't be achieved, the permanent pacemaker is inserted by a transthoracic approach in the operating room using general anesthesia. The pacing electrode is attached to the epicardial surface of the right or left ventricle and the pulse generator implanted in a subcutaneous pocket.

## Classification of pacemakers

Pacemakers are classified with a universal five-letter coding system used to describe the expected function of the device according to the site of the pacing lead and the mode of pacing. The first three letters describe basic operations, whereas the last two refer to more sophisticated features incorporated into some permanent pacemakers. The five-letter coding system is explained below:

■ The first letter refers to the chamber paced: A = atrium; V = ventricle; D = dual (both atrium and ventricle); O = none.

■ The second letter refers to the chamber where intrinsic electrical activity is sensed: A = atrium; V = ventricle; D = dual (both atrium and ventricle); O = none.

■ The third letter refers to the pacemaker response after it senses intrinsic electrical activity: I = inhibited — When intrinsic electrical activity is sensed the pacemaker is inhibited (won't fire). T = triggered — A pacemaker stimulus is triggered in response to a sensed event. For example, a sensed P wave may trigger the delivery of a stimulus into the ventricle. D = dual — This setting combines triggered pacing and inhibition. O = none.

■ The fourth letter refers to programmable functions or the ability to alter pacing parameters using an external device.

■ The fifth letter refers to special antitachycardia functions.

The most commonly used pacing modes are VVI and DDD. Single-chamber ventricular demand pacing (VVI) is the most commonly used mode of pacing with temporary transvenous wires because it's the quickest and easiest method of pacing in an emergency. This pacemaker paces and senses only in the ventricle and is inhibited only by ventricular activity. In other words, when ventricular activity is sensed, the pacemaker is inhibited (it withholds a pacing stimulus), but when ventricular activity isn't sensed, the pacemaker discharges impulses at a preset rate. Further discussion and ECG tracings will focus on the temporary transvenous ventricular demand pacemaker (VVI).

## Pacemaker terms

Basic functions of all pacemakers include the ability to sense, fire, and capture. *Sensing* means that the pulse generator is able to "see" intrinsic patient beats. *Firing* means that the pulse generator has delivered a stimulus to the heart. *Capturing* means that the heart has responded to the stimulus. Most difficulties encountered with cardiac pacing result from abnormalities in sensing, firing, capturing, or any combination of these. Most of these difficulties can be traced to parameter settings, battery failure, problems at the interface of the catheter tip and endocardium, or problems with generator or lead integrity (loose connections, break in pacing catheter, and so forth).

### Ventricular capture

Ventricular capture indicates that the ventricle has responded to a pacing stimulus (see Figure 10-4, complex A). This is reflected on the ECG tracing by a stimulus artifact (a spike) followed by a wide QRS complex. Ventricular pacing causes sequential depolarization instead of synchronous depolarization. This means that one ventricle (usually the right)

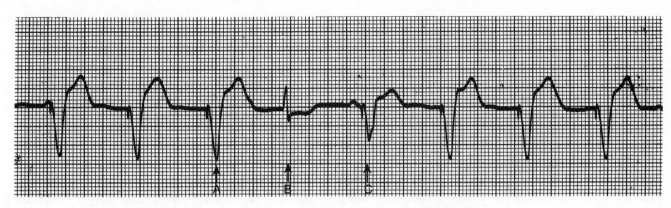

**Figure 10-4.** Ventricular capture (complex A), native beat (complex B), and fusion beat (complex C).

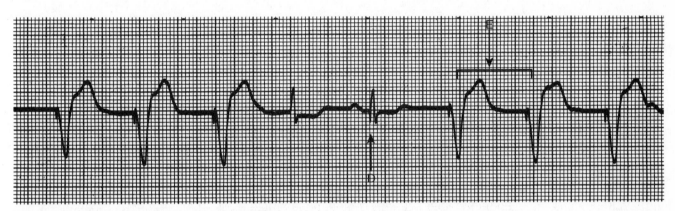

**Figure 10-5.** Pseudofusion beat (complex D) and automatic interval (complex E).

will be depolarized before the other. The prolonged depolarization time results in a wide QRS complex.

### Native beat

A native beat (also called *intrinsic beat*) is produced by the patient's own electrical conduction system. This beat is shown in Figure 10-4, complex B.

### Fusion beat

A fusion beat (see Figure 10-4, complex C) occurs when the pacemaker fires an electrical impulse at the same time that the patient's normal electrical impulse has activated the ventricles. The two forces simultaneously depolarize the ventricles, resulting in a fusion beat. The fusion beat has the characteristics of both pacemaker and patient forces, although one usually dominates the other. The resulting complex is different in configuration and height from that caused by either force alone. Fusion beats are normal.

### Pseudofusion beat

A pseudofusion beat (see Figure 10-5, complex D) occurs when a pacemaker spike falls within the QRS complex of a native beat but doesn't alter the height or configuration of the complex. The pacing stimulus had no effect on depo-

larization because the ventricle was already fully stimulated by the intrinsic beat. Pseudofusion beats are normal.

### Automatic interval

The automatic interval (see Figure 10-5, complex E) refers to the heart rate at which the pacemaker is set. This interval is measured from one pacing spike to the next consecutive pacing spike.

### Pacemaker rhythm

Pacemaker rhythm (see Figure 10-6) occurs when the heart's rhythm is completely pacemaker induced. This is reflected by an ECG tracing in which no patient beats are seen and all QRS complexes are induced by the pacemaker.

## Pacemaker malfunctions

The most common malfunctions associated with the temporary transvenous ventricular demand pacemaker involve failure to capture and undersensing. These malfunctions are discussed below.

### Failure to capture

Failure to capture (see Figure 10-7) means that the ventricles failed to respond to a pacing stimulus. This is reflected

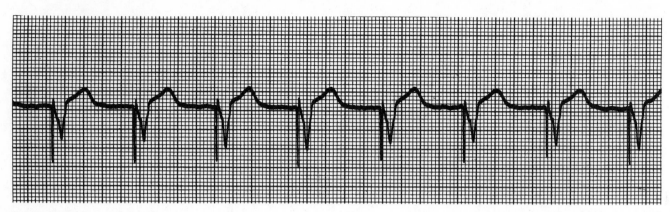

**Figure 10-6.** Pacemaker rhythm.

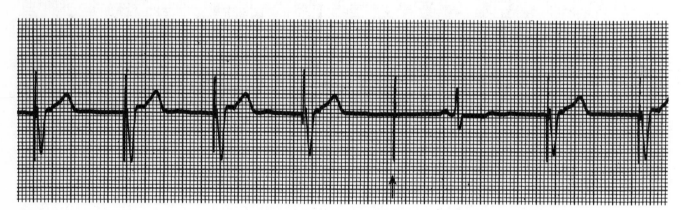

**Figure 10-7.** Loss of capture.

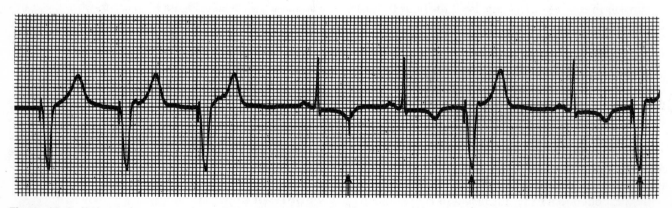

**Figure 10-8.** Undersensing.

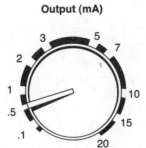

**Output (mA)**

The output (mA) dial controls
the amount of electrical energy
delivered to the myocardium.
Turning the dial to a higher number
increases the mA.

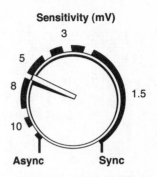

**Sensitivity (mV)**

The sensitivity (mV) dial controls
the ability of the generator to sense
intrinsic activity. Turning the dial to
a low number increases the sensitivity.
Turning the dial to a high number
decreases the sensitivity.

**Figure 10-9.** Output (mA) and sensitivity (mV) dials on a temporary pulse generator.

---

on the ECG tracing by a pacing spike that occurs on time (at the automatic interval rate), but isn't followed by a QRS complex. Failure to capture is common with temporary pacemakers and typically results from:

■ Problems with interface between catheter tip and endocardium – Capture can't occur if the lead is dislodged. The electrode tip must be in contact with the endocardium for the electrical stimulus to cause depolarization. Also, capture usually can't occur if the catheter tip lies in infarcted tissue. The electrode tip must be in contact with healthy endocardium that is capable of responding to the electrical stimulus.

■ Increase in stimulation threshold – The minimum amount of current required to cause a ventricular response is called "threshold" and is determined during pacemaker insertion. The milliamperes (mA) dial is usually set at two times the insertion threshold. Over a period of days, inflammation or fibrosis of tissue surrounding the catheter tip may raise the stimulation threshold, resulting in failure to capture. Effective capture is usually regained by turning the mA dial clockwise to a higher number (see Figure 10-9). Table 10-1 summarizes the causes and appropriate interventions for failure to capture.

## Undersensing

Undersensing (see Figure 10-8) occurs when the pulse generator doesn't sense the patient's intrinsic beats. This problem is reflected on the ECG by a pacing spike that occurs

**Table 10-1.**
## Failure to capture

| Causes | Interventions |
|---|---|
| Electrical milliamperes (mA) set too low | ■ Increase the mA setting on pulse generator until consistent capture is achieved. Increasing the mA is achieved by turning the mA dial clockwise to a higher number. |
| Dislodgement of lead or pacing lead positioned in infarcted tissue | ■ Do overpenetrated chest x-ray to determine catheter position. ■ If catheter is out of position, a temporary intervention is to place patient on left side (gravity may allow catheter to contact endocardium). ■ Physician may need to reposition pacing catheter. |

**Table 10-2.**
## Undersensing

| Causes | Interventions |
|---|---|
| Sensitivity setting too low | ■ Increase sensitivity on pulse generator by turning the sensitivity dial clockwise to a lower number. |
| Dislodgement of lead or pacing lead positioned in infarcted tissue | ■ Do overpenetrated chest X-ray to determine catheter position. ■ If catheter is out of position, a temporary intervention is to place patient on left side (gravity may allow catheter to contact endocardium). ■ The pacemaker may be turned off until the physician can assess the problem if: – initial interventions had no effect – patient's heart rate is adequate – the pacing spike is falling in the T wave, and there is a great potential for lethal arrhythmias to be induced. ■ Physician may need to reposition pacing catheter. |
| Pacer set on asynchronous (fixed-rate) mode | ■ Turn sensitivity dial to synchronous (demand) mode. |

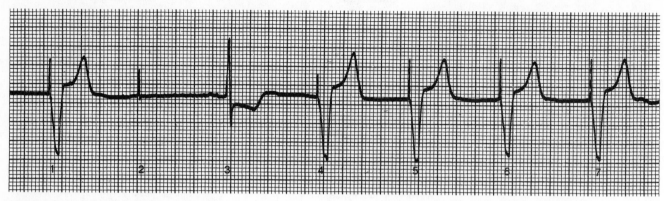

**Figure 10-10.** Pacemaker analysis strip #1.

■ The automatic interval can be measured from beat #4 to beat #5. Mark automatic interval on index card. The heart rate is 63 beats/minute.

■ Beat #2 can be analyzed by placing left mark on index card on spike of beat just before it; beat #2 matches right mark on index card; beat #2 occurs on time but does not cause ventricular depolarization so it indicates failure to capture.

■ Beat #3 is a native beat and does not need analyzing.

■ Beat #4 can be analyzed by placing left mark on R wave of native QRS just before it; beat #4 matches right mark on index card; beat #4 occurs on time and causes ventricular depolarization, indicating ventricular capture beat.

■ Beats #5, #6, and #7 are all analyzed by placing left mark on spikes immediately preceding each beat to be analyzed; all occur on time and cause ventricular depolarization, indicating ventricular capture beats.

■ Interpretation: Failure to capture (one occurrence).

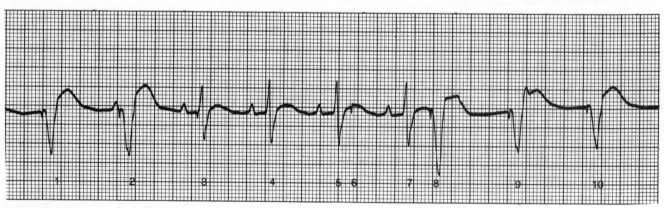

**Figure 10-11.** Pacemaker analysis strip #2.

■ The automatic interval can be measured from beat #1 to beat #2. The heart rate is 72 beats/minute.

■ Beat #2 can be analyzed by placing left mark on index card on spike of beat immediately before it; beat #2 matches right mark on index card; beat #2 occurs on time and causes ventricular depolarization indicating ventricular capture beat.

■ Beat #3 is a native beat (note spike at beginning of R wave); place left mark on spike of beat immediately before it; beat #3 matches right mark; beat #3 has a spike in it and is different from the other native beats (#4, #5, #7) in height so this represents a fusion beat.

■ Beats #4 and #5 are native beats and do not need analyzing.

■ Beat #6 can be analyzed by placing left mark on R wave of native beat just before it; beat #6 occurs much earlier than right mark; beat #6 indicates that the generator did not sense preceding beat and represents undersensing problem.

■ Beat #7 is a native beat.

■ Beat #8 can be analyzed by placing left mark on R wave of native beat just before it; beat #8 occurs much earlier than right mark; beat #8 indicates the generator did not sense preceding beat and represents an undersensing problem. (*Note:* Beat #6 represents an undersensing problem without capture while beat #8 represents an undersensing problem with capture.)

■ Beat #9 can be analyzed by placing left mark on spike of beat just before it; beat #9 matches right mark; beat #9 occurs on time and causes ventricular depolarization indicating ventricular capture beat.

■ Beat #10 can be analyzed by placing left mark on spike of beat just before it; beat #10 matches right mark; beat #10 occurs on time and causes ventricular depolarization indicating ventricular capture beat.

■ Interpretation: Undersensing malfunction (two occurrences).

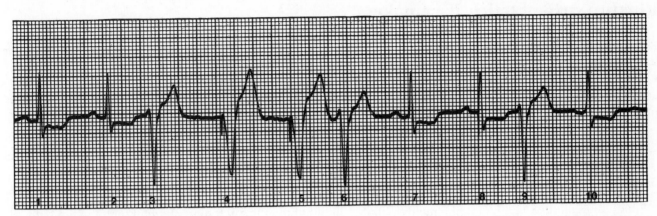

**Figure 10-12.** Pacemaker analysis strip #3.
- The automatic interval can be measured from beat #4 to beat #5. Mark automatic interval on index card. The pacing rate is 79 beats/minute.
- The first three beats are patient produced (native beats or intrinsic beats) and don't need analyzing.
- Beat #4 can be analyzed by placing left mark on index card on R wave of native QRS just before it; beat #4 matches right mark on index card; beat #4 occurs on time and causes ventricular depolarization, indicating ventricular capture beat.
- Beat #5 can be analyzed by placing left mark on index card on spike of paced beat; beat #5 matches right mark on index card; beat #5 occurs on time and causes ventricular depolarization, indicating ventricular capture beat.
- Beats #6 through #10 are patient-produced beats.
- Beat #8 has a pacing spike at the beginning of the QRS complex that doesn't alter the QRS configuration, indicating a pseudo fusion beat.
- Interpretation: Normal pacemaker function.

earlier than it should after a native or paced beat. Ventricular capture may or may not occur. Under normal circumstances the generator senses the beat before it and doesn't fire a stimulus until the time indicated by the automatic interval setting. Undersensing typically results from:

- **Problems with interface between catheter tip and endocardium** – The pacing catheter may be out of place or lying in infracted tissue.
- **Sensitivity setting set too low (Figure 10-9)** – High sensitivity settings (low number on sensitivity dial) instruct the pacemaker to sense virtually all intrinsic activity (even low-voltage signals), whereas low sensitivity settings (high number on sensitivity dial) instruct the pacemaker to virtually ignore all intrinsic activity (even high-voltage signals). Increasing the pacemaker's sensitivity (by turning the sensitivity dial clockwise to a lower number) allows it to see smaller signals and may solve the problem.
- **Pacemaker set on asynchronous (fixed-rate) mode** – In the asynchronous mode the sensing circuit is off. This problem can be corrected by turning the sensitivity dial to synchronous (demand) mode.

## Analyzing pacemaker rhythm strips (ventricular demand type)

When analyzing pacemaker rhythm strips, you will again need to use either calipers or an index card. I have found the following steps to be helpful.
- **Step 1** – Place an index card (or caliper) above two consecutively paced beats. Mark on the index card the interval from one pacing spike to the next. This is called the *automatic interval* and indicates the heart rate at which the pacemaker is set. The automatic interval measurement will assist you in determining if the pacemaker fired on time, too early, too late, or not at all.
- **Step 2** – Start on left side of rhythm strip. Each pacing spike should be analyzed systematically to assess if the pacemaker is functioning appropriately.
- **Step 3** – Identify the pacing spike to be analyzed (only one spike should be analyzed at a time). Using marked index card (step 1), place left mark on spike of paced beat or R wave of native beat immediately preceding pacing spike being analyzed. Observe the relationship of the spike being analyzed to the right mark on the index card. If the spike being analyzed coincides with the right mark, the possible answers include:
  - ventricular capture beat (normal)
  - fusion beat (normal)
  - pseudofusion beat (normal)
  - failure to capture (abnormal).

If the spike being analyzed occurs earlier than the right mark, the answer is undersensing malfunction (abnormal).

Study Figures 10-10 through 10-12. These strips have been analyzed for you.

# Rhythm strip practice: Pacemakers

For each of the following rhythm strips:
- Determine the automatic interval.
- Using the automatic interval measurement as a guide, analyze each pacing spike or beat with a spike for pacemaker malfunction.

- Interpret the strip as normal pacemaker function or as one of the pacer malfunctions (failure to capture or under-sensing malfunction).

All pacemaker strips are lead II unless otherwise noted. Check your answers with the answer key in the appendix.

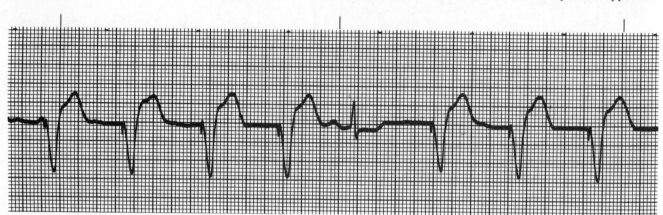

**Strip 10-1.** Automatic interval rate: _____
Analysis: _____
Interpretation: _____

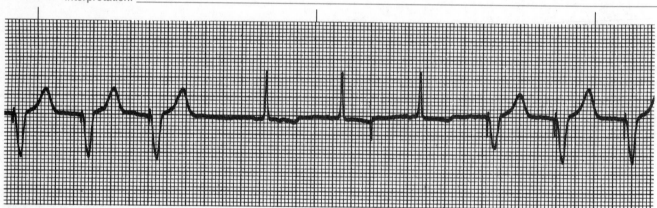

**Strip 10-2.** Automatic interval rate: _____
Analysis: _____
Interpretation: _____

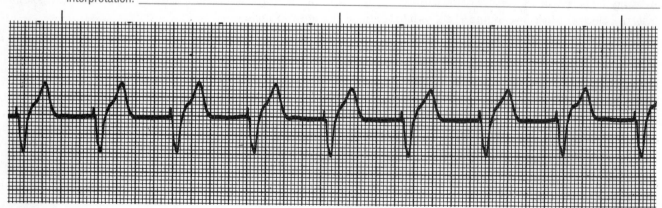

**Strip 10-3.** Automatic interval rate: _____
Analysis: _____
Interpretation: _____

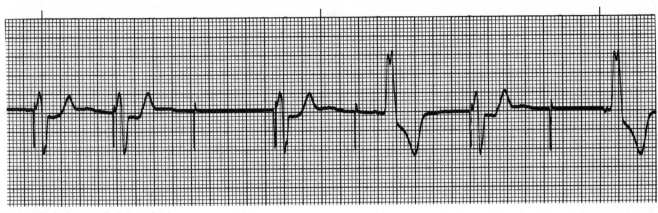

**Strip 10-4.** Automatic interval rate: _____

Analysis: _____

Interpretation: _____

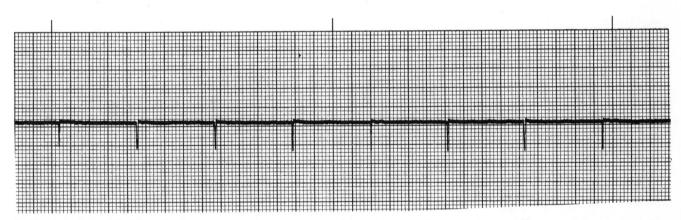

**Strip 10-5.** Automatic interval rate: _____

Analysis: _____

Interpretation: _____

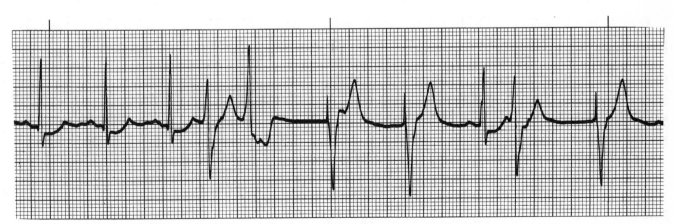

**Strip 10-6.** Automatic interval rate: _____

Analysis: _____

Interpretation: _____

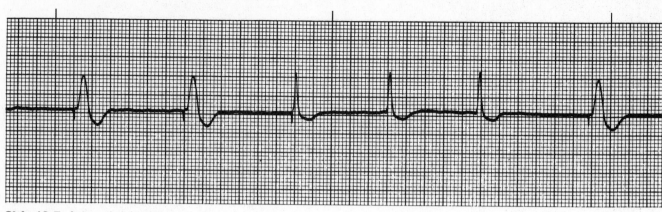

**Strip 10-7.** Automatic interval rate: _____

Analysis: _____

Interpretation: _____

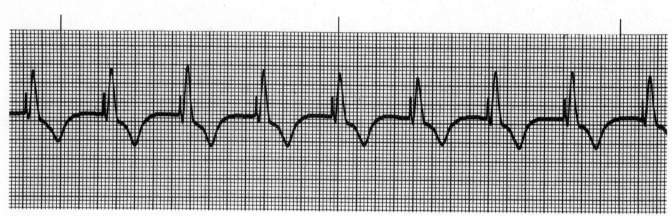

**Strip 10-8.** Automatic interval rate: _____

Analysis: _____

Interpretation: _____

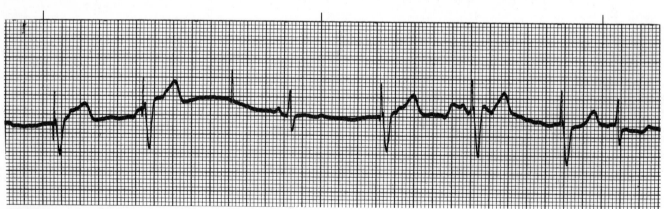

**Strip 10-9.** Automatic interval rate: _____

Analysis: _____

Interpretation: _____

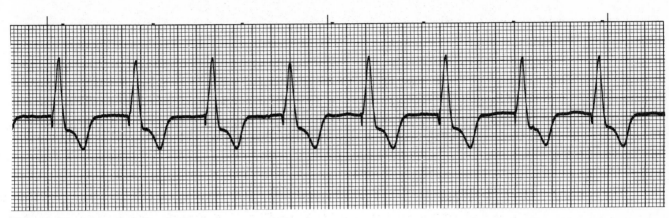

**Strip 10-10.** Automatic interval rate: _____

Analysis: _____

Interpretation: _____

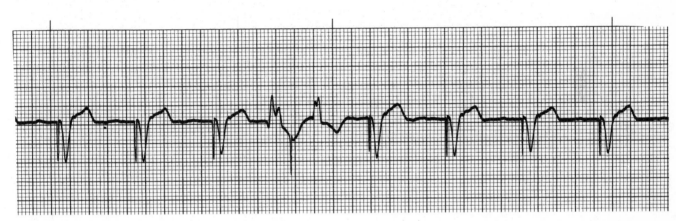

**Strip 10-11.** Automatic interval rate: _____

Analysis: _____

Interpretation: _____

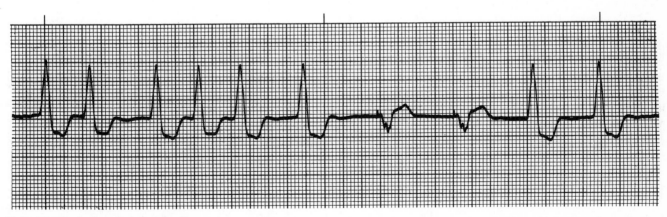

**Strip 10-12.** Automatic interval rate: _____

Analysis: _____

Interpretation: _____

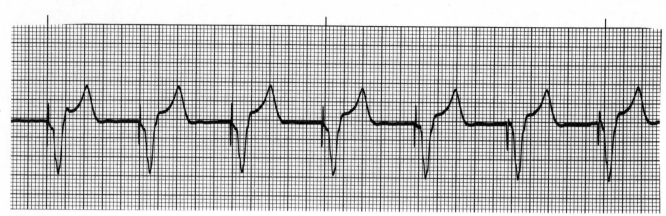

**Strip 10-13.** Automatic interval rate: _____

Analysis: _____

Interpretation: _____

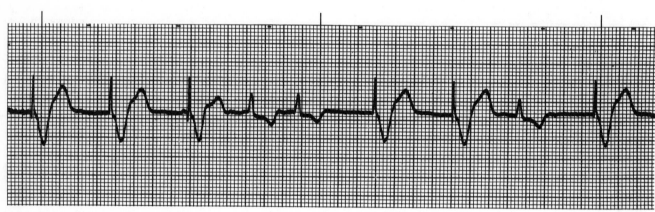

**Strip 10-14.** Automatic interval rate: _____

Analysis: _____

Interpretation: _____

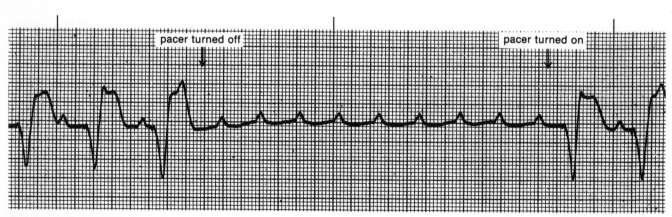

**Strip 10-15.** Automatic interval rate: _____

Analysis: _____

Interpretation: _____

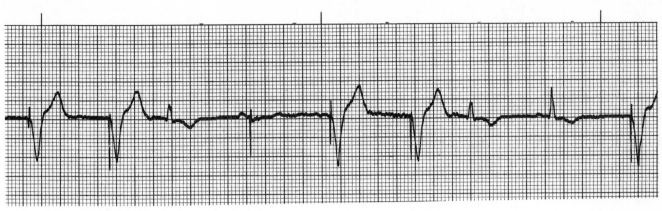

**Strip 10-16.** Automatic interval rate: _____

Analysis: _____

Interpretation: _____

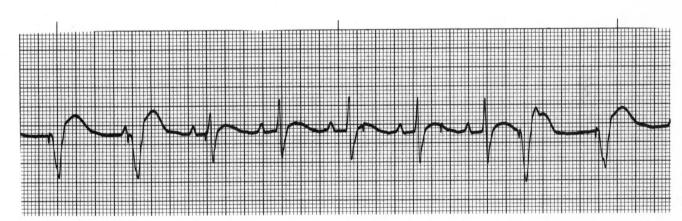

**Strip 10-17.** Automatic interval rate: _____

Analysis: _____

Interpretation: _____

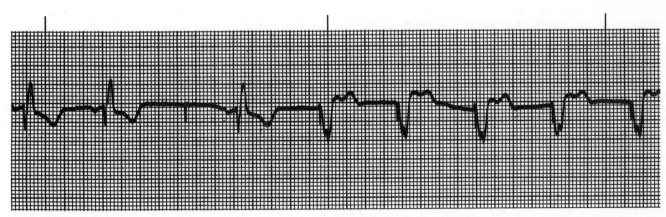

**Strip 10-18.** Automatic interval rate: _____

Analysis: _____

Interpretation: _____

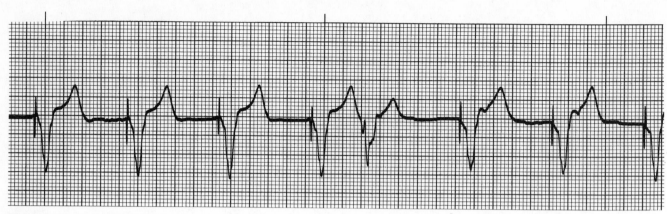

**Strip 10-19.** Automatic interval rate: _____

Analysis: _____

Interpretation: _____

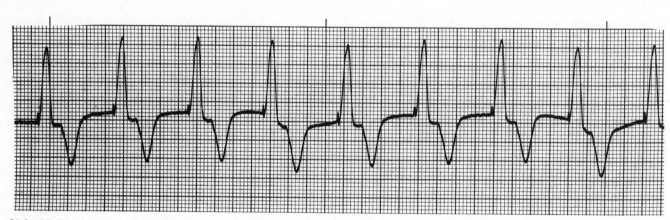

**Strip 10-20.** Automatic interval rate: _____

Analysis: _____

Interpretation: _____

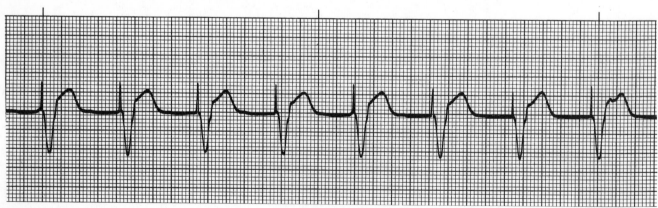

**Strip 10-21.** Automatic interval rate: _____

Analysis: _____

Interpretation: _____

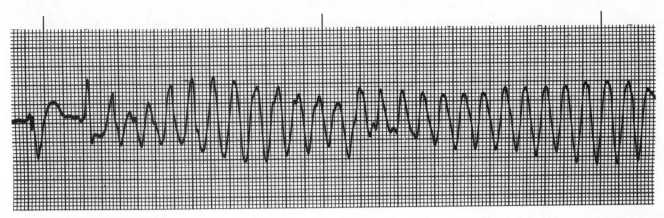

**Strip 10-22.** Automatic interval rate: _____

              Analysis: _____

              Interpretation: _____

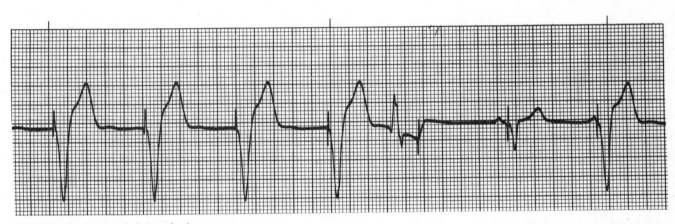

**Strip 10-23.** Automatic interval rate: _____

              Analysis: _____

              Interpretation: _____

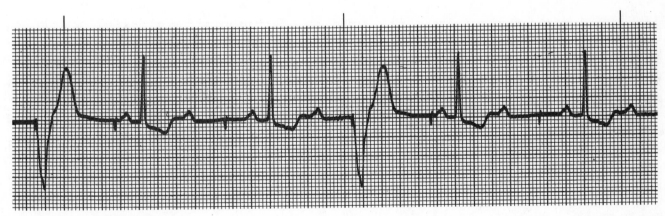

**Strip 10-24.** Automatic interval rate: _____

              Analysis: _____

              Interpretation: _____

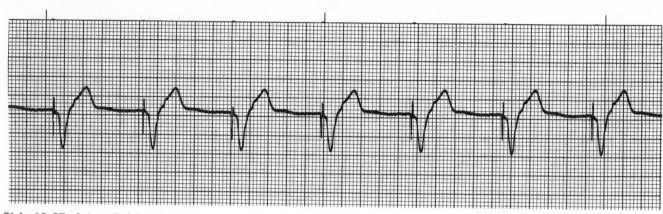

**Strip 10-25.** Automatic interval rate: _____

　　　　　　　Analysis: _____

　　　　　　　Interpretation: _____

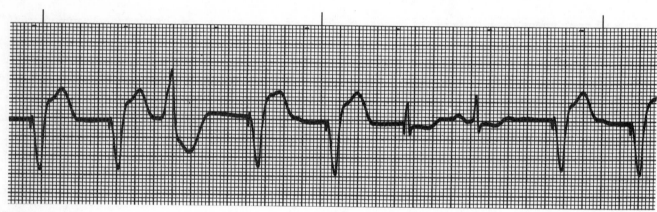

**Strip 10-26.** Automatic interval rate: _____

　　　　　　　Analysis: _____

　　　　　　　Interpretation: _____

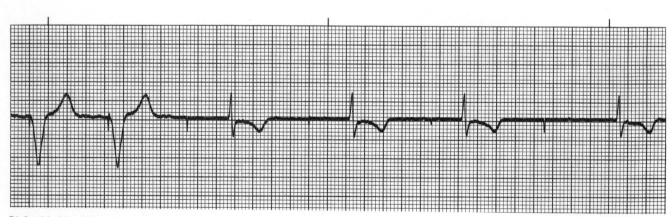

**Strip 10-27.** Automatic interval rate: _____

　　　　　　　Analysis: _____

　　　　　　　Interpretation: _____

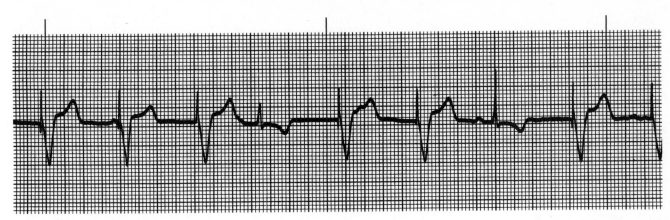

**Strip 10-28.** Automatic interval rate: _____

Analysis: _____

Interpretation: _____

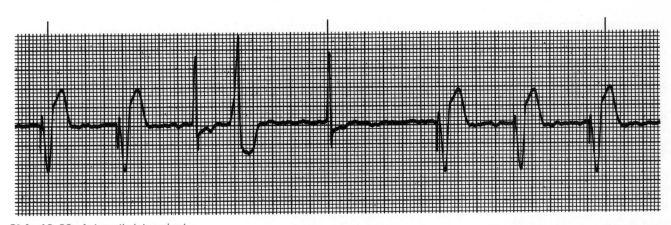

**Strip 10-29.** Automatic interval rate: _____

Analysis: _____

Interpretation: _____

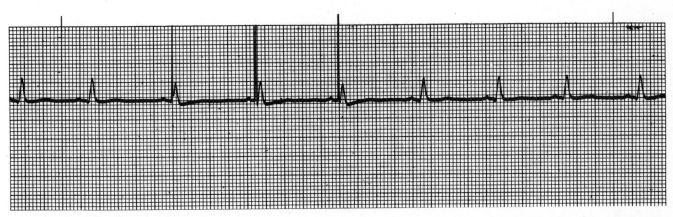

**Strip 10-30.** Automatic interval rate: _____

Analysis: _____

Interpretation: _____

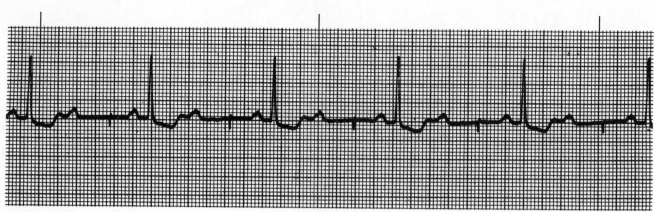

**Strip 10-31.** Automatic interval rate: _____

Analysis: _____

Interpretation: _____

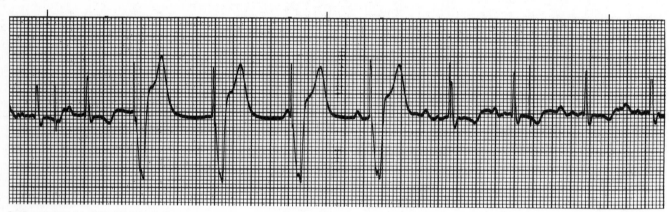

**Strip 10-32.** Automatic interval rate: _____

Analysis: _____

Interpretation: _____

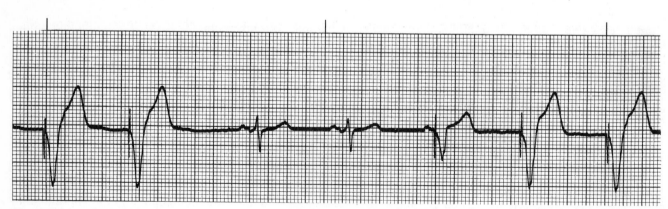

**Strip 10-33.** Automatic interval rate: _____

Analysis: _____

Interpretation: _____

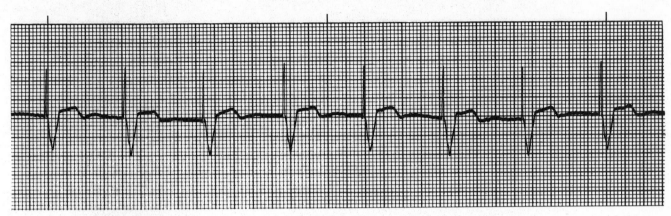

**Strip 10-34.** Automatic interval rate: _____

　　　　　　　 Analysis: _____

　　　　　　　 Interpretation: _____

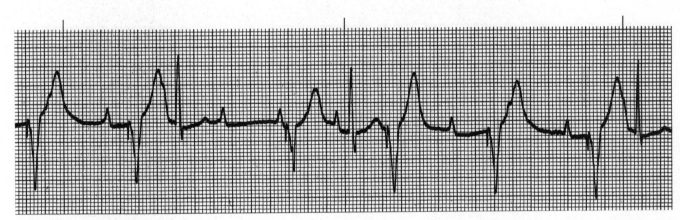

**Strip 10-35.** Automatic interval rate: _____

　　　　　　　 Analysis: _____

　　　　　　　 Interpretation: _____

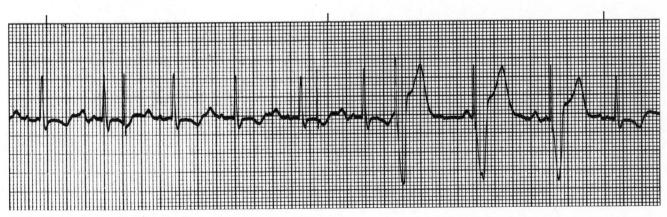

**Strip 10-36.** Automatic interval rate: _____

　　　　　　　 Analysis: _____

　　　　　　　 Interpretation: _____

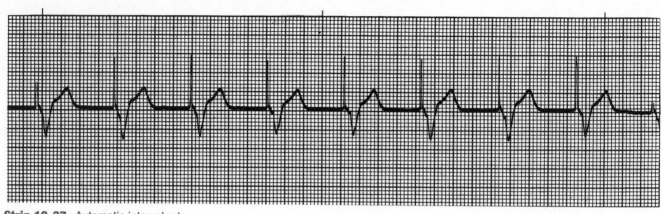

**Strip 10-37.** Automatic interval rate: _____

Analysis: _____

Interpretation: _____

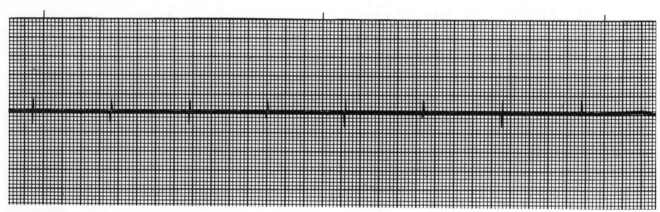

**Strip 10-38.** Automatic interval rate: _____

Analysis: _____

Interpretation: _____

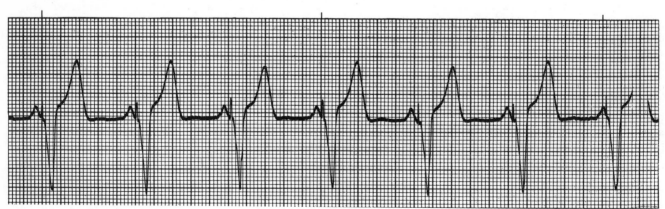

**Strip 10-39.** Automatic interval rate: _____

Analysis: _____

Interpretation: _____

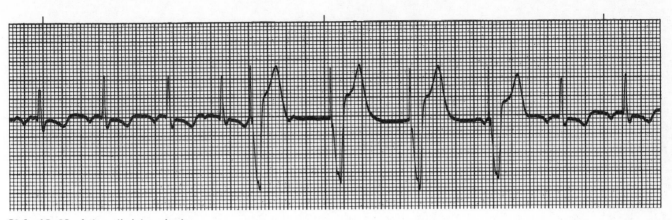

**Strip 10-40.** Automatic interval rate: _____

Analysis: _____

Interpretation: _____

# 11 Posttest

# Posttest: All rhythm groups

For each of the following rhythm strips:
- determine the rhythm regularity, ventricular rate and, if it differs from the ventricular rate, the atrial rate
- identify and examine the P waves
- measure the duration of the PR interval and the QRS complex
- interpret the rhythm.

For pacemaker strips, determine the automatic interval. Using the automatic interval measurement, analyze each pacing spike or beat with a spike for pacemaker malfunction. Interpret the rhythm as normal pacemaker function or one of the pacer malfunctions (failure to capture or undersensing malfunction).

All strips are lead II unless otherwise noted. Check your answers with the answer key in the appendix.

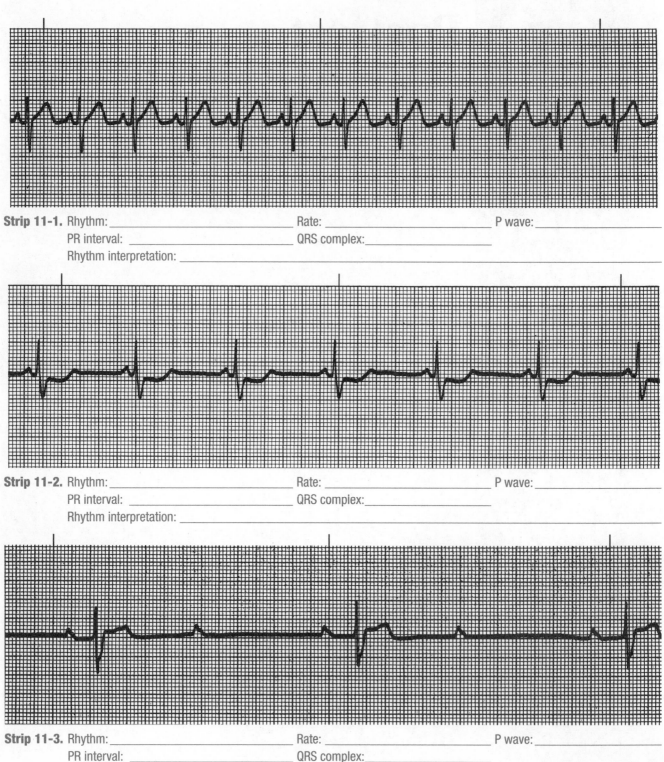

**Strip 11-1.** Rhythm: _____ Rate: _____ P wave: _____

PR interval: _____ QRS complex: _____

Rhythm interpretation: _____

**Strip 11-2.** Rhythm: _____ Rate: _____ P wave: _____

PR interval: _____ QRS complex: _____

Rhythm interpretation: _____

**Strip 11-3.** Rhythm: _____ Rate: _____ P wave: _____

PR interval: _____ QRS complex: _____

Rhythm interpretation: _____

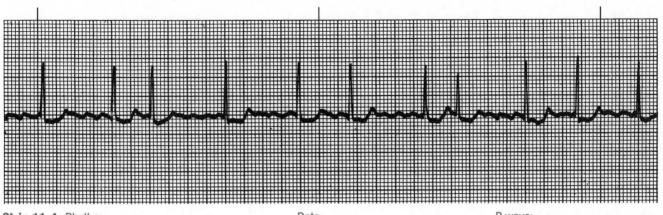

**Strip 11-4.** Rhythm: _____ Rate: _____ P wave: _____

PR interval: _____ QRS complex: _____

Rhythm interpretation: _____

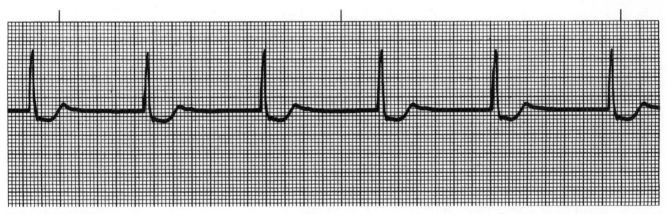

**Strip 11-5.** Rhythm: _____ Rate: _____ P wave: _____

PR interval: _____ QRS complex: _____

Rhythm interpretation: _____

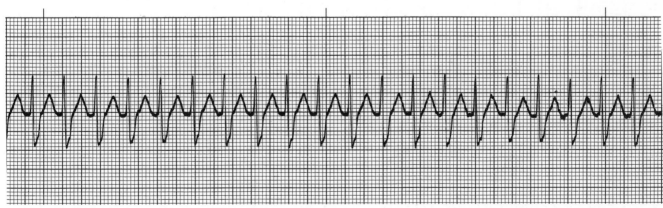

**Strip 11-6.** Rhythm: _____ Rate: _____ P wave: _____

PR interval: _____ QRS complex: _____

Rhythm interpretation: _____

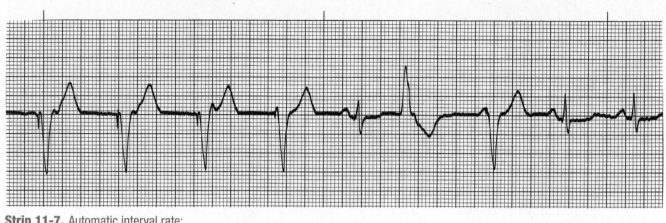

**Strip 11-7.** Automatic interval rate: _____

Analysis: _____

Interpretation: _____

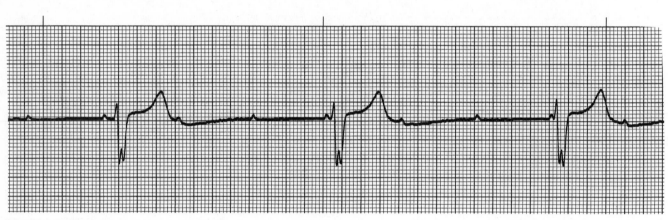

**Strip 11-8.** Rhythm: _____ Rate: _____ P wave: _____

PR interval: _____ QRS complex: _____

Rhythm interpretation: _____

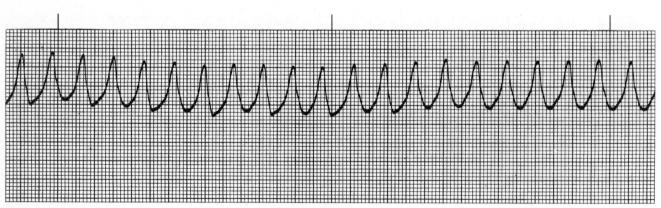

**Strip 11-9.** Rhythm: _____ Rate: _____ P wave: _____

PR interval: _____ QRS complex: _____

Rhythm interpretation: _____

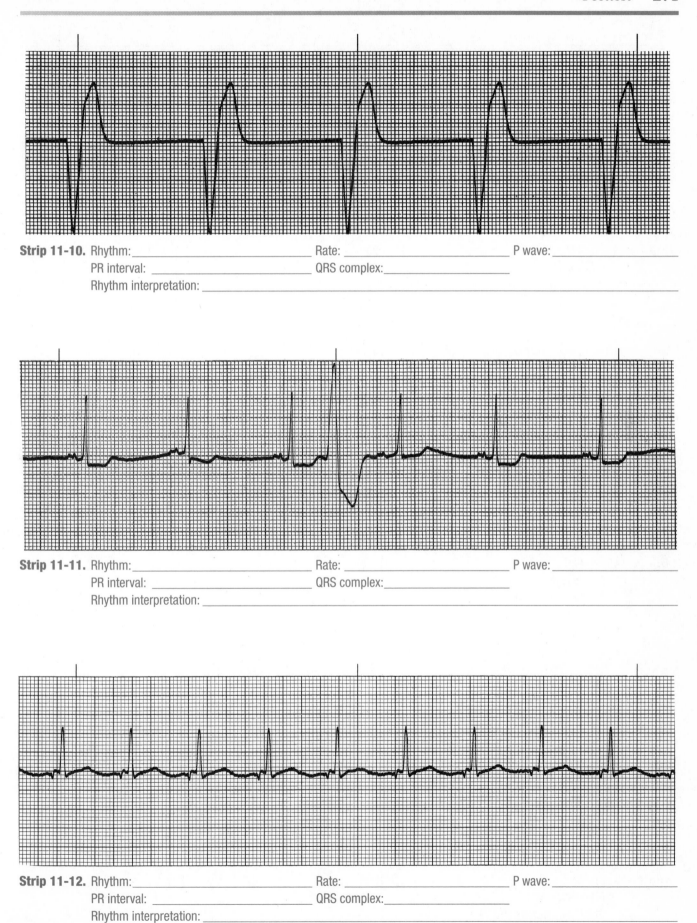

**Strip 11-10.** Rhythm:_____ Rate:_____ P wave:_____

PR interval: _____ QRS complex:_____

Rhythm interpretation: _____

**Strip 11-11.** Rhythm:_____ Rate:_____ P wave:_____

PR interval: _____ QRS complex:_____

Rhythm interpretation: _____

**Strip 11-12.** Rhythm:_____ Rate:_____ P wave:_____

PR interval: _____ QRS complex:_____

Rhythm interpretation: _____

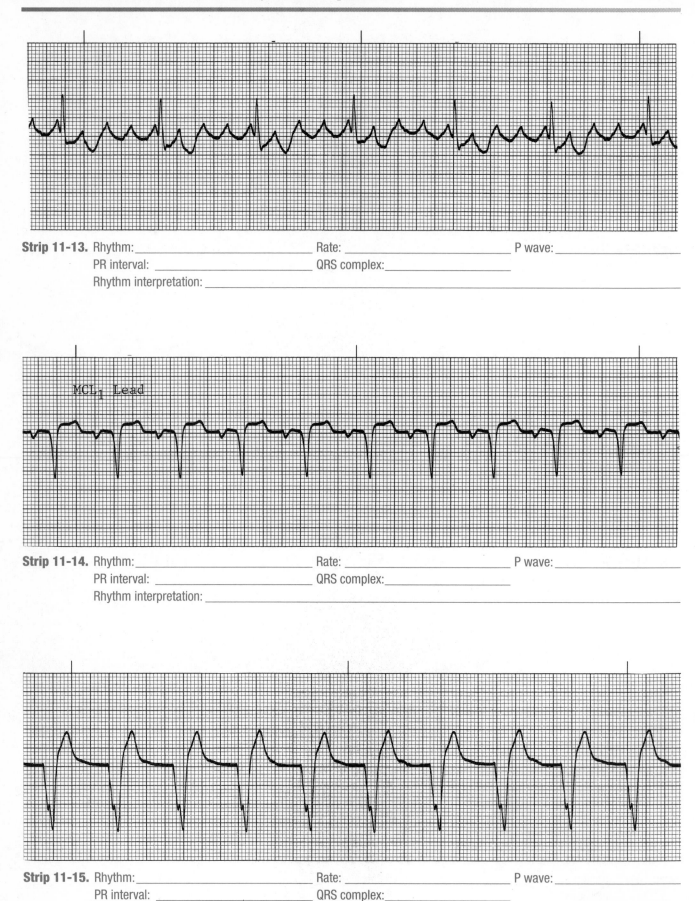

**Strip 11-13.** Rhythm:_____ Rate:_____ P wave:_____

PR interval:_____ QRS complex:_____

Rhythm interpretation:_____

MCL₁ Lead

**Strip 11-14.** Rhythm:_____ Rate:_____ P wave:_____

PR interval:_____ QRS complex:_____

Rhythm interpretation:_____

**Strip 11-15.** Rhythm:_____ Rate:_____ P wave:_____

PR interval:_____ QRS complex:_____

Rhythm interpretation:_____

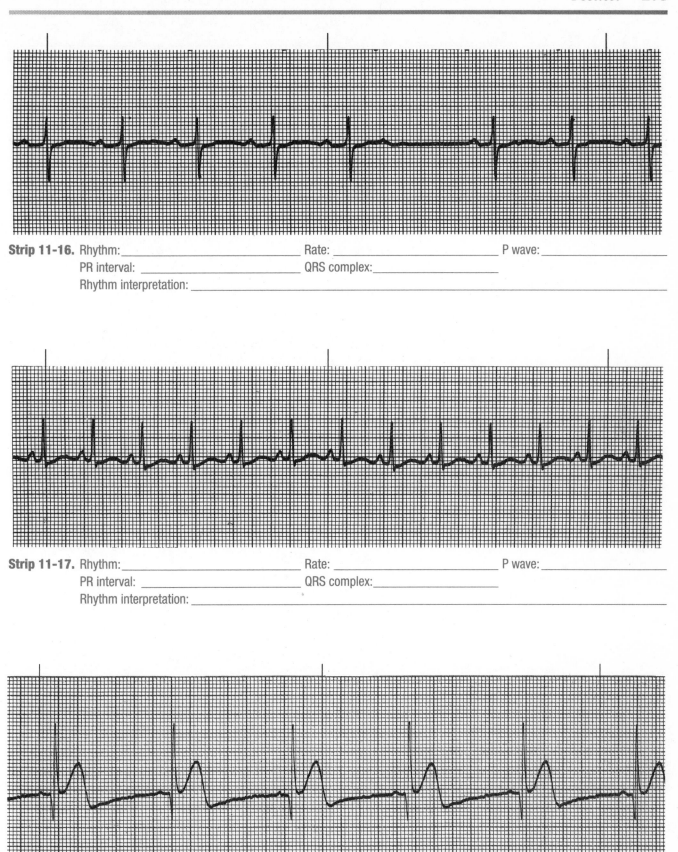

**Strip 11-16.** Rhythm:_____ Rate:_____ P wave:_____

PR interval: _____ QRS complex:_____

Rhythm interpretation: _____

**Strip 11-17.** Rhythm:_____ Rate:_____ P wave:_____

PR interval: _____ QRS complex:_____

Rhythm interpretation: _____

**Strip 11-18.** Rhythm:_____ Rate:_____ P wave:_____

PR interval: _____ QRS complex:_____

Rhythm interpretation: _____

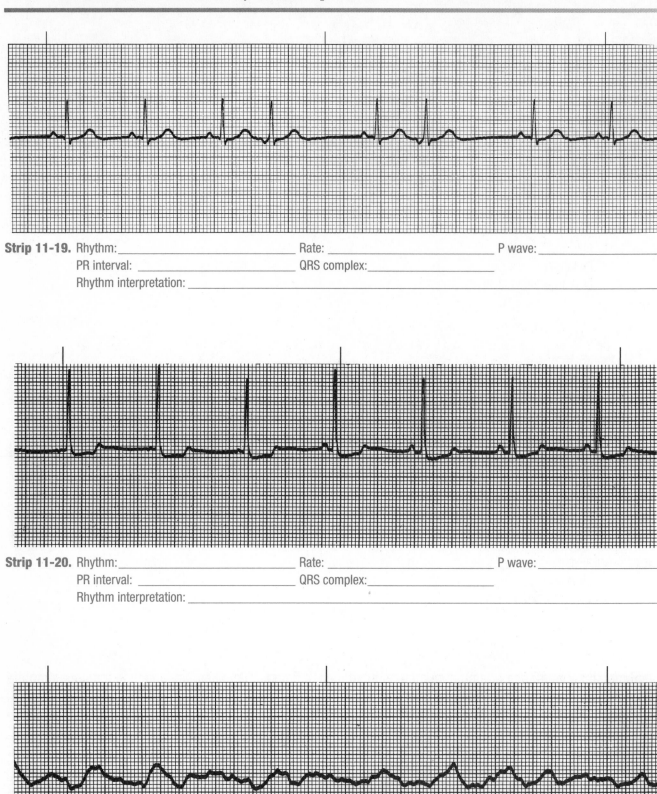

**Strip 11-19.** Rhythm:_____ Rate:_____ P wave:_____
PR interval:_____ QRS complex:_____
Rhythm interpretation:_____

**Strip 11-20.** Rhythm:_____ Rate:_____ P wave:_____
PR interval:_____ QRS complex:_____
Rhythm interpretation:_____

**Strip 11-21.** Rhythm:_____ Rate:_____ P wave:_____
PR interval:_____ QRS complex:_____
Rhythm interpretation:_____

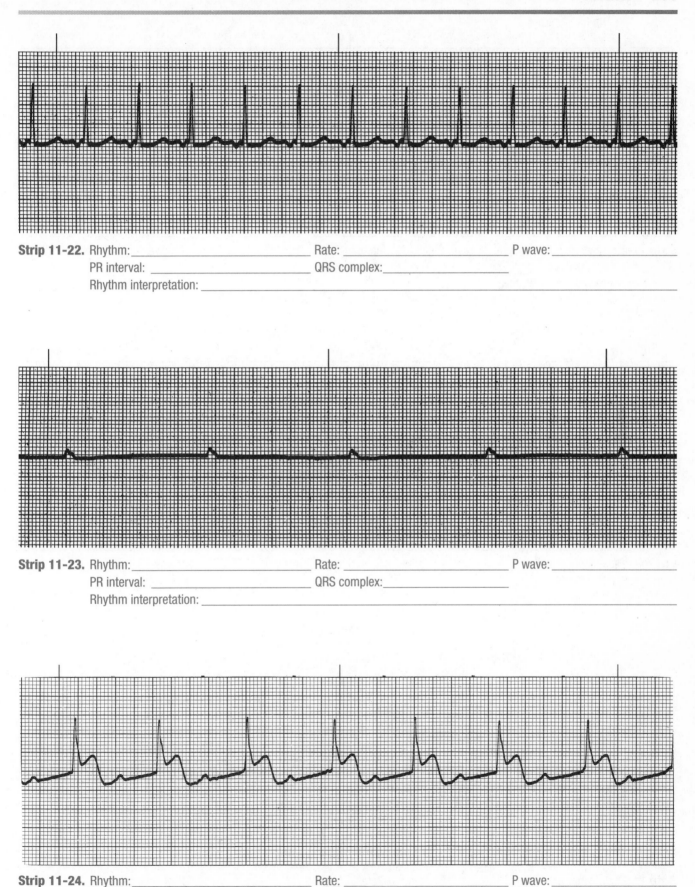

**Strip 11-22.** Rhythm:_____ Rate:_____ P wave:_____
PR interval:_____ QRS complex:_____
Rhythm interpretation:_____

**Strip 11-23.** Rhythm:_____ Rate:_____ P wave:_____
PR interval:_____ QRS complex:_____
Rhythm interpretation:_____

**Strip 11-24.** Rhythm:_____ Rate:_____ P wave:_____
PR interval:_____ QRS complex:_____
Rhythm interpretation:_____

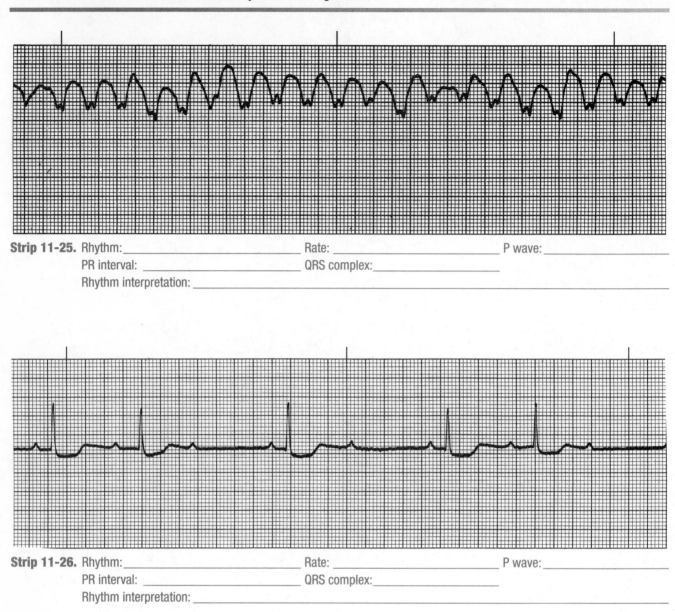

**Strip 11-25.** Rhythm:_____ Rate: _____ P wave: _____

PR interval: _____ QRS complex:_____

Rhythm interpretation: _____

**Strip 11-26.** Rhythm:_____ Rate: _____ P wave: _____

PR interval: _____ QRS complex:_____

Rhythm interpretation: _____

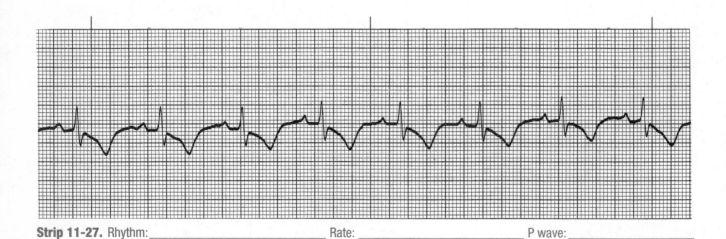

**Strip 11-27.** Rhythm:_____ Rate: _____ P wave: _____

PR interval: _____ QRS complex:_____

Rhythm interpretation: _____

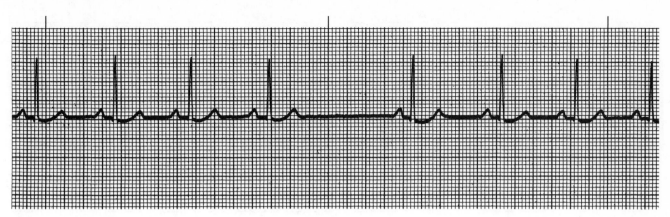

**Strip 11-28.** Rhythm:_____ Rate:_____ P wave:_____
PR interval:_____ QRS complex:_____
Rhythm interpretation:_____

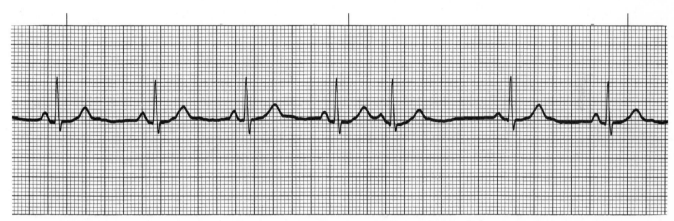

**Strip 11-29.** Rhythm:_____ Rate:_____ P wave:_____
PR interval:_____ QRS complex:_____
Rhythm interpretation:_____

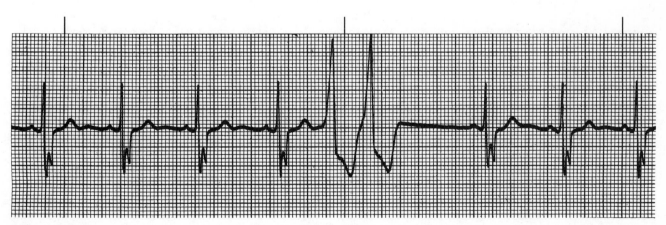

**Strip 11-30.** Rhythm:_____ Rate:_____ P wave:_____
PR interval:_____ QRS complex:_____
Rhythm interpretation:_____

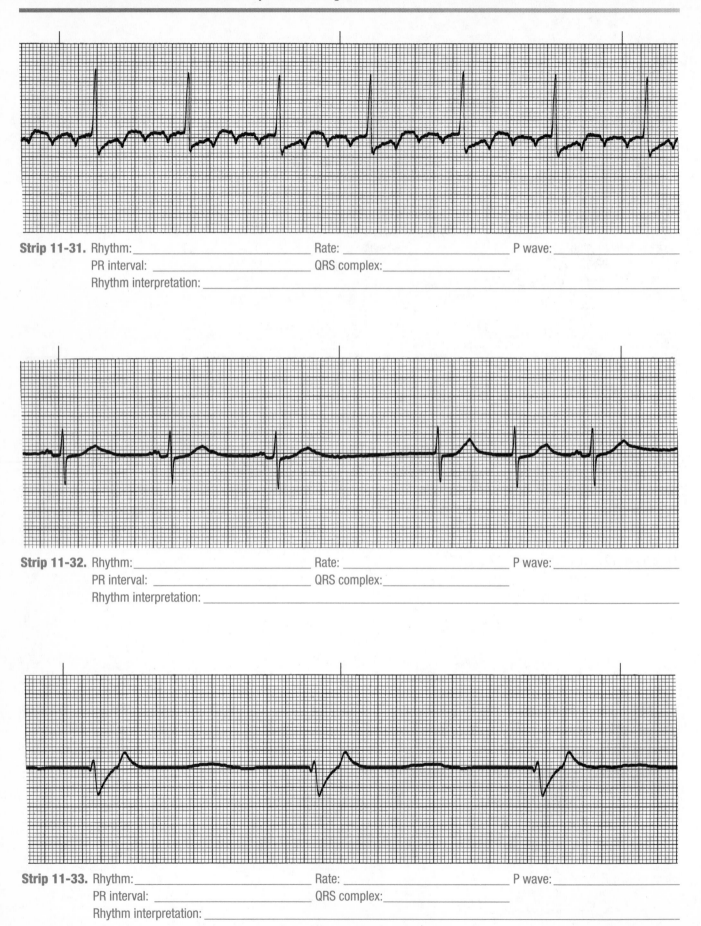

**Strip 11-31.** Rhythm:_____ Rate:_____ P wave:_____

PR interval: _____ QRS complex:_____

Rhythm interpretation: _____

**Strip 11-32.** Rhythm:_____ Rate:_____ P wave:_____

PR interval: _____ QRS complex:_____

Rhythm interpretation: _____

**Strip 11-33.** Rhythm:_____ Rate:_____ P wave:_____

PR interval: _____ QRS complex:_____

Rhythm interpretation: _____

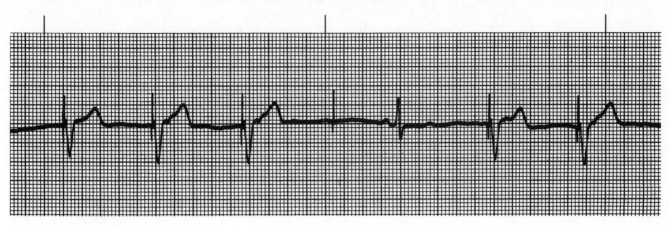

**Strip 11-34.** Automatic interval rate: _____

Analysis: _____

Interpretation: _____

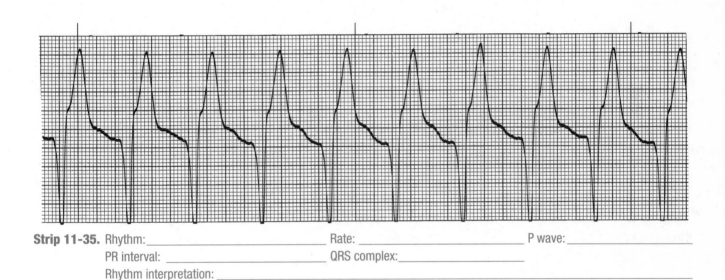

**Strip 11-35.** Rhythm:_____ Rate: _____ P wave: _____

PR interval: _____ QRS complex:_____

Rhythm interpretation: _____

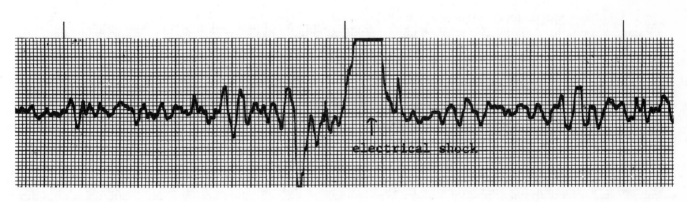

electrical shock

**Strip 11-36.** Rhythm:_____ Rate: _____ P wave: _____

PR interval: _____ QRS complex:_____

Rhythm interpretation: _____

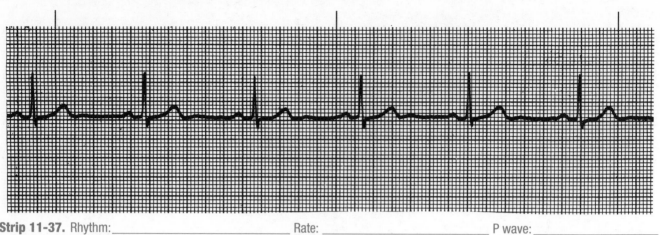

**Strip 11-37.** Rhythm:_____ Rate:_____ P wave:_____
PR interval: _____ QRS complex:_____
Rhythm interpretation: _____

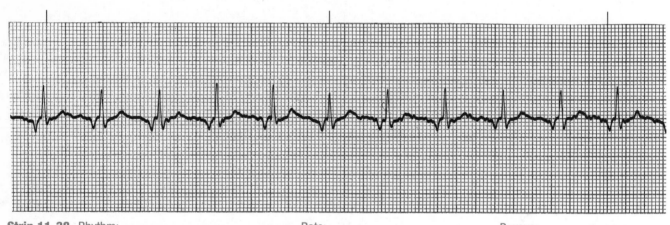

**Strip 11-38.** Rhythm:_____ Rate:_____ P wave:_____
PR interval: _____ QRS complex:_____
Rhythm interpretation: _____

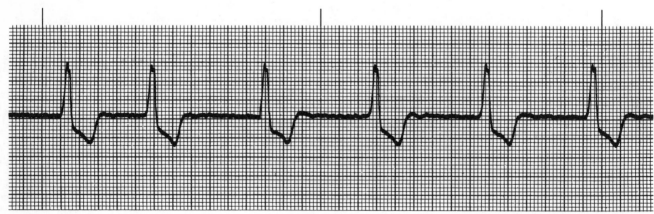

**Strip 11-39.** Rhythm:_____ Rate:_____ P wave:_____
PR interval: _____ QRS complex:_____
Rhythm interpretation: _____

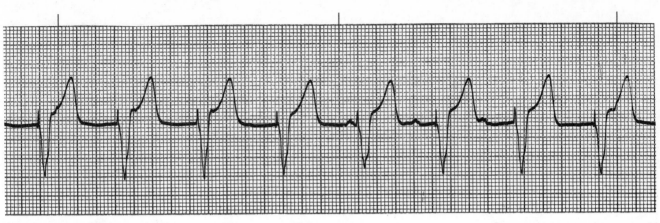

**Strip 11-40.** Rhythm:_____ Rate:_____ P wave:_____
PR interval:_____ QRS complex:_____
Rhythm interpretation:_____

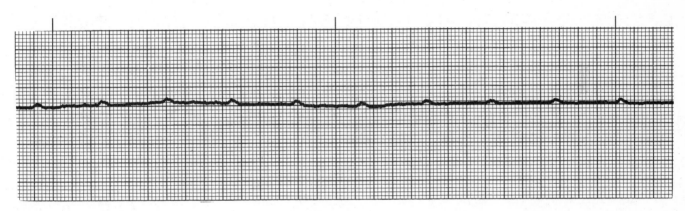

**Strip 11-41.** Rhythm:_____ Rate:_____ P wave:_____
PR interval:_____ QRS complex:_____
Rhythm interpretation:_____

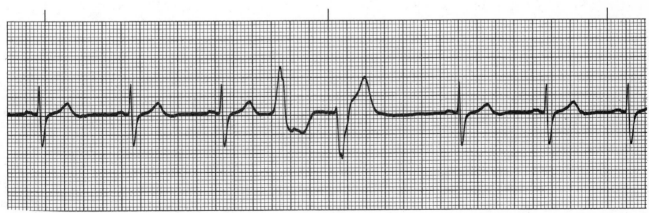

**Strip 11-42.** Rhythm:_____ Rate:_____ P wave:_____
PR interval:_____ QRS complex:_____
Rhythm interpretation:_____

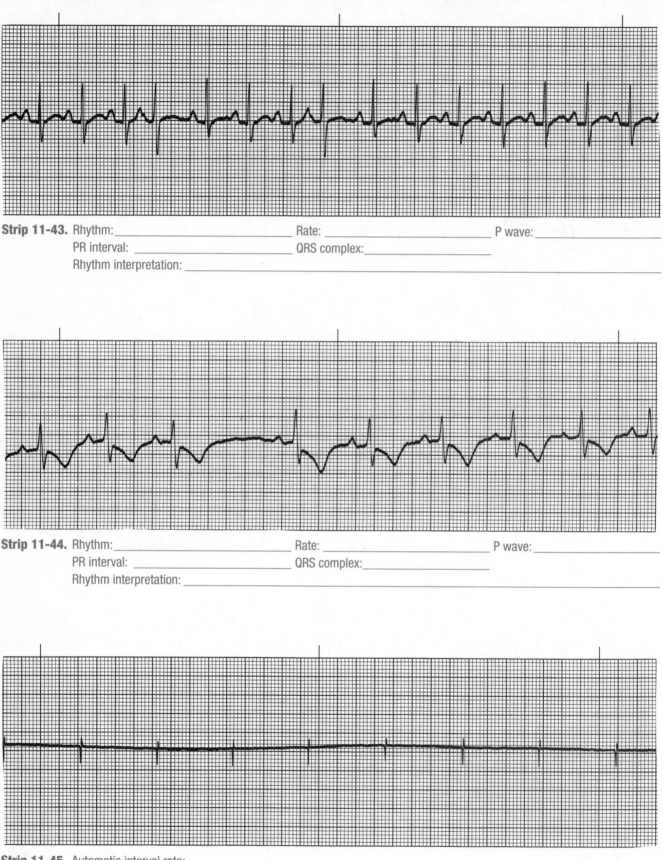

**Strip 11-43.** Rhythm:_____ Rate:_____ P wave:_____

PR interval:_____ QRS complex:_____

Rhythm interpretation:_____

**Strip 11-44.** Rhythm:_____ Rate:_____ P wave:_____

PR interval:_____ QRS complex:_____

Rhythm interpretation:_____

**Strip 11-45.** Automatic interval rate:_____

Analysis:_____

Interpretation:_____

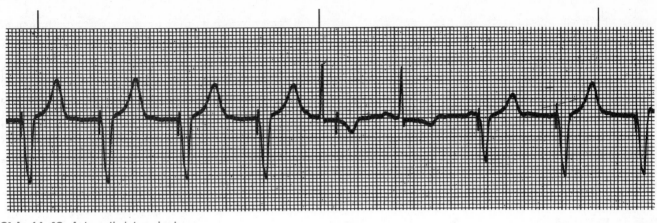

**Strip 11-46.** Automatic interval rate: _____

Analysis: _____

Interpretation: _____

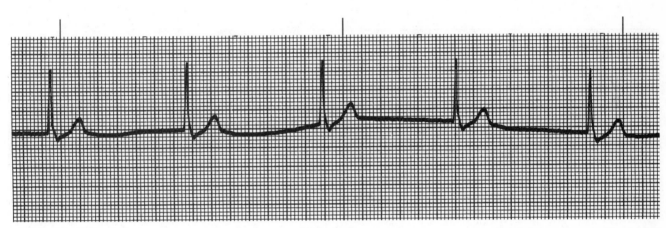

**Strip 11-47.** Rhythm: _____ Rate: _____ P wave: _____

PR interval: _____ QRS complex: _____

Rhythm interpretation: _____

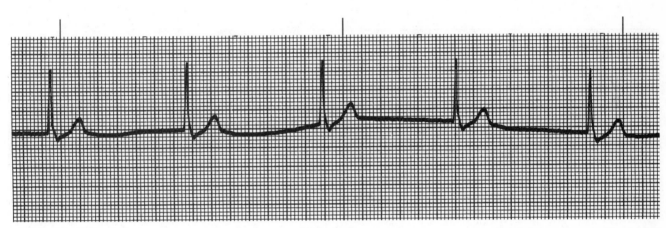

**Strip 11-48.** Rhythm: _____ Rate: _____ P wave: _____

PR interval: _____ QRS complex: _____

Rhythm interpretation: _____

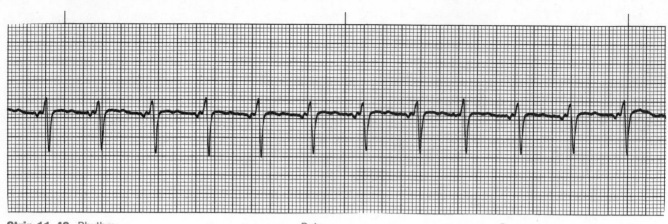

**Strip 11-49.** Rhythm:_____ Rate:_____ P wave:_____
PR interval:_____ QRS complex:_____
Rhythm interpretation:_____

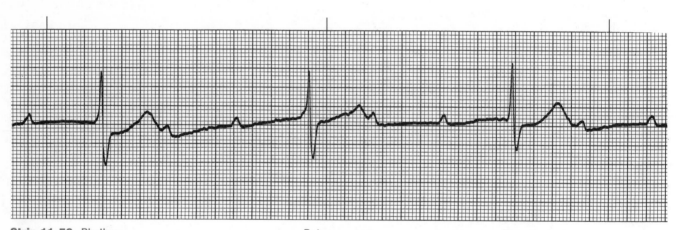

**Strip 11-50.** Rhythm:_____ Rate:_____ P wave:_____
PR interval:_____ QRS complex:_____
Rhythm interpretation:_____

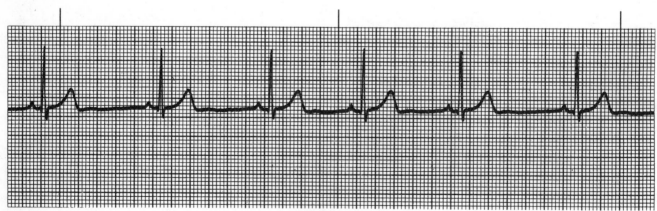

**Strip 11-51.** Rhythm:_____ Rate:_____ P wave:_____
PR interval:_____ QRS complex:_____
Rhythm interpretation:_____

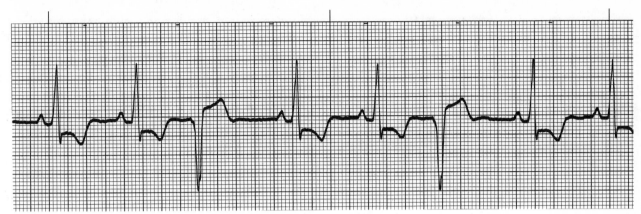

**Strip 11-52.** Rhythm:_____ Rate: _____ P wave: _____

PR interval: _____ QRS complex:_____

Rhythm interpretation: _____

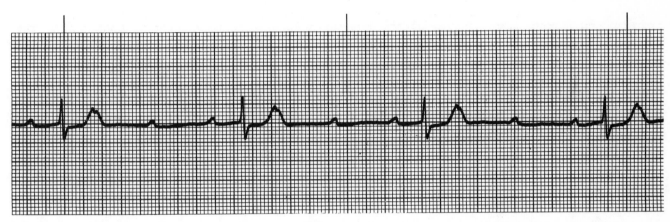

**Strip 11-53.** Rhythm:_____ Rate: _____ P wave: _____

PR interval: _____ QRS complex:_____

Rhythm interpretation: _____

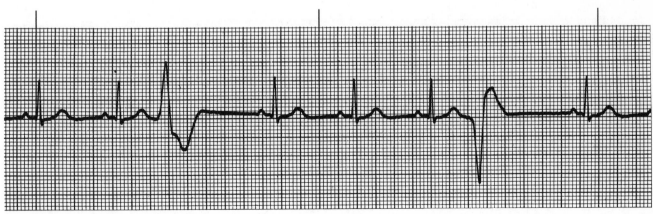

**Strip 11-54.** Rhythm:_____ Rate: _____ P wave: _____

PR interval: _____ QRS complex:_____

Rhythm interpretation: _____

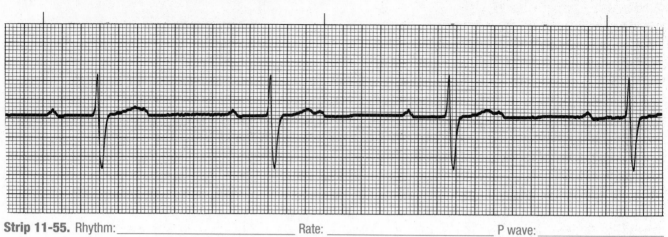

**Strip 11-55.** Rhythm:_____ Rate:_____ P wave:_____
PR interval: _____ QRS complex:_____
Rhythm interpretation: _____

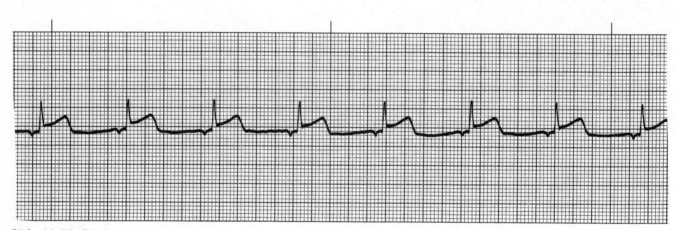

**Strip 11-56.** Rhythm:_____ Rate:_____ P wave:_____
PR interval: _____ QRS complex:_____
Rhythm interpretation: _____

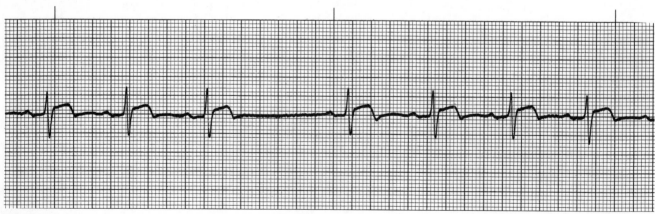

**Strip 11-57.** Rhythm:_____ Rate:_____ P wave:_____
PR interval: _____ QRS complex:_____
Rhythm interpretation: _____

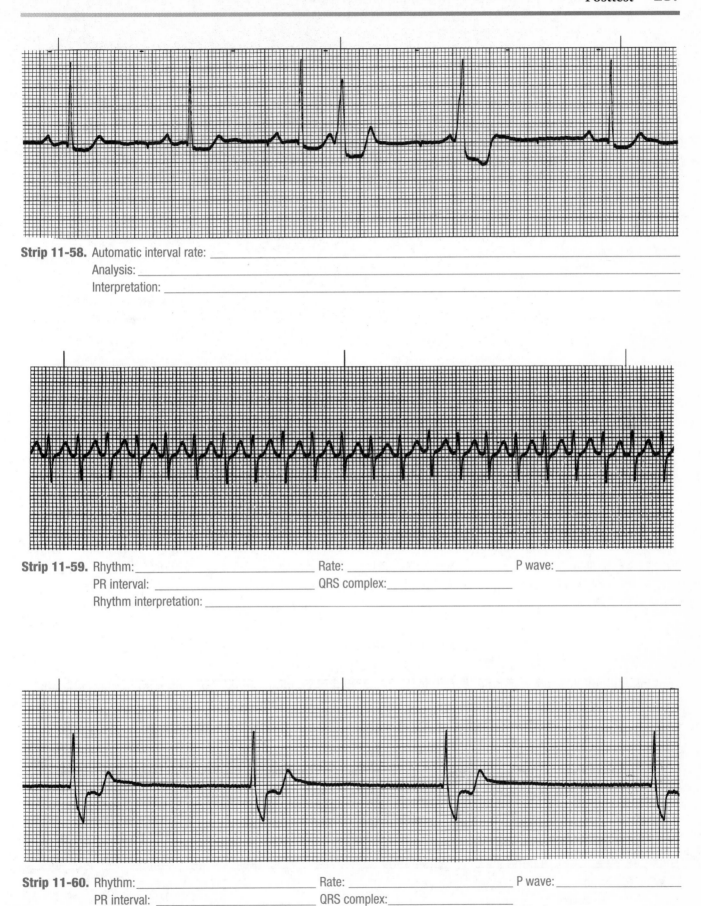

**Strip 11-58.** Automatic interval rate: _____

Analysis: _____

Interpretation: _____

**Strip 11-59.** Rhythm:_____ Rate: _____ P wave: _____

PR interval: _____ QRS complex:_____

Rhythm interpretation: _____

**Strip 11-60.** Rhythm:_____ Rate: _____ P wave: _____

PR interval: _____ QRS complex:_____

Rhythm interpretation: _____

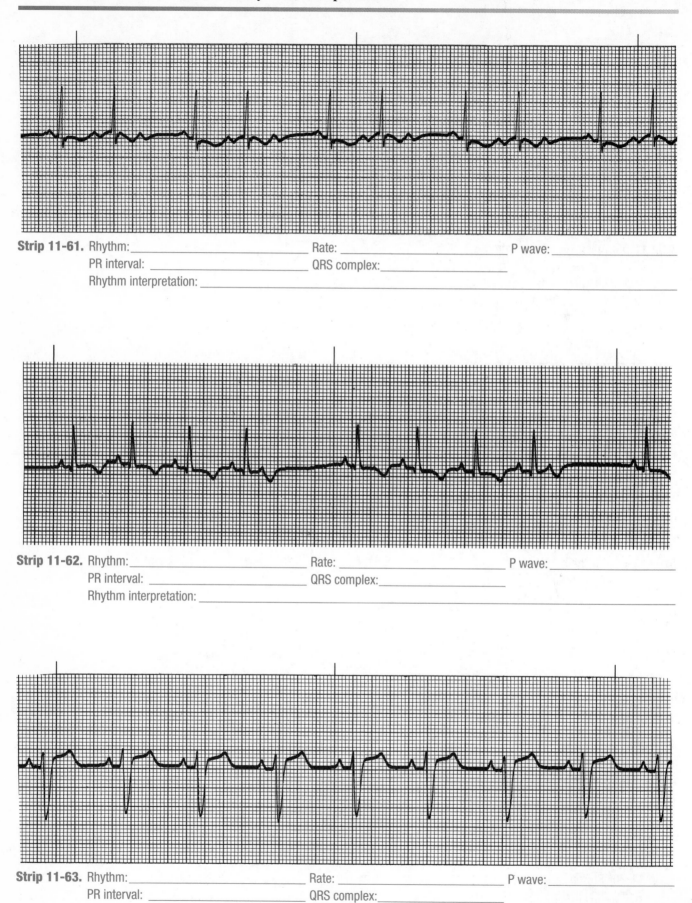

**Strip 11-61.** Rhythm:_____ Rate:_____ P wave:_____

PR interval:_____ QRS complex:_____

Rhythm interpretation:_____

**Strip 11-62.** Rhythm:_____ Rate:_____ P wave:_____

PR interval:_____ QRS complex:_____

Rhythm interpretation:_____

**Strip 11-63.** Rhythm:_____ Rate:_____ P wave:_____

PR interval:_____ QRS complex:_____

Rhythm interpretation:_____

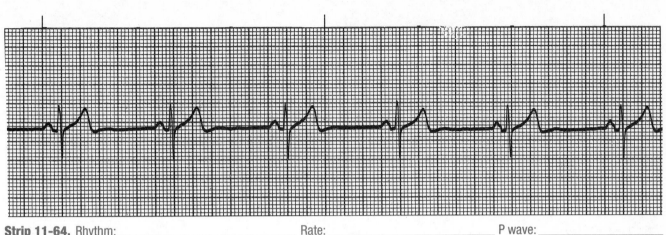

**Strip 11-64.** Rhythm:_____ Rate: _____ P wave: _____

PR interval: _____ QRS complex:_____

Rhythm interpretation: _____

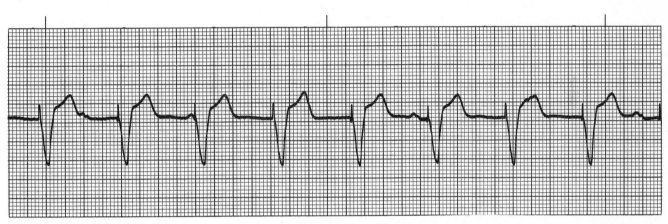

**Strip 11-65.** Automatic interval rate: _____

Analysis: _____

Interpretation: _____

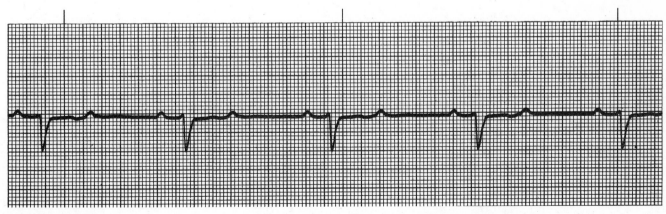

**Strip 11-66.** Rhythm:_____ Rate: _____ P wave: _____

PR interval: _____ QRS complex:_____

Rhythm interpretation: _____

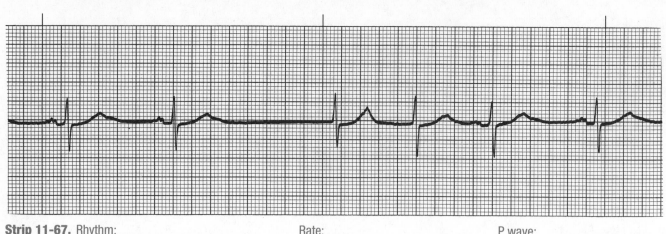

**Strip 11-67.** Rhythm:_____ Rate: _____ P wave:_____

PR interval: _____ QRS complex:_____

Rhythm interpretation: _____

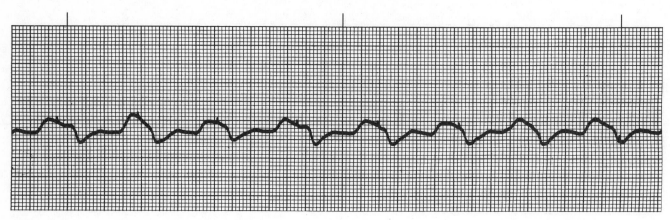

**Strip 11-68.** Automatic interval rate: _____

Analysis: _____

Interpretation: _____

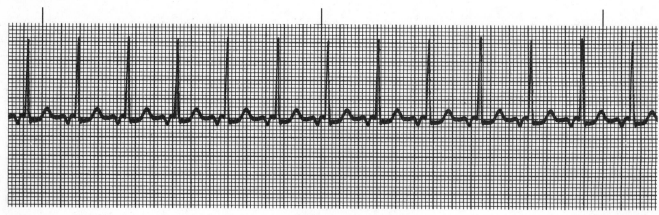

**Strip 11-69.** Rhythm:_____ Rate: _____ P wave:_____

PR interval: _____ QRS complex:_____

Rhythm interpretation: _____

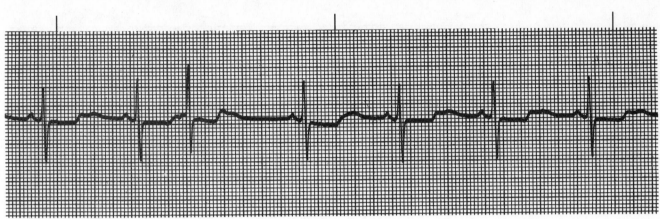

**Strip 11-70.** Rhythm:_____ Rate: _____ P wave: _____

PR interval: _____ QRS complex:_____

Rhythm interpretation: _____

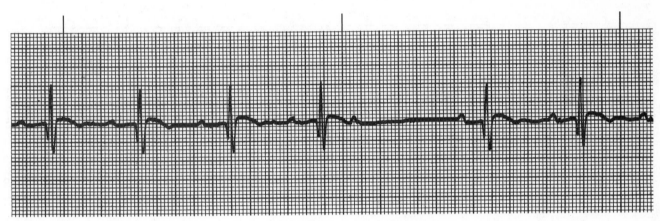

**Strip 11-71.** Rhythm:_____ Rate: _____ P wave: _____

PR interval: _____ QRS complex:_____

Rhythm interpretation: _____

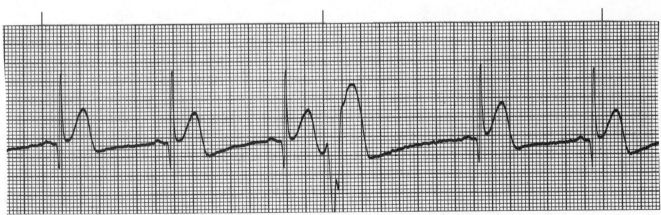

**Strip 11-72.** Rhythm:_____ Rate: _____ P wave: _____

PR interval: _____ QRS complex:_____

Rhythm interpretation: _____

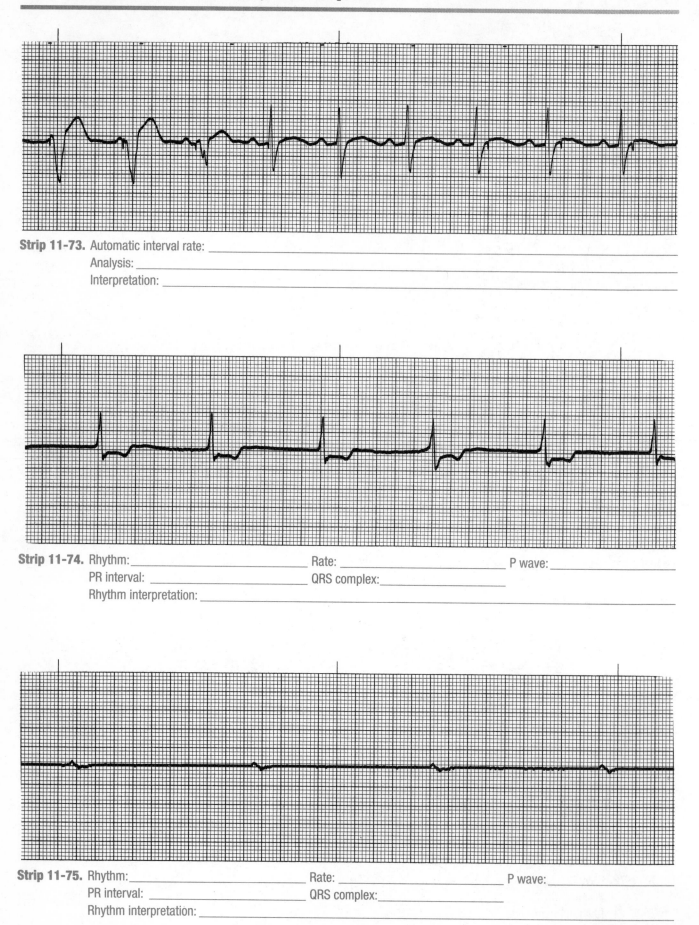

**Strip 11-73.** Automatic interval rate: _____

Analysis: _____

Interpretation: _____

**Strip 11-74.** Rhythm: _____ Rate: _____ P wave: _____

PR interval: _____ QRS complex: _____

Rhythm interpretation: _____

**Strip 11-75.** Rhythm: _____ Rate: _____ P wave: _____

PR interval: _____ QRS complex: _____

Rhythm interpretation: _____

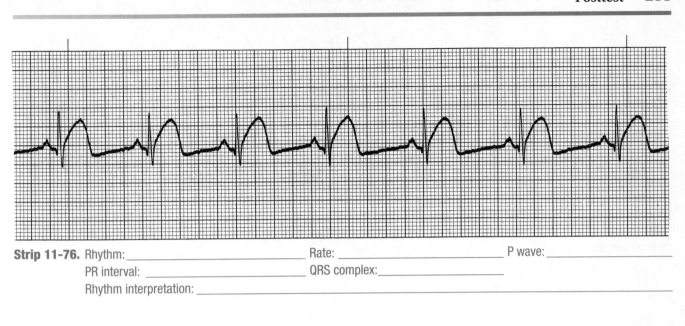

**Strip 11-76.** Rhythm:_____ Rate:_____ P wave:_____

PR interval:_____ QRS complex:_____

Rhythm interpretation:_____

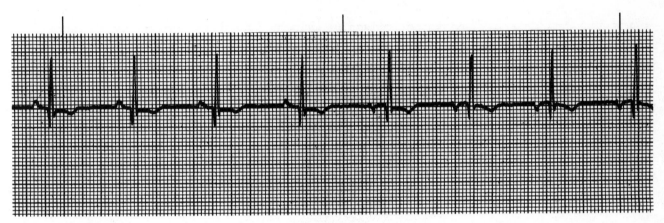

**Strip 11-77.** Rhythm:_____ Rate:_____ P wave:_____

PR interval:_____ QRS complex:_____

Rhythm interpretation:_____

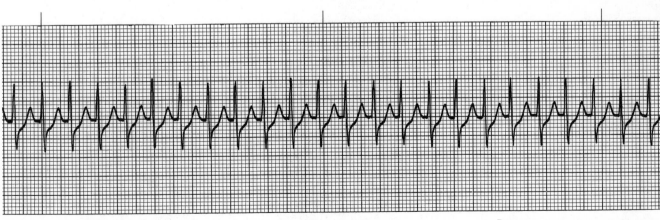

**Strip 11-78.** Rhythm:_____ Rate:_____ P wave:_____

PR interval:_____ QRS complex:_____

Rhythm interpretation:_____

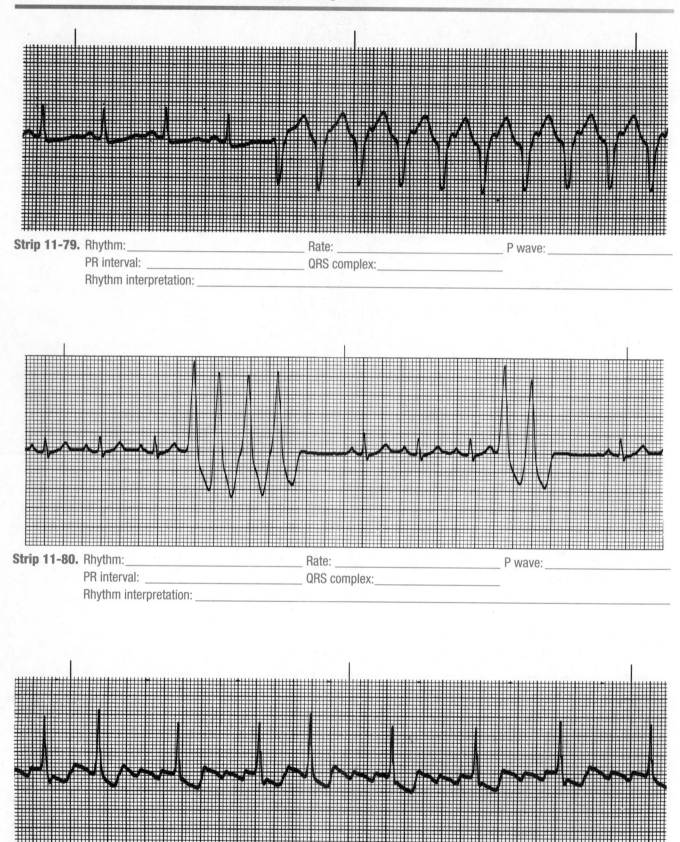

**Strip 11-79.** Rhythm:_____ Rate:_____ P wave:_____
PR interval:_____ QRS complex:_____
Rhythm interpretation:_____

**Strip 11-80.** Rhythm:_____ Rate:_____ P wave:_____
PR interval:_____ QRS complex:_____
Rhythm interpretation:_____

**Strip 11-81.** Rhythm:_____ Rate:_____ P wave:_____
PR interval:_____ QRS complex:_____
Rhythm interpretation:_____

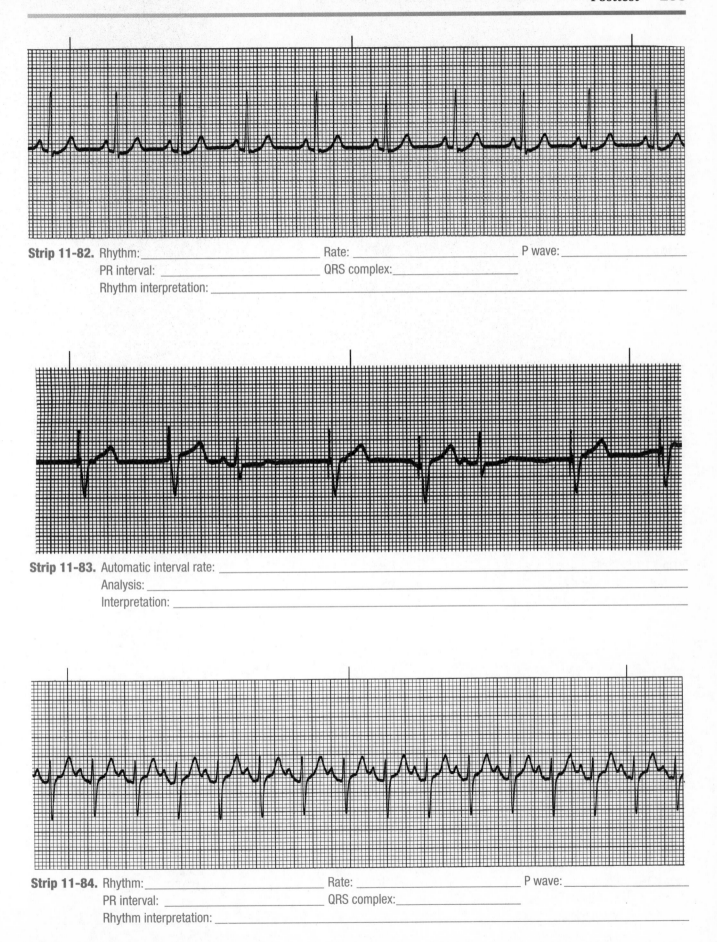

**Strip 11-82.** Rhythm:_____ Rate: _____ P wave: _____

PR interval: _____ QRS complex:_____

Rhythm interpretation: _____

**Strip 11-83.** Automatic interval rate: _____

Analysis: _____

Interpretation: _____

**Strip 11-84.** Rhythm:_____ Rate: _____ P wave: _____

PR interval: _____ QRS complex:_____

Rhythm interpretation: _____

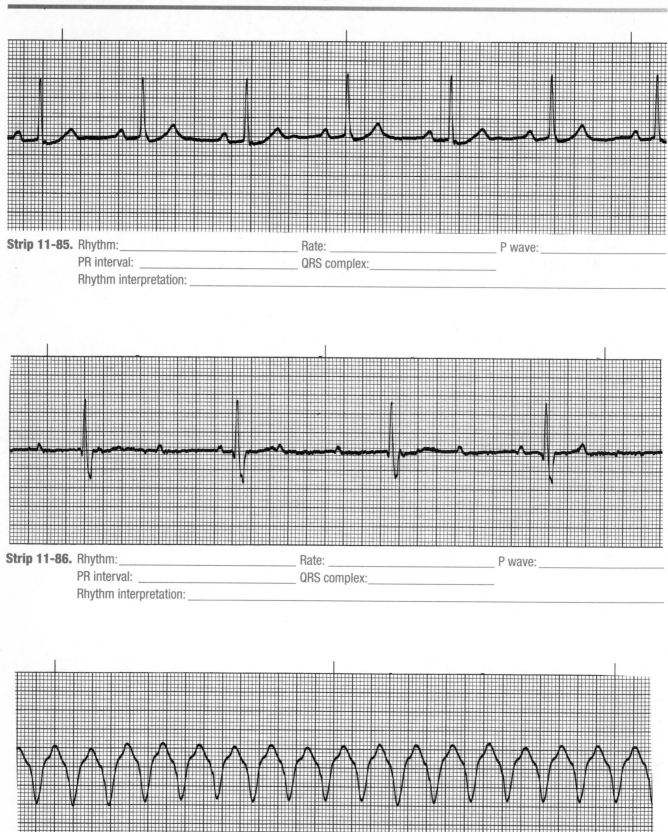

**Strip 11-85.** Rhythm:_____ Rate:_____ P wave:_____

PR interval:_____ QRS complex:_____

Rhythm interpretation:_____

**Strip 11-86.** Rhythm:_____ Rate:_____ P wave:_____

PR interval:_____ QRS complex:_____

Rhythm interpretation:_____

**Strip 11-87.** Rhythm:_____ Rate:_____ P wave:_____

PR interval:_____ QRS complex:_____

Rhythm interpretation:_____

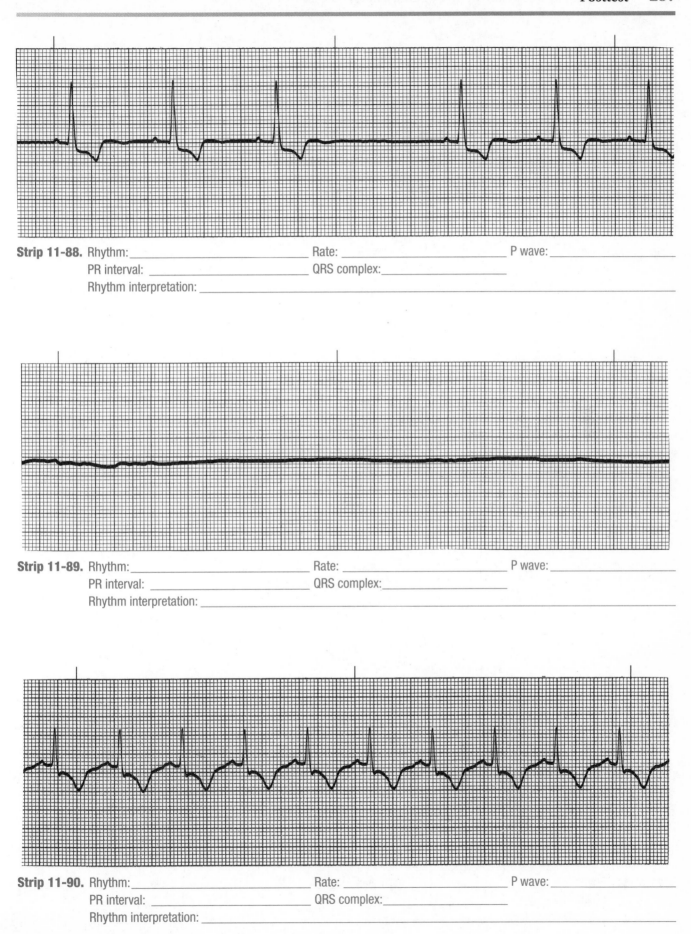

**Strip 11-88.** Rhythm:_____ Rate: _____ P wave: _____
PR interval: _____ QRS complex:_____
Rhythm interpretation: _____

**Strip 11-89.** Rhythm:_____ Rate: _____ P wave: _____
PR interval: _____ QRS complex:_____
Rhythm interpretation: _____

**Strip 11-90.** Rhythm:_____ Rate: _____ P wave: _____
PR interval: _____ QRS complex:_____
Rhythm interpretation: _____

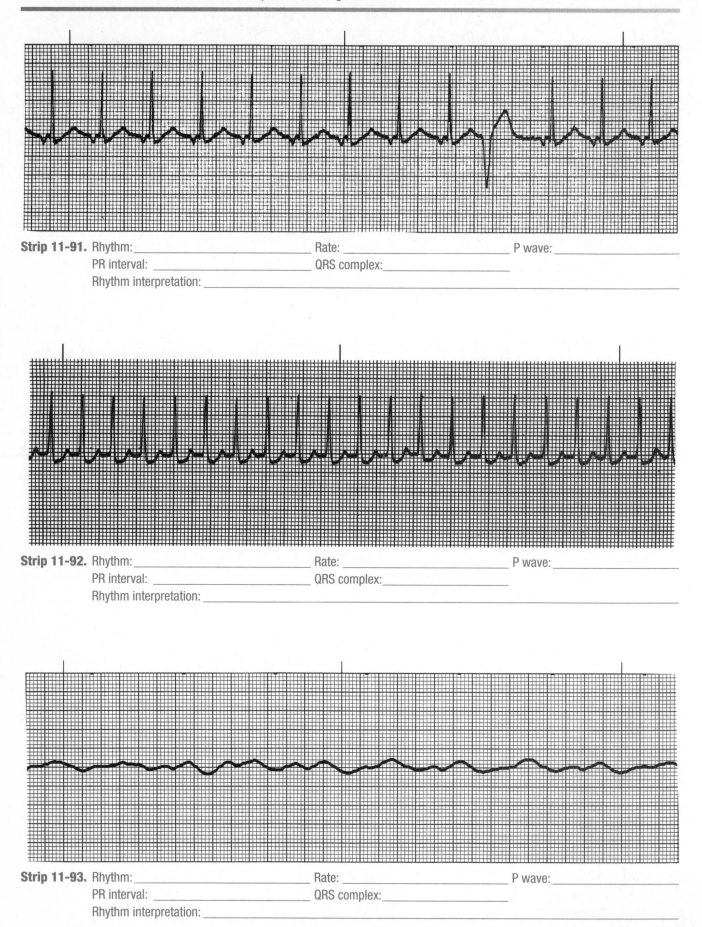

**Strip 11-91.** Rhythm:_____ Rate:_____ P wave:_____

PR interval:_____ QRS complex:_____

Rhythm interpretation:_____

**Strip 11-92.** Rhythm:_____ Rate:_____ P wave:_____

PR interval:_____ QRS complex:_____

Rhythm interpretation:_____

**Strip 11-93.** Rhythm:_____ Rate:_____ P wave:_____

PR interval:_____ QRS complex:_____

Rhythm interpretation:_____

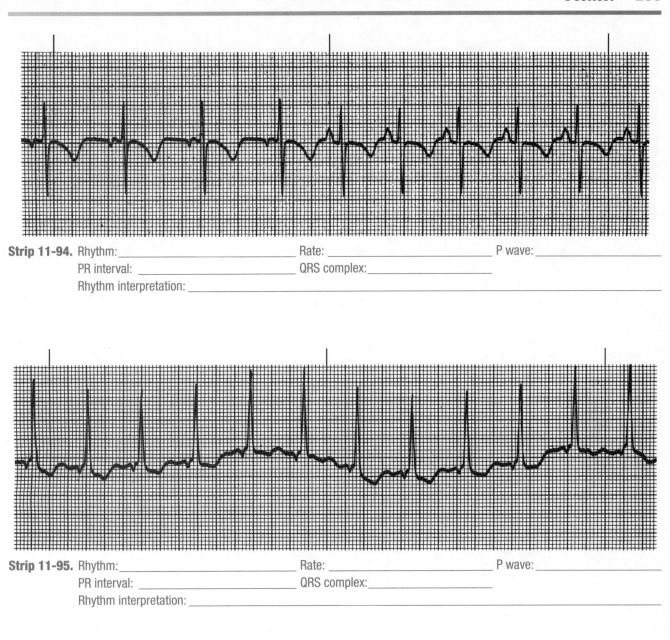

**Strip 11-94.** Rhythm: _____ Rate: _____ P wave: _____

PR interval: _____ QRS complex: _____

Rhythm interpretation: _____

**Strip 11-95.** Rhythm: _____ Rate: _____ P wave: _____

PR interval: _____ QRS complex: _____

Rhythm interpretation: _____

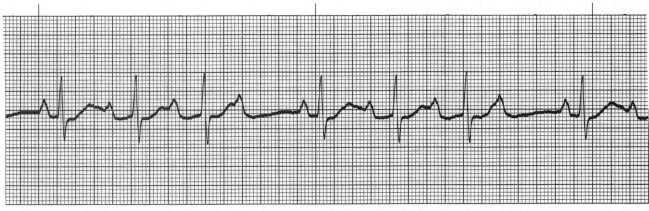

**Strip 11-96.** Rhythm: _____ Rate: _____ P wave: _____

PR interval: _____ QRS complex: _____

Rhythm interpretation: _____

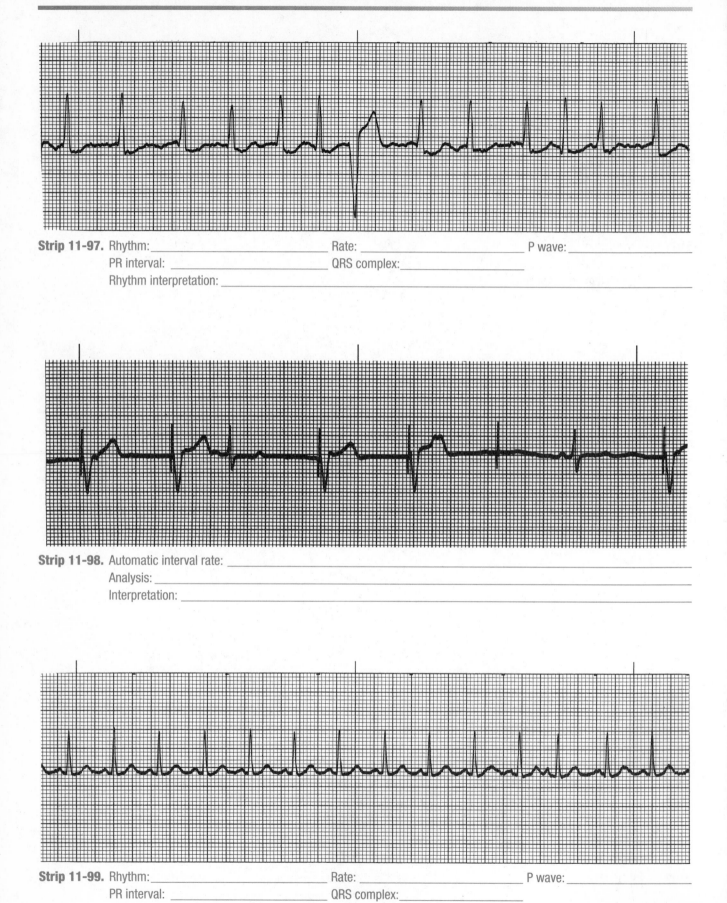

**Strip 11-97.** Rhythm:_____ Rate: _____ P wave: _____
PR interval: _____ QRS complex:_____
Rhythm interpretation: _____

**Strip 11-98.** Automatic interval rate: _____
Analysis: _____
Interpretation: _____

**Strip 11-99.** Rhythm:_____ Rate: _____ P wave: _____
PR interval: _____ QRS complex:_____
Rhythm interpretation: _____

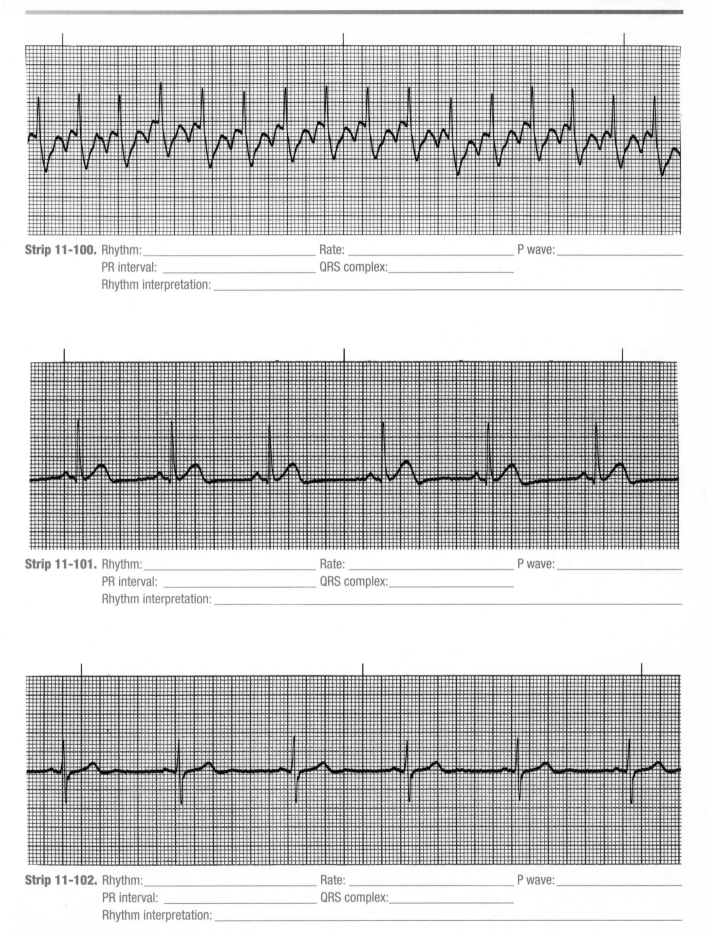

**Strip 11-100.** Rhythm:_____ Rate:_____ P wave:_____

PR interval:_____ QRS complex:_____

Rhythm interpretation:_____

**Strip 11-101.** Rhythm:_____ Rate:_____ P wave:_____

PR interval:_____ QRS complex:_____

Rhythm interpretation:_____

**Strip 11-102.** Rhythm:_____ Rate:_____ P wave:_____

PR interval:_____ QRS complex:_____

Rhythm interpretation:_____

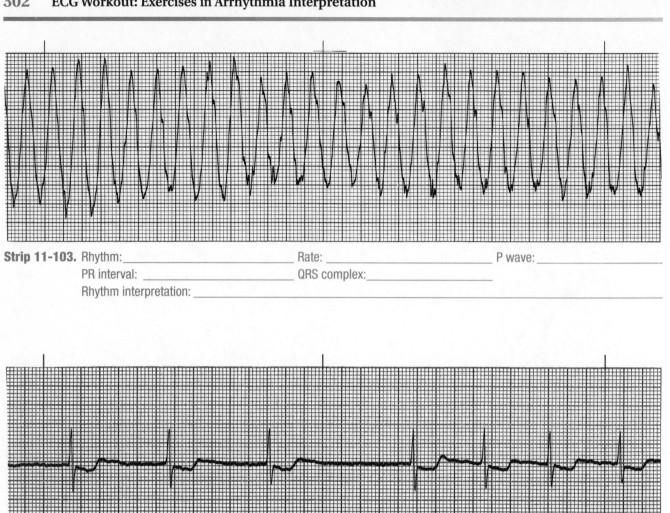

**Strip 11-103.** Rhythm:_____ Rate:_____ P wave:_____
PR interval:_____ QRS complex:_____
Rhythm interpretation:_____

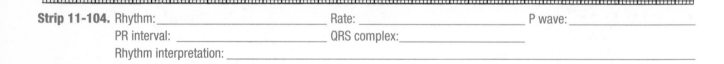

**Strip 11-104.** Rhythm:_____ Rate:_____ P wave:_____
PR interval:_____ QRS complex:_____
Rhythm interpretation:_____

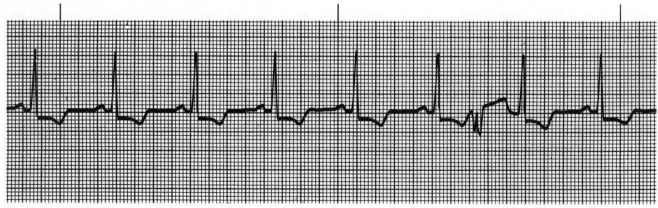

**Strip 11-105.** Rhythm:_____ Rate:_____ P wave:_____
PR interval:_____ QRS complex:_____
Rhythm interpretation:_____

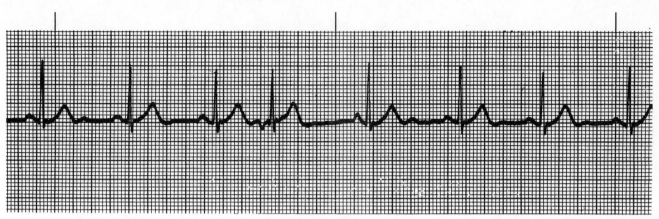

**Strip 11-106.** Rhythm:_____ Rate: _____ P wave: _____

PR interval: _____ QRS complex:_____

Rhythm interpretation: _____

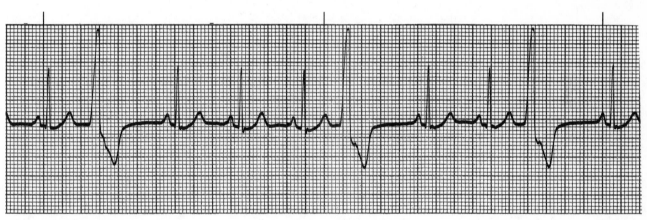

**Strip 11-107.** Rhythm:_____ Rate: _____ P wave: _____

PR interval: _____ QRS complex:_____

Rhythm interpretation: _____

# Answer key to Chapter 3

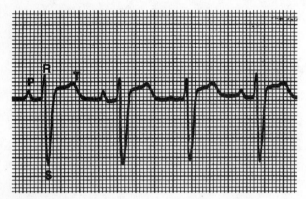

Strip 3-1.

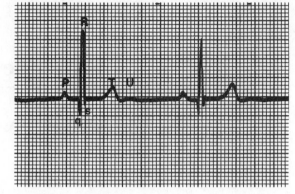

Strip 3-2.

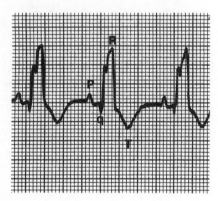

Strip 3-3.

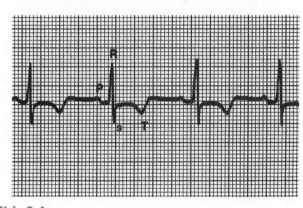

Strip 3-4.

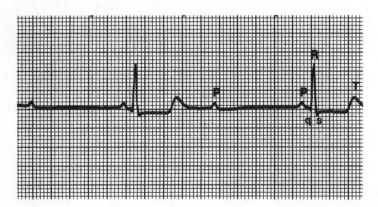

Strip 3-5.

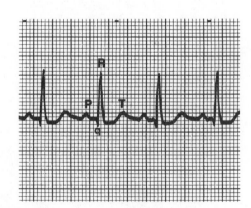

Strip 3-6.

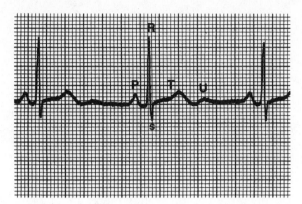

**Strip 3-7.**

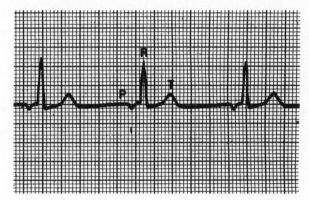

**Strip 3-8.**

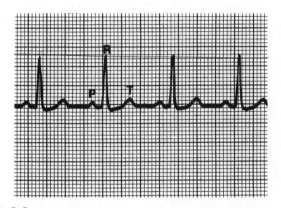

**Strip 3-9.**

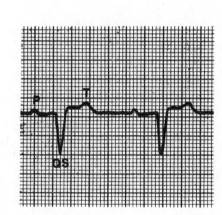

**Strip 3-10.**

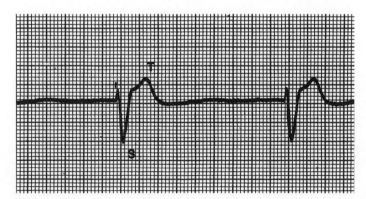

**Strip 3-11.**

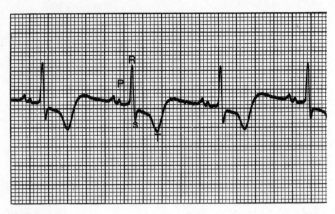

**Strip 3-12.**

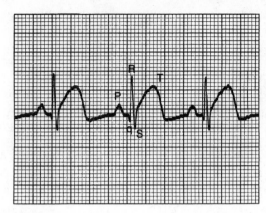

**Strip 3-13.**

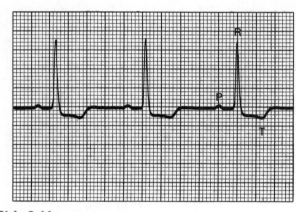

**Strip 3-14.**

# Answer key to Chapters 5 through 11

**Strip 5-1**
Rhythm: Regular
Rate: 79 beats/minute
P waves: Sinus
PR interval: 0.14 to 0.16 second
QRS complex: 0.06 to 0.08 second
Comment: An inverted T wave is present.

**Strip 5-2**
Rhythm: Regular
Rate: 45 beats/minute
P waves: Sinus
PR interval: 0.14 to 0.16 second
QRS complex: 0.08 second
Comment: A small U wave is seen after the T wave.

**Strip 5-3**
Rhythm: Regular
Rate: 88 beats/minute
P waves: Sinus
PR interval: 0.20 second
QRS complex: 0.08 to 0.10 second
Comment: A depressed ST segment and biphasic T wave
are present.

**Strip 5-4**
Rhythm: Irregular
Rate: 50 beats/minute
P waves: Sinus
PR interval: 0.16 to 0.18 second
QRS complex: 0.04 second

**Strip 5-5**
Rhythm: Regular
Rate: 50 beats/minute
P waves: Sinus
PR interval: 0.18 to 0.20 second
QRS complex: 0.06 to 0.08 second
Comment: An elevated ST segment is present.

**Strip 5-6**
Rhythm: Regular
Rate: 136 beats/minute
P waves: Sinus
PR interval: 0.14 to 0.16 second
QRS complex: 0.06 to 0.08 second

**Strip 5-7**
Rhythm: Regular
Rate: 68 beats/minute
P waves: Sinus
PR interval: 0.16 to 0.18 second
QRS complex: 0.12 to 0.14 second
Comment: A U wave is present.

**Strip 5-8**
Rhythm: Irregular
Rate: 50 beats/minute
P waves: Sinus
PR interval: 0.12 to 0.14 second
QRS complex: 0.06 to 0.08 second
Comment: An elevated ST segment and inverted T wave
are present.

**Strip 5-9**
Rhythm: Regular
Rate: 94 beats/minute
P waves: Sinus
PR interval: 0.14 to 0.16 second
QRS complex: 0.06 to 0.08 second
Comment: A depressed ST segment is present.

**Strip 5-10**
Rhythm: Regular
Rate: 58 beats/minute
P waves: Sinus
PR interval: 0.16 to 0.18 second
QRS complex: 0.14 to 0.16 second

**Strip 5-11**
Rhythm: Regular
Rate: 56 beats/minute
P waves: Sinus
PR interval: 0.24 to 0.26 second
QRS complex: 0.04 to 0.06 second

**Strip 6-1**
Rhythm: Regular
Rate: 44 beats/minute
P waves: Sinus
PR interval: 0.20 second
QRS complex: 0.10 second
Rhythm interpretation: Sinus bradycardia; an elevated ST
segment and a U wave are present.

**Strip 6-2**
Rhythm: Regular
Rate: 68 beats/minute
P waves: Sinus
PR interval: 0.16 to 0.18 second
QRS complex: 0.06 to 0.08 second
Rhythm interpretation: Normal sinus rhythm; ST-segment depression and T-wave inversion are present.

**Strip 6-3**
Rhythm: Regular
Rate: 79 beats/minute
P waves: Sinus
PR interval: 0.14 to 0.16 second
QRS complex: 0.06 to 0.08 second
Rhythm interpretation: Normal sinus rhythm

**Strip 6-4**
Rhythm: Regular
Rate: 107 beats/minute
P waves: Sinus
PR interval: 0.12 to 0.16 second
QRS complex: 0.06 to 0.08 second
Rhythm interpretation: Sinus tachycardia; ST-segment depression and T-wave inversion are present.

**Strip 6-5**
Rhythm: Regular
Rate: 58 beats/minute
P waves: Sinus
PR interval: 0.16 to 0.18 second
QRS complex: 0.06 to 0.08 second
Rhythm interpretation: Sinus bradycardia; a U wave is present.

**Strip 6-6**
Rhythm: Regular (basic rhythm); irregular during pause
Rate: 100 beats/minute (basic rhythm)
P waves: Sinus (basic rhythm); absent during pause
PR interval: 0.16 to 0.20 second
QRS complex: 0.08 to 0.10 second (basic rhythm)
Rhythm interpretation: Normal sinus rhythm with sinus block; ST-segment depression and T-wave inversion are present.

**Strip 6-7**
Rhythm: Regular
Rate: 54 beats/minute
P waves: Sinus (notched P waves usually indicate left atrial hypertrophy)
PR interval: 0.14 to 0.16 second
QRS complex: 0.06 to 0.08 second
Rhythm interpretation: Sinus bradycardia; a U wave is present.

**Strip 6-8**
Rhythm: Irregular
Rate: 50 beats/minute
P waves: Sinus
PR interval: 0.20 second
QRS complex: 0.06 to 0.08 second
Rhythm interpretation: Sinus arrhythmia with a bradycardic rate; a U wave is present.

**Strip 6-9**
Rhythm: Regular (basic rhythm); irregular during pause
Rate: 58 beats/minute (basic rhythm)
P waves: Sinus (basic rhythm); absent during pause
PR interval: 0.14 to 0.18 second (basic rhythm); absent during pause
QRS complex: 0.08 to 0.10 second (basic rhythm); absent during pause
Rhythm interpretation: Sinus bradycardia with sinus arrest; a depressed ST segment and an inverted T wave are present.

**Strip 6-10**
Rhythm: Regular
Rate: 125 beats/minute
P waves: Sinus
PR interval: 0.12 to 0.14 second
QRS complex: 0.06 to 0.08 second
Rhythm interpretation: Sinus tachycardia

**Strip 6-11**
Rhythm: Regular
Rate: 63 beats/minute
P waves: Sinus
PR interval: 0.18 to 0.20 second
QRS complex: 0.08 second
Rhythm interpretation: Normal sinus rhythm; a U wave is present.

**Strip 6-12**
Rhythm: Regular
Rate: 47 beats/minute
P waves: Sinus
PR interval: 0.18 to 0.20 second
QRS complex: 0.08 second
Rhythm interpretation: Sinus bradycardia; an elevated ST segment is present.

**Strip 6-13**
Rhythm: Irregular
Rate: 80 beats/minute
P waves: Sinus
PR interval: 0.12 to 0.14 second
QRS complex: 0.08 second
Rhythm interpretation: Sinus arrhythmia

Strip 6-14
Rhythm: Regular
Rate: 63 beats/minute
P waves: Sinus
PR interval: 0.18 to 0.20 second
QRS complex: 0.08 to 0.10 second
Rhythm interpretation: Normal sinus rhythm; ST-segment depression and T-wave inversion are present.

Strip 6-15
Rhythm: Regular (basic rhythm); irregular during pause
Rate: 84 beats/minute (basic rhythm); slows to 56 beats/minute after a pause (temporary rate suppression may occur after a pause in the basic rhythm)
P waves: Sinus (basic rhythm); absent during pause
PR interval: 0.16 to 0.18 second (basic rhythm); absent during pause
QRS complex: 0.08 to 0.10 second (basic rhythm); absent during pause
Rhythm interpretation: Normal sinus rhythm with sinus arrest; rate suppression is present after the pause.

Strip 6-16
Rhythm: Regular
Rate: 115 beats/minute
P waves: Sinus
PR interval: 0.16 to 0.18 second
QRS complex: 0.06 to 0.08 second
Rhythm interpretation: Sinus tachycardia; a depressed ST segment and an inverted T wave are present.

Strip 6-17
Rhythm: Regular
Rate: 52 beats/minute
P waves: Sinus
PR interval: 0.16 to 0.18 second
QRS complex: 0.08 to 0.10 second
Rhythm interpretation: Sinus bradycardia

Strip 6-18
Rhythm: Irregular
Rate: 60 beats/minute
P waves: Sinus
PR interval: 0.16 to 0.18 second
QRS complex: 0.08 to 0.10 second
Rhythm interpretation: Sinus arrhythmia

Strip 6-19
Rhythm: Regular
Rate: 79 beats/minute
P waves: Sinus
PR interval: 0.16 to 0.20 second
QRS complex: 0.06 second
Rhythm interpretation: Normal sinus rhythm

Strip 6-20
Rhythm: Regular (basic rhythm); irregular during pause
Rate: 88 beats/minute (basic rhythm)
P waves: Sinus (basic rhythm); absent during pause
PR interval: 0.14 to 0.16 second (basic rhythm)
QRS complex: 0.08 second (basic rhythm)
Rhythm interpretation: Normal sinus rhythm with sinus block; a U wave is present.

Strip 6-21
Rhythm: Regular
Rate: 150 beats/minute
P waves: Sinus
PR interval: 0.12 second
QRS complex: 0.06 second
Rhythm interpretation: Sinus tachycardia

Strip 6-22
Rhythm: Regular
Rate: 60 beats/minute
P waves: Sinus
PR interval: 0.12 second
QRS complex: 0.08 second
Rhythm interpretation: Normal sinus rhythm; T-wave inversion is present.

Strip 6-23
Rhythm: Irregular
Rate: 60 beats/minute
P waves: Sinus
PR interval: 0.16 second
QRS complex: 0.08 second
Rhythm interpretation: Sinus arrhythmia

Strip 6-24
Rhythm: Regular (basic rhythm); irregular during pause
Rate: 60 beats/minute (basic rhythm); slows to 47 beats/minute after a pause (temporary rate suppression can occur after a pause in the basic rhythm)
P waves: Sinus (basic rhythm); absent during pause
PR interval: 0.16 to 0.18 second (basic rhythm); absent during pause
QRS complex: 0.06 to 0.08 second (basic rhythm); absent during pause
Rhythm interpretation: Normal sinus rhythm with sinus arrest

Strip 6-25
Rhythm: Regular
Rate: 125 beats/minute
P waves: Sinus
PR interval: 0.12 to 0.14 second
QRS complex: 0.04 to 0.06 second
Rhythm interpretation: Sinus tachycardia

Strip 6-26
Rhythm: Regular
Rate: 35 beats/minute
P waves: Sinus
PR interval: 0.14 to 0.16 second
QRS complex: 0.10 second
Rhythm interpretation: Marked sinus bradycardia

Strip 6-27
Rhythm: Regular (basic rhythm); irregular during pause
Rate: 72 beats/minute (basic rhythm)
P waves: Sinus (basic rhythm); absent during pause
PR interval: 0.14 to 0.16 second (basic rhythm); absent during pause
QRS complex: 0.08 to 0.10 second (basic rhythm); absent during pause
Rhythm interpretation: Normal sinus rhythm with sinus block

Strip 6-28
Rhythm: Irregular
Rate: 60 beats/minute
P waves: Sinus
PR interval: 0.12 to 0.14 second
QRS complex: 0.10 second
Rhythm interpretation: Sinus arrhythmia; a U wave is present.

Strip 6-29
Rhythm: Regular
Rate: 65 beats/minute
P waves: Sinus
PR interval: 0.20 second
QRS complex: 0.08 to 0.10 second
Rhythm interpretation: Normal sinus rhythm; ST segment depression and T wave inversion are present.

Strip 6-30
Rhythm: Regular (basic rhythm); irregular during pause
Rate: 68 beats/minute (basic rhythm); slows to 63 beats/minute after a pause (temporary rate suppression can occur after a pause in the basic rhythm; after several cycles the rate returns to the basic rate)
P waves: Sinus (basic rhythm); absent during pause
PR interval: 0.16 second (basic rhythm); absent during pause
QRS complex: 0.06 to 0.08 second (basic rhythm); absent during pause
Rhythm interpretation: Normal sinus rhythm with sinus arrest; a U wave is present.

Strip 6-31
Rhythm: Regular
Rate: 56 beats/minute
P waves: Sinus
PR interval: 0.12 to 0.14 second
QRS complex: 0.08 to 0.10 second
Rhythm interpretation: Sinus bradycardia; T-wave inversion is present.

Strip 6-32
Rhythm: Irregular
Rate: 60 beats/minute
P waves: Sinus
PR interval: 0.14 to 0.16 second
QRS complex: 0.06 to 0.08 second
Rhythm interpretation: Sinus arrhythmia

Strip 6-33
Rhythm: Regular
Rate: 115 beats/minute
P waves: Sinus
PR interval: 0.16 to 0.18 second
QRS complex: 0.06 to 0.08 second
Rhythm interpretation: Sinus tachycardia

Strip 6-34
Rhythm: Regular
Rate: 88 beats/minute
P waves: Sinus
PR interval: 0.18 to 0.20 second
QRS complex: 0.08 second
Rhythm interpretation: Normal sinus rhythm; ST-segment depression is present.

Strip 6-35
Rhythm: Irregular
Rate: 60 beats/minute
P waves: Sinus
PR interval: 0.14 to 0.16 second
QRS complex: 0.06 to 0.08 second
Rhythm interpretation: Sinus arrhythmia

Strip 6-36
Rhythm: Regular
Rate: 41 beats/minute
P waves: Sinus
PR interval: 0.16 to 0.18 second
QRS complex: 0.06 to 0.08 second
Rhythm interpretation: Sinus bradycardia; ST-segment depression is present.

Strip 6-37
Rhythm: Regular (basic rhythm); irregular during pause
Rate: 88 beats/minute (basic rhythm)
P waves: Sinus
PR interval: 0.20 second
QRS complex: 0.06 to 0.08 second
Rhythm interpretation: Normal sinus rhythm with sinus arrest; ST-segment depression is present.

Strip 6-38
Rhythm: Regular
Rate: 107 beats/minute
P waves: Sinus
PR interval: 0.16 to 0.18 second
QRS complex: 0.06 to 0.08 second
Rhythm interpretation: Sinus tachycardia

Strip 6-39
Rhythm: Regular
Rate: 107 beats/minute
P waves: Sinus
PR interval: 0.16 to 0.18 second
QRS complex: 0.06 to 0.08 second
Rhythm interpretation: Sinus tachycardia; ST-segment elevation is present.

Strip 6-40
Rhythm: Regular
Rate: 54 beats/minute
P waves: Sinus (notched P waves usually indicate left atrial hypertrophy)
PR interval: 0.16 to 0.20 second
QRS complex: 0.06 to 0.08 second
Rhythm interpretation: Sinus bradycardia

Strip 6-41
Rhythm: Regular
Rate: 94 beats/minute
P waves: Sinus (negative P waves are normal in lead $MCL_1$)
PR interval: 0.18 to 0.20 second
QRS complex: 0.08 to 0.10 second (negative QRS complexes are normal in lead $MCL_1$)
Rhythm interpretation: Normal sinus rhythm

Strip 6-42
Rhythm: Irregular
Rate: 40 beats/minute
P waves: Sinus
PR interval: 0.18 to 0.20 second
QRS complex: 0.06 to 0.08 second
Rhythm interpretation: Sinus arrhythmia with a bradycardic rate

Strip 6-43
Rhythm: Regular (basic rhythm); irregular during pause
Rate: 63 beats/minute (basic rhythm)
P waves: Sinus (basic rhythm); absent during pause
PR interval: 0.18 to 0.20 second (basic rhythm); absent during pause
QRS complex: 0.04 to 0.06 second (basic rhythm); absent during pause
Rhythm interpretation: Normal sinus rhythm with sinus arrest; ST-segment depression is present.

Strip 6-44
Rhythm: Irregular
Rate: 60 beats/minute
P waves: Sinus
PR interval: 0.12 to 0.14 second
QRS complex: 0.08 to 0.10 second
Rhythm interpretation: Sinus arrhythmia; ST-segment elevation is present.

Strip 6-45
Rhythm: Regular
Rate: 27 beats/minute
P waves: Sinus
PR interval: 0.14 to 0.16 second
QRS complex: 0.08 to 0.10 second
Rhythm interpretation: Sinus bradycardia with extremely slow rate; ST-segment depression is present.

Strip 6-46
Rhythm: Irregular
Rate: 50 beats/minute
P waves: Sinus
PR interval: 0.12 to 0.14 second
QRS complex: 0.06 to 0.08 second
Rhythm interpretation: Sinus arrhythmia with a bradycardic rate

Strip 6-47
Rhythm: Regular
Rate: 136 beats/minute
P waves: Sinus
PR interval: 0.12 to 0.14 second
QRS complex: 0.06 to 0.08 second
Rhythm interpretation: Sinus tachycardia

Strip 6-48
Rhythm: Irregular
Rate: 70 beats/minute
P waves: Sinus
PR interval: 0.16 to 0.20 second
QRS complex: 0.04 to 0.06 second
Rhythm interpretation: Sinus arrhythmia; a U wave is present.

Strip 6-49
Rhythm: Regular
Rate: 52 beats/minute
P waves: Sinus
PR interval: 0.12 second
QRS complex: 0.08 second
Rhythm interpretation: Sinus bradycardia

Strip 6-50
Rhythm: Regular
Rate: 60 beats/minute
P waves: Sinus
PR interval: 0.16 to 0.18 second
QRS complex: 0.08 second
Rhythm interpretation: Normal sinus rhythm; an elevated
ST segment is present.

Strip 6-51
Rhythm: Regular
Rate: 107 beats/minute
P waves: Sinus
PR interval: 0.12 to 0.14 second
QRS complex: 0.06 to 0.08 second
Rhythm interpretation: Sinus tachycardia

Strip 6-52
Rhythm: Regular (basic rhythm); irregular during pause
Rate: 60 beats/minute (basic rhythm); slows to 31 beats/
minute after a pause; temporary rate suppression is com-
mon after a pause in the basic rhythm
P waves: Sinus
PR interval: 0.16 to 0.20 second
QRS complex: 0.06 to 0.08 second
Rhythm interpretation: Normal sinus rhythm with sinus
arrest; ST-segment depression and T-wave inversion are
present.

Strip 6-53
Rhythm: Irregular
Rate: 50 beats/minute
P waves: Sinus
PR interval: 0.14 to 0.16 second
QRS complex: 0.06 to 0.08 second
Rhythm interpretation: Sinus arrhythmia with a brady-
cardic rate

Strip 6-54
Rhythm: Regular (basic rhythm); irregular during pause
Rate: 94 beats/minute (basic rhythm); rate slows to 54
beats/minute after a pause (temporary rate suppression
can occur after a pause in the basic rhythm)
P waves: Sinus (basic rhythm); absent during pause
PR interval: 0.16 to 0.18 second (basic rhythm); absent
during pause
QRS complex: 0.08 to 0.10 second
Rhythm interpretation: Normal sinus rhythm with sinus
block

Strip 6-55
Rhythm: Regular
Rate: 65 beats/minute
P waves: Sinus
PR interval: 0.16 to 0.18 second
QRS complex: 0.06 second
Rhythm interpretation: Normal sinus rhythm

Strip 6-56
Rhythm: Regular
Rate: 125 beats/minute
P waves: Sinus
PR interval: 0.16 second
QRS complex: 0.08 second
Rhythm interpretation: Sinus tachycardia; ST-segment
depression is present.

Strip 6-57
Rhythm: Irregular
Rate: 40 beats/minute
P waves: Sinus
PR interval: 0.16 to 0.18 second
QRS complex: 0.08 second
Rhythm interpretation: Sinus arrhythmia with a brady-
cardic rate; a U wave is present.

Strip 6-58
Rhythm: Regular
Rate: 72 beats/minute
P waves: Sinus
PR interval: 0.16 to 0.20 second
QRS complex: 0.06 to 0.08 second
Rhythm interpretation: Normal sinus rhythm; ST-
segment depression and T-wave inversion are present.

Strip 6-59
Rhythm: Regular
Rate: 50 beats/minute
P waves: Sinus
PR interval: 0.20 second
QRS complex: 0.06 to 0.08 second
Rhythm interpretation: Sinus bradycardia; ST-segment
depression and T-wave inversion are present.

**Strip 6-60**
Rhythm: Regular (basic rhythm); irregular during pause
Rate: 88 beats/minute (basic rhythm)
P waves: Sinus (basic rhythm); absent during pause
PR interval: 0.14 to 0.20 second (basic rhythm); absent during pause
QRS complex: 0.08 to 0.10 second (basic rhythm); absent during pause
Rhythm interpretation: Normal sinus rhythm with sinus block; ST-segment depression is present.

**Strip 6-61**
Rhythm: Regular
Rate: 72 beats/minute
P waves: Sinus
PR interval: 0.12 to 0.14 second
QRS complex: 0.06 to 0.08 second
Rhythm interpretation: Normal sinus rhythm; an inverted T wave is present.

**Strip 6-62**
Rhythm: Regular
Rate: 125 beats/minute
P waves: Sinus
PR interval: 0.12 second
QRS complex: 0.04 second
Rhythm interpretation: Sinus tachycardia; ST-segment depression is present.

**Strip 6-63**
Rhythm: Regular
Rate: 44 beats/minute
P waves: Sinus
PR interval: 0.18 to 0.20 second
QRS complex: 0.06 to 0.08 second
Rhythm interpretation: Sinus bradycardia; a U wave is present.

**Strip 6-64**
Rhythm: Regular
Rate: 79 beats/minute
P waves: Sinus
PR interval: 0.14 to 0.16 second
QRS complex: 0.04 to 0.06 second
Rhythm interpretation: Normal sinus rhythm; T-wave inversion is present.

**Strip 6-65**
Rhythm: Regular
Rate: 107 beats/minute
P waves: Sinus
PR interval: 0.18 to 0.20 second
QRS complex: 0.08 to 0.10 second
Rhythm interpretation: Sinus tachycardia; an elevated ST segment is present.

**Strip 6-66**
Rhythm: Regular
Rate: 100 beats/minute
P waves: Sinus
PR interval: 0.20 second
QRS complex: 0.08 second
Rhythm interpretation: Normal sinus rhythm; an extremely elevated ST segment is present.

**Strip 6-67**
Rhythm: Regular
Rate: 44 beats/minute
P waves: Sinus
PR interval: 0.14 to 0.16 second
QRS complex: 0.08 second
Rhythm interpretation: Sinus bradycardia; a U wave is present.

**Strip 6-68**
Rhythm: Regular
Rate: 88 beats/minute
P waves: Sinus
PR interval: 0.18 to 0.20 second
QRS complex: 0.06 to 0.08 second
Rhythm interpretation: Normal sinus rhythm; a depressed ST segment is present.

**Strip 6-69**
Rhythm: Regular
Rate: 136 beats/minute
P waves: Sinus
PR interval: 0.14 to 0.16 second
QRS complex: 0.08 second
Rhythm interpretation: Sinus tachycardia; an elevated ST segment is present.

**Strip 6-70**
Rhythm: Regular (basic rhythm); irregular during pause
Rate: 56 beats/minute (basic rhythm); slows to 50 beats/minute after a pause (temporary rate suppression can occur after a pause in the basic rhythm; after several cycles the rate returns to the basic rate)
P waves: Sinus (basic rhythm); absent during pause
PR interval: 0.14 to 0.16 second (basic rhythm); absent during pause
QRS complex: 0.08 to 0.10 second (basic rhythm); absent during pause
Rhythm interpretation: Sinus bradycardia with sinus arrest

**Strip 6-71**
Rhythm: Regular
Rate: 115 beats/minute
P waves: Sinus
PR interval: 0.14 to 0.16 second
QRS complex: 0.08 to 0.10 second
Rhythm interpretation: Sinus tachycardia; ST-segment depression is present.

**Strip 6-72**
Rhythm: Regular
Rate: 79 beats/minute
P waves: Sinus
PR interval: 0.14 to 0.16 second
QRS complex: 0.06 to 0.08 second
Rhythm interpretation: Normal sinus rhythm; a depressed ST segment and a biphasic T wave are present

**Strip 6-73**
Rhythm: Regular
Rate: 54 beats/minute
P waves: Sinus
PR interval: 0.14 to 0.16 second
QRS complex: 0.06 to 0.08 second
Rhythm interpretation: Sinus bradycardia; an elevated ST segment is present

**Strip 6-74**
Rhythm: Regular
Rate: 94 beats/minute
P waves: Sinus
PR interval: 0.16 second
QRS complex: 0.08 to 0.10 second
Rhythm interpretation: Normal sinus rhythm; ST-segment depression and a biphasic T wave are present.

**Strip 6-75**
Rhythm: Regular
Rate: 94 beats/minute
P waves: Sinus
PR interval: 0.16 to 0.20 second
QRS complex: 0.06 to 0.08 second
Rhythm interpretation: Normal sinus rhythm

**Strip 6-76**
Rhythm: Regular
Rate: 125 beats/minute
P waves: Sinus
PR interval: 0.12 second
QRS complex: 0.06 to 0.08 second
Rhythm interpretation: Sinus tachycardia

**Strip 6-77**
Rhythm: Regular
Rate: 79 beats/minute
P waves: Sinus
PR interval: 0.18 to 0.20 second
QRS complex: 0.06 to 0.08 second
Rhythm interpretation: Normal sinus rhythm; an elevated ST segment is present.

**Strip 6-78**
Rhythm: Regular
Rate: 58 beats/minute
P waves: Sinus
PR interval: 0.16 to 0.18 second
QRS complex: 0.06 to 0.08 second
Rhythm interpretation: Sinus bradycardia; an elevated ST segment and a U wave are present.

**Strip 6-79**
Rhythm: Regular (basic rhythm); irregular during pause
Rate: 107 beats/minute (basic rhythm); slows to 94 beats/minute for one cycle after a pause (temporary rate suppression can occur after a pause in the basic rhythm)
P waves: Sinus in basic rhythm; absent during pause
PR interval: 0.16 to 0.20 second (basic rhythm); absent during pause
QRS complex: 0.10 second (basic rhythm); absent during pause
Rhythm interpretation: Sinus tachycardia with sinus block; baseline artifact is present.

**Strip 6-80**
Rhythm: Regular
Rate: 84 beats/minute
P waves: Sinus
PR interval: 0.16 second
QRS complex: 0.06 second
Rhythm interpretation: Normal sinus rhythm; T-wave inversion is present.

**Strip 6-81**
Rhythm: Regular
Rate: 56 beats/minute
P waves: Sinus
PR interval: 0.16 to 0.18 second
QRS complex: 0.06 to 0.08 second
Rhythm interpretation: Sinus bradycardia; T-wave inversion is present.

**Strip 6-82**
Rhythm: Regular
Rate: 125 beats/minute
P waves: Sinus
PR interval: 0.16 to 0.18 second
QRS complex: 0.04 to 0.06 second
Rhythm interpretation: Sinus tachycardia

**Strip 6-83**
Rhythm: Irregular (basic rhythm)
Rate: 60 beats/minute (basic rhythm)
P waves: Sinus
PR interval: 0.20 second (basic rhythm); absent during pause
QRS complex: 0.06 to 0.08 second (basic rhythm); absent during pause
Rhythm interpretation: Sinus arrhythmia with sinus pause (with an irregular basic rhythm it's impossible to distinguish sinus arrest from sinus block, so the rhythm is interpreted using the broad term *sinus pause*); ST-segment depression is present.

**Strip 6-84**
Rhythm: Regular
Rate: 79 beats/minute
P waves: Sinus
PR interval: 0.12 second
QRS complex: 0.06 to 0.08 second
Rhythm interpretation: Normal sinus rhythm; an elevated ST segment is present.

**Strip 6-85**
Rhythm: Regular
Rate: 136 beats/minute
P waves: Sinus
PR interval: 0.14 to 0.16 second
QRS complex: 0.06 to 0.08 second
Rhythm interpretation: Sinus tachycardia

**Strip 6-86**
Rhythm: Regular
Rate: 54 beats/minute
P waves: Sinus
PR interval: 0.16 second
QRS complex: 0.06 to 0.08 second
Rhythm interpretation: Sinus bradycardia

**Strip 6-87**
Rhythm: Regular (basic rhythm); irregular during pause
Rate: 84 beats/minute (basic rhythm); slows to 75 beats/minute for one cycle after the pause (temporary rate suppression is common after a pause in the basic rhythm)
P waves: Sinus (basic rhythm); absent during pause
PR interval: 0.16 to 0.18 second (basic rhythm); absent during pause
QRS complex: 0.06 to 0.08 second (basic rhythm); absent during pause
Rhythm interpretation: Normal sinus rhythm with sinus arrest

**Strip 6-88**
Rhythm: Regular
Rate: 100 beats/minute
P waves: Sinus
PR interval: 0.12 to 0.14 second
QRS complex: 0.08 to 0.10 second
Rhythm interpretation: Normal sinus rhythm; an elevated ST segment is present.

**Strip 6-89**
Rhythm: Regular
Rate: 54 beats/minute
P waves: Sinus
PR interval: 0.18 to 0.20 second
QRS complex: 0.06 to 0.08 second
Rhythm interpretation: Sinus bradycardia; an elevated ST segment and T wave inversion are present.

**Strip 6-90**
Rhythm: Regular (basic rhythm); irregular during pause
Rate: 72 beats/minute (basic rhythm); slows to 68 beats/minute for two cycles after a pause (temporary rate suppression can occur after a pause in the basic rhythm)
P waves: Sinus (basic rhythm); absent during pause
PR interval: 0.12 to 0.14 second (basic rhythm); absent during pause
QRS complex: 0.06 to 0.08 second (basic rhythm); absent during pause
Rhythm interpretation: Normal sinus rhythm with sinus arrest; T-wave inversion is present.

**Strip 6-91**
Rhythm: Regular
Rate: 65 beats/minute
P waves: Sinus
PR interval: 0.14 to 0.16 second
QRS complex: 0.06 to 0.08 second
Rhythm interpretation: Normal sinus rhythm; a U wave is present.

Strip 6-92
Rhythm: Regular
Rate: 63 beats/minute
P waves: Sinus
PR interval: 0.18 to 0.20 second
QRS complex: 0.08 to 0.10 second
Rhythm interpretation: Normal sinus rhythm; ST-segment depression and T-wave inversion are present.

Strip 6-93
Rhythm: Regular (basic rhythm); irregular during pause
Rate: 79 beats/minute (basic rhythm); slows to 72 beats/minute after a pause (temporary rate suppression can occur after a pause in the basic rhythm)
P waves: Sinus (basic rhythm); absent during pause
PR interval: 0.20 second (basic rhythm); absent during pause
QRS complex: 0.08 to 0.10 second (basic rhythm); absent during pause
Rhythm interpretation: Normal sinus rhythm with sinus arrest; ST-segment depression and T-wave inversion are present.

Strip 6-94
Rhythm: Regular
Rate: 150 beats/minute
P waves: Sinus
PR interval: 0.12 second
QRS complex: 0.04 to 0.06 second
Rhythm interpretation: Sinus tachycardia

Strip 6-95
Rhythm: Regular
Rate: 136 beats/minute
P waves: Sinus
PR interval: 0.12 second
QRS complex: 0.06 to 0.08 second
Rhythm interpretation: Sinus tachycardia

Strip 6-96
Rhythm: Irregular
Rate: 50 beats/minute
P waves: Sinus
PR interval: 0.14 to 0.16 second
QRS complex: 0.08 second
Rhythm interpretation: Sinus arrhythmia with a bradycardic rate

Strip 6-97
Rhythm: Irregular
Rate: 40 beats/minute
P waves: Sinus
PR interval: 0.18 to 0.20 second
QRS complex: 0.06 to 0.08 second
Rhythm interpretation: Sinus arrhythmia with a bradycardic rate and sinus pause (With an irregular basic rhythm it's impossible to distinguish sinus arrest from sinus block, so the rhythm is interpreted using the broad term *sinus pause*.)

Strip 6-98
Rhythm: Regular
Rate: 136 beats/minute
P waves: Sinus
PR interval: 0.14 to 0.16 second
QRS complex: 0.08 to 0.10 second
Rhythm interpretation: Sinus tachycardia; ST-segment elevation is present.

Strip 6-99
Rhythm: Irregular
Rate: 50 beats/minute
P waves: Sinus
PR interval: 0.14 to 0.16 second
QRS complex: 0.08 to 0.10 second
Rhythm interpretation: Sinus arrhythmia with a bradycardic rate

Strip 7-1
Rhythm: Irregular
Rate: 60 beats/minute (ventricular); atrial not measurable
P waves: Fibrillation waves present
PR interval: Not measurable
QRS complex: 0.06 to 0.08 second
Rhythm interpretation: Atrial fibrillation; ST-segment depression is present.

Strip 7-2
Rhythm: Regular
Rate: 188 beats/minute
P waves: Hidden in T waves
PR interval: Not measurable
QRS complex: 0.06 to 0.08 second
Rhythm interpretation: Paroxysmal atrial tachycardia

## Strip 7-3

Rhythm: Regular (basic rhythm); irregular (PACs)
Rate: 94 beats/minute (basic rhythm)
P waves: Sinus (basic rhythm); premature and abnormal (PACs)
PR interval: 0.12 second (basic rhythm); 0.14 second (PACs)
QRS complex: 0.08 to 0.10 second (basic rhythm and PACs)
Rhythm interpretation: Normal sinus rhythm with two PACs (fourth and eighth complexes); ST-segment depression is present.

## Strip 7-4

Rhythm: Irregular
Rate: 100 beats/minute
P waves: Vary in size, shape, and position
PR interval: 0.12 second
QRS complex: 0.06 to 0.08 second
Rhythm interpretation: Wandering atrial pacemaker

## Strip 7-5

Rhythm: Regular (basic rhythm); irregular (PAC)
Rate: 125 beats/minute (basic rhythm)
P waves: Sinus (basic rhythm); premature and pointed (PAC)
PR interval: 0.12 second (basic rhythm)
QRS complex: 0.04 to 0.06 second (basic rhythm)
Rhythm interpretation: Sinus tachycardia with one PAC (eighth complex)

## Strip 7-6

Rhythm: Regular
Rate: 167 beats/minute
P waves: Pointed, abnormal
PR interval: 0.14 to 0.16 second
QRS complex: 0.06 to 0.08 second
Rhythm interpretation: Paroxysmal atrial tachycardia; ST-segment depression is present.

## Strip 7-7

Rhythm: Regular (basic rhythm); irregular (nonconducted PAC)
Rate: 88 beats/minute (basic rhythm)
P waves: Sinus (basic rhythm); premature and abnormal (nonconducted PAC)
PR interval: 0.16 second
QRS complex: 0.06 to 0.08 second
Rhythm interpretation: Normal sinus rhythm with nonconducted PAC (after the seventh QRS complex); ST-segment depression is present.

## Strip 7-8

Rhythm: Irregular
Rate: 320 beats/minute (atrial); 120 beats/minute (ventricular)
P waves: Flutter waves present (varying ratios)
PR interval: Not measurable
QRS complex: 0.06 to 0.08 second
Rhythm interpretation: Atrial flutter with variable AV conduction

## Strip 7-9

Rhythm: Irregular
Rate: 70 beats/minute
P waves: Vary in size, shape, and direction
PR interval: 0.12 to 0.14 second
QRS complex: 0.06 to 0.08 second
Rhythm interpretation: Wandering atrial pacemaker

## Strip 7-10

Rhythm: Irregular
Rate: 60 beats/minute (ventricular); atrial not measurable
P waves: Fibrillatory waves present
PR interval: Not measurable
QRS complex: 0.04 to 0.06 second
Rhythm interpretation: Atrial fibrillation

## Strip 7-11

Rhythm: Regular (basic rhythm); irregular (PAC)
Rate: 72 beats/minute (basic rhythm)
P waves: Sinus (basic rhythm); premature and pointed (PAC)
PR interval: 0.18 to 0.20 second (basic rhythm)
QRS complex: 0.06 to 0.08 second (basic rhythm)
Rhythm interpretation: Normal sinus rhythm with one PAC (sixth complex)

## Strip 7-12

Rhythm: Regular
Rate: 237 beats/minute (atrial); 79 beats/minute (ventricular)
P waves: Three flutter waves to each QRS complex
PR interval: Not necessary to measure
QRS complex: 0.04 second
Rhythm interpretation: Atrial flutter with 3:1 AV conduction

## Strip 7-13

Rhythm: Regular (basic rhythm); irregular (PAC)
Rate: 107 beats/minute (basic rhythm)
P waves: Sinus (basic rhythm); premature and pointed P wave without a QRS complex after the fifth QRS complex
PR interval: 0.18 to 0.20 second
QRS complex: 0.04 to 0.06 second
Rhythm interpretation: Sinus tachycardia with one nonconducted PAC (after the fifth QRS complex)

## Strip 7-14

Rhythm: Irregular
Rate: 110 beats/minute (ventricular); atrial not measurable
P waves: Fibrillatory waves present
PR interval: Not measurable
QRS complex: 0.06 to 0.08 second
Rhythm interpretation: Atrial fibrillation; some flutter waves are noted.

## Strip 7-15

Rhythm: Regular (both rhythms)
Rate: 167 beats/minute (first rhythm); 100 beats/minute (second rhythm)
P waves: Obscured in T waves (first rhythm); sinus (second rhythm)
PR interval: Not measurable (first rhythm); 0.16 to 0.18 second (second rhythm)
QRS complex: 0.08 second (both rhythms)
Rhythm interpretation: Paroxysmal atrial tachycardia converting to normal sinus rhythm

## Strip 7-16

Rhythm: Regular
Rate: 300 beats/minute (atrial); 100 beats/minute (ventricular)
P waves: Three flutter waves before each QRS complex
PR interval: Not measurable
QRS complex: 0.08 second
Rhythm interpretation: Atrial flutter with 3:1 AV conduction

## Strip 7-17

Rhythm: Irregular
Rate: 40 beats/minute
P waves: Fibrillatory waves
PR interval: Not measurable
QRS complex: 0.08 second
Rhythm interpretation: Atrial fibrillation

## Strip 7-18

Rhythm: Irregular
Rate: 320 beats/minute (atrial); 90 beats/minute (ventricular)
P waves: Flutter waves (varying ratios)
PR interval: Not discernible
QRS complex: 0.04 to 0.06 second
Rhythm interpretation: Atrial flutter with variable AV conduction

## Strip 7-19

Rhythm: Regular (basic rhythm); irregular (PACs and nonconducted PACs)
Rate: 84 beats/minute (basic rhythm)
P waves: Sinus (basic rhythm); premature and abnormal (PACs and nonconducted PACs)
PR interval: 0.16 second (basic rhythm)
QRS complex: 0.06 to 0.08 second (basic rhythm and PACs)
Rhythm interpretation: Normal sinus rhythm with two PACs (third and ninth complexes) and two nonconducted PACs (after the fourth and fifth complexes)

## Strip 7-20

Rhythm: Regular
Rate: 167 beats/minute
P waves: Pointed and abnormal
PR interval: 0.16 to 0.18 second
QRS complex: 0.06 to 0.08 second
Rhythm interpretation: Paroxysmal atrial tachycardia

## Strip 7-21

Rhythm: Regular (basic rhythm); irregular (nonconducted PAC)
Rate: 75 beats/minute (basic rhythm); slows to 72 beats/minute for two cycles after a pause (temporary rate suppression is common after a pause in the underlying rhythm)
P waves: Sinus (basic rhythm); premature and pointed without QRS complex after the third QRS complex
PR interval: 0.16 second
QRS complex: 0.08 second
Rhythm interpretation: Normal sinus rhythm with one nonconducted PAC (after the third QRS complex); a U wave is present.

## Strip 7-22

Rhythm: Regular
Rate: 232 beats/minute (atrial); 58 beats/minute (ventricular)
P waves: Four flutter waves to each QRS complex
PR interval: Not measurable
QRS complex: 0.06 to 0.08 second
Rhythm interpretation: Atrial flutter with 4:1 AV conduction

Strip 7-23
Rhythm: Regular (basic rhythm); irregular with pause
Rate: 79 beats/minute (basic rhythm)
P waves: Sinus (basic rhythm); premature and abnormal without QRS complex after the fourth QRS complex
PR interval: 0.16 to 0.18 second (basic rhythm)
QRS complex: 0.06 to 0.08 second (basic rhythm)
Rhythm interpretation: Normal sinus rhythm with one nonconducted PAC (after the fourth QRS complex); ST-segment depression and T-wave inversion are present.

Strip 7-24
Rhythm: Irregular
Rate: 170 beats/minute (ventricular); atrial not measurable
P waves: Fibrillatory waves present
PR interval: Not measurable
QRS complex: 0.06 to 0.08 second
Rhythm interpretation: Atrial fibrillation

Strip 7-25
Rhythm: Regular
Rate: 84 beats/minute
P waves: Vary in size, shape, and position
PR interval: 0.12 to 0.14 second
QRS complex: 0.06 to 0.08 second
Rhythm interpretation: Wandering atrial pacemaker; T-wave inversion is present.

Strip 7-26
Rhythm: Regular (basic rhythm); irregular (PAC)
Rate: 68 beats/minute (basic rhythm)
P waves: Sinus (basic rhythm); premature and inverted (PAC)
PR interval: 0.12 to 0.14 second (basic rhythm); 0.12 second (PAC)
QRS complex: 0.06 to 0.08 second (basic rhythm); 0.08 second (PAC)
Rhythm interpretation: Normal sinus rhythm with one PAC (fourth complex); a U wave is present.

Strip 7-27
Rhythm: Regular
Rate: 232 beats/minute (atrial); 58 beats/minute (ventricular)
P waves: Four flutter waves to each QRS complex
PR interval: Not measurable
QRS complex: 0.06 to 0.08 second
Rhythm interpretation: Atrial flutter with 4:1 AV conduction

Strip 7-28
Rhythm: Regular (basic rhythm); irregular (PACs)
Rate: 42 beats/minute (basic rhythm; measured between the fifth and sixth complexes)
P waves: Sinus (basic rhythm); premature and abnormal (PACs)
PR interval: 0.12 to 0.14 second (basic rhythm); 0.16 second (PACs)
QRS complex: 0.08 to 0.10 second
Rhythm interpretation: Sinus bradycardia with four PACs (second, fourth, seventh, and ninth complexes)

Strip 7-29
Rhythm: Regular
Rate: 150 beats/minute
P waves: Obscured in preceding T wave
PR interval: Not measurable
QRS complex: 0.08 second
Rhythm interpretation: Paroxysmal atrial tachycardia

Strip 7-30
Rhythm: Regular
Rate: 272 beats/minute (atrial); 136 beats/minute (ventricular)
P waves: Two flutter waves to each QRS complex
PR interval: Not measurable
QRS complex: 0.06 second
Rhythm interpretation: Atrial flutter with 2:1 AV conduction

Strip 7-31
Rhythm: Regular (basic rhythm); irregular (PACs and atrial fibrillation)
Rate: 68 beats/minute (basic rhythm); 140 beats/minute (atrial fibrillation)
P waves: Sinus (basic rhythm); premature and abnormal (PACs); fibrillation waves (atrial fibrillation)
PR interval: 0.12 to 0.14 second (basic rhythm)
QRS complex: 0.08 to 0.10 second
Rhythm interpretation: Normal sinus rhythm with two PACs (second and fifth complex); last PAC initiates atrial fibrillation; ST-segment depression is present.

Strip 7-32
Rhythm: Regular (basic rhythm); irregular (nonconducted PAC)
Rate: 94 beats/minute (basic rhythm); slows to 84 beats/minute for one cycle after a pause (temporary rate suppression can occur after a pause in the basic rhythm)
P waves: Sinus (basic rhythm); premature, abnormal P wave without a QRS complex hidden in T wave after the seventh QRS complex
PR interval: 0.16 to 0.18 second
QRS complex: 0.06 to 0.08 second
Rhythm interpretation: Normal sinus rhythm with one nonconducted PAC (after the seventh QRS complex)

Strip 7-33
Rhythm: Regular (basic rhythm); irregular (PAC)
Rate: 47 beats/minute (basic rhythm)
P waves: Sinus (basic rhythm); premature and pointed (PAC)
PR interval: 0.18 to 0.20 second
QRS complex: 0.08 second
Rhythm interpretation: Sinus bradycardia with one PAC (fifth complex); a U wave is present.

Strip 7-34
Rhythm: Irregular
Rate: 50 beats/minute (ventricular); atrial not measurable
P waves: Fibrillatory waves present
PR interval: Not measurable
QRS complex: 0.06 to 0.08 second
Rhythm interpretation: Atrial fibrillation; ST-segment depression and T-wave inversion are present.

Strip 7-35
Rhythm: Regular
Rate: 188 beats/minute
P waves: Obscured in T waves
PR interval: Unmeasurable
QRS complex: 0.04 to 0.08 second
Rhythm interpretation: Paroxysmal atrial tachycardia; ST-segment depression is present.

Strip 7-36
Rhythm: Irregular
Rate: 50 beats/minute
P waves: Vary in size, shape, or direction across strip
PR interval: 0.12 to 0.16 second
QRS complex: 0.04 to 0.06 second
Rhythm interpretation: Wandering atrial pacemaker

Strip 7-37
Rhythm: Irregular
Rate: 260 beats/minute (atrial); 70 beats/minute (ventricular)
P waves: Flutter waves (varying ratios)
PR interval: Not measurable
QRS complex: 0.08 second
Rhythm interpretation: Atrial flutter with variable AV conduction

Strip 7-38
Rhythm: Regular
Rate: 150 beats/minute
P waves: Obscured in T wave
PR interval: Not measurable
QRS complex: 0.04 to 0.06 second
Rhythm interpretation: Paroxysmal atrial tachycardia; ST-segment depression is present.

Strip 7-39
Rhythm: Regular (basic rhythm); irregular (PAC)
Rate: 136 beats/minute (basic rhythm)
P waves: Sinus (basic rhythm); premature and pointed (PAC)
PR interval: 0.16 to 0.18 (basic rhythm); 0.18 second (PAC)
QRS complex: 0.06 to 0.08 second (basic rhythm); 0.06 second (PAC)
Rhythm interpretation: Sinus tachycardia with one PAC (eleventh complex)

Strip 7-40
Rhythm: Irregular
Rate: 130 beats/minute (ventricular); atrial not measurable
P waves: Fibrillatory waves present
PR interval: Not measurable
QRS complex: 0.04 to 0.06 second
Rhythm interpretation: Atrial fibrillation (uncontrolled rate)

Strip 7-41
Rhythm: Regular (basic rhythm); irregular (nonconducted PAC)
Rate: 79 beats/minute (basic rhythm)
P waves: Sinus (basic rhythm); premature, abnormal P wave hidden in the T wave after the seventh QRS complex
PR interval: 0.20 second
QRS complex: 0.08 to 0.10 second
Rhythm interpretation: Normal sinus rhythm with one nonconducted PAC (hidden in the T wave after the seventh QRS complex); a U wave is present.

## Strip 7-42

Rhythm: Regular (basic rhythm); irregular (nonconducted PAC)
Rate: 72 beats/minute
P waves: Sinus; one premature, abnormal P wave without a QRS complex (after the fifth QRS complex)
PR interval: 0.16 second
QRS complex: 0.08 second
Rhythm interpretation: Normal sinus rhythm with one nonconducted PAC (after the fifth QRS complex); T-wave inversion is present.

## Strip 7-43

Rhythm: Regular
Rate: 68 beats/minute
P waves: Vary in size, shape, and position
PR interval: 0.12 second
QRS complex: 0.06 to 0.08 second
Rhythm interpretation: Wandering atrial pacemaker; ST-segment depression is present.

## Strip 7-44

Rhythm: Regular
Rate: 272 beats/minute (atrial); 136 beats/minute (ventricular)
P waves: Two flutter waves to each QRS complex
PR interval: Not measurable
QRS complex: 0.06 to 0.08 second
Rhythm interpretation: Atrial flutter with 2:1 AV conduction

## Strip 7-45

Rhythm: Regular
Rate: 188 beats/minute
P waves: Hidden in T waves
PR interval: Not measurable
QRS complex: 0.04 to 0.06 second
Rhythm interpretation: Paroxysmal atrial tachycardia; ST-segment depression is present.

## Strip 7-46

Rhythm: Regular (basic rhythm); irregular (premature beat)
Rate: 79 beats/minute (basic rhythm)
P waves: Sinus (basic rhythm); premature and pointed (PAC)
PR interval: 0.14 to 0.16 second (basic rhythm); 0.12 second (PAC)
QRS complex: 0.06 to 0.08 second
Rhythm interpretation: Normal sinus rhythm with one PAC (fifth complex)

## Strip 7-47

Rhythm: Regular (basic rhythm); irregular (PAC)
Rate: 84 beats/minute (basic rhythm)
P waves: Sinus; premature and pointed (PAC)
PR interval: 0.14 to 0.16 (basic rhythm); 0.16 second (PAC)
QRS complex: 0.06 to 0.08 second (basic rhythm); 0.08 second (PAC)
Rhythm interpretation: Normal sinus rhythm with one PAC (seventh complex); ST-segment depression is present.

## Strip 7-48

Rhythm: Irregular
Rate: 40 beats/minute
P waves: Fibrillatory waves present
PR interval: Not measurable
QRS complex: 0.08 second
Rhythm interpretation: Atrial fibrillation (controlled rate)

## Strip 7-49

Rhythm: Irregular
Rate: 280 beats/minute (atrial); 50 beats/minute (ventricular)
P waves: Flutter waves present (varying ratios)
PR interval: Not measurable
QRS complex: 0.06 to 0.08 second
Rhythm interpretation: Atrial flutter with variable AV conduction

## Strip 7-50

Rhythm: Irregular
Rate: 300 beats/minute (atrial); 100 beats/minute (ventricular)
P waves: Flutter waves (varying ratios)
PR interval: Not measurable
QRS complex: 0.04 to 0.06 second
Rhythm interpretation: Atrial flutter with variable AV conduction

## Strip 7-51

Rhythm: Regular
Rate: 150 beats/minute
P waves: Hidden in T waves
PR interval: Not measurable
QRS complex: 0.08 to 0.10 second
Rhythm interpretation: Paroxysmal atrial tachycardia

**Strip 7-52**

Rhythm: Regular (basic rhythm); irregular (nonconducted PACs)

Rate: 88 beats/minute (basic rhythm); slows to 79 beats/minute after each nonconducted PAC (temporary rate suppression is common after a pause in the basic rhythm)

P waves: Sinus (basic rhythm); two premature abnormal P waves without a QRS complex after the fifth and seventh QRS complexes

PR interval: 0.18 to 0.20 second

QRS complex: 0.06 to 0.08 second

Rhythm interpretation: Normal sinus rhythm with two nonconducted PACs (after the fifth and seventh QRS complexes)

**Strip 7-53**

Rhythm: Irregular

Rate: 70 beats/minute

P waves: Fibrillatory waves

PR interval: Not measurable

QRS complex: 0.06 to 0.08 second

Rhythm interpretation: Atrial fibrillation; ST-segment depression is present.

**Strip 7-54**

Rhythm: Regular (basic rhythm); irregular (PAC)

Rate: 94 beats/minute (basic rhythm)

P waves: Sinus (basic rhythm); premature and pointed (PAC)

PR interval: 0.12 to 0.16 second

QRS complex: 0.06 to 0.08 second

Rhythm interpretation: Normal sinus rhythm with one PAC (eighth complex); ST-segment depression is present.

**Strip 7-55**

Rhythm: Irregular

Rate: 140 beats/minute (ventricular); atrial not measurable

P waves: Fibrillatory waves on the first part of the strip; sinus P waves on the last part of the strip

PR interval: Not measurable on the first part of the strip; 0.14 second (with the two sinus beats on the last part of the strip)

QRS complex: 0.04 to 0.06 second

Rhythm interpretation: Atrial fibrillation converting to a sinus rhythm (one PAC after the first sinus beat)

**Strip 7-56**

Rhythm: Regular (basic rhythm); irregular (PAC)

Rate: 84 beats/minute (basic rhythm)

P waves: Sinus (basic rhythm); premature and pointed (PAC)

PR interval: 0.12 to 0.14 second (basic rhythm); 0.12 second (PAC)

QRS complex: 0.06 to 0.08 second (basic rhythm); 0.08 second (PAC)

Rhythm interpretation: Normal sinus rhythm with one PAC (fifth complex); baseline artifact is present (baseline artifact shouldn't be confused with atrial fibrillation)

**Strip 7-57**

Rhythm: Regular

Rate: 225 beats/minute (atrial); 75 beats/minute (ventricular)

P waves: Three flutter waves to each QRS complex

PR interval: Not measurable

QRS complex: 0.06 to 0.08 second

Rhythm interpretation: Atrial flutter with 3:1 AV conduction

**Strip 7-58**

Rhythm: Regular (basic rhythm); irregular (nonconducted PACs)

Rate: 88 beats/minute (basic rhythm); rate slows to 72 beats/minute after a pause (temporary rate suppression is common after a pause in the basic rhythm)

P waves: Sinus (basic rhythm); premature, abnormal P wave without a QRS complex hidden in the T wave after the seventh QRS complex

PR interval: 0.12 to 0.14 second (basic rhythm)

QRS complex: 0.08 to 0.10 second

Rhythm interpretation: Normal sinus rhythm with one nonconducted PAC (after the seventh QRS complex)

**Strip 7-59**

Rhythm: Irregular

Rate: 70 beats/minute

P waves: Vary in size, shape, and direction

PR interval: 0.14 to 0.16 second

QRS complex: 0.06 to 0.08 second

Rhythm interpretation: Wandering atrial pacemaker; T-wave inversion is present.

**Strip 7-60**

Rhythm: Irregular

Rate: 300 beats/minute (atrial); 80 beats/minute (ventricular)

P waves: Flutter waves present before each QRS complex (varying ratios)

PR interval: Not measurable

QRS complex: 0.04 to 0.06 second

Rhythm interpretation: Atrial flutter with variable AV conduction

Strip 7-61
Rhythm: Irregular
Rate: 50 beats/minute
P waves: Fibrillatory waves present
PR interval: Not measurable
QRS complex: 0.06 to 0.08 second
Rhythm interpretation: Atrial fibrillation; some flutter waves present

Strip 7-62
Rhythm: Regular (basic rhythm); irregular (PAC)
Rate: 58 beats/minute (basic rhythm)
P waves: Sinus (basic rhythm); premature, abnormal P wave (PAC)
PR interval: 0.16 to 0.18 second (basic rhythm)
QRS complex: 0.06 to 0.08 second
Rhythm interpretation: Sinus bradycardia with one PAC (fifth complex); a U wave is present.

Strip 7-63
Rhythm: Irregular
Rate: 80 beats/minute (ventricular); atrial not measurable
P waves: Fibrillatory waves present
PR interval: Not measurable
QRS complex: 0.04 to 0.06 second
Rhythm interpretation: Atrial fibrillation; ST-segment depression is present.

Strip 7-64
Rhythm: Regular
Rate: 214 beats/minute
P waves: Hidden in T waves
PR interval: Not measurable
QRS complex: 0.08 second
Rhythm interpretation: Paroxysmal atrial tachycardia

Strip 7-65
Rhythm: Regular (basic rhythm); irregular (PAC)
Rate: 52 beats/minute (basic rhythm)
P waves: Sinus (basic rhythm); premature, pointed P wave associated with PAC hidden in the T wave after the fourth QRS complex
PR interval: 0.16 to 0.18 second
QRS complex: 0.06 to 0.08 second
Rhythm interpretation: Sinus bradycardia with one PAC (fifth complex); a U wave is present.

Strip 7-66
Rhythm: Regular (basic rhythm); irregular (nonconducted PAC)
Rate: 75 beats/minute (basic rhythm)
P waves: Sinus (basic rhythm); premature, abnormal P wave hidden in the T wave after the fourth QRS complex
PR interval: 0.20 second
QRS complex: 0.06 to 0.08 second
Rhythm interpretation: Normal sinus rhythm with one nonconducted PAC (after the fourth QRS complex); a U wave is present.

Strip 7-67
Rhythm: Regular (off by two squares)
Rate: 79 beats/minute
P waves: Vary in size, shape, and direction
PR interval: 0.12 to 0.18 second
QRS complex: 0.08 to 0.10 second
Rhythm interpretation: Wandering atrial pacemaker

Strip 7-68
Rhythm: Regular
Rate: 150 beats/minute
P waves: Hidden in preceding T waves
PR interval: Not measurable
QRS complex: 0.04 to 0.06 second
Rhythm interpretation: Paroxysmal atrial tachycardia; ST-segment depression is present.

Strip 7-69
Rhythm: Irregular
Rate: 250 beats/minute (atrial); 70 beats/minute (ventricular)
P waves: Flutter waves before each QRS complex (varying ratios)
PR interval: Not measurable
QRS complex: 0.06 to 0.08 second
Rhythm interpretation: Atrial flutter with variable AV conduction

Strip 7-70
Rhythm: Irregular
Rate: 130 beats/minute (ventricular); atrial not measurable
P waves: Fibrillatory waves; some flutter waves
PR interval: Not measurable
QRS complex: 0.04 second
Rhythm interpretation: Atrial fibrillation; ST-segment depression is present.

Strip 7-71
Rhythm: Regular (basic rhythm); irregular (PACs)
Rate: 88 beats/minute (basic rhythm)
P waves: Sinus (basic rhythm); premature and abnormal (PACs)
PR interval: 0.14 to 0.16 second (basic rhythm)
QRS complex: 0.06 to 0.08 second
Rhythm interpretation: Normal sinus rhythm with paired PACs (third and fourth complexes)

Strip 7-72
Rhythm: Regular
Rate: 54 beats/minute
P waves: Varying in size and shape
PR interval: 0.12
QRS complex: 0.08 to 0.10 second
Rhythm interpretation: Wandering atrial pacemaker; ST-segment depression is present.

Strip 7-73
Rhythm: Regular
Rate: 272 beats/minute (atrial); 136 beats/minute (ventricular)
P waves: Two flutter waves to each QRS complex
PR interval: Not measurable
QRS complex: 0.08 second
Rhythm interpretation: Atrial flutter with 2:1 AV conduction

Strip 7-74
Rhythm: Regular (basic rhythm); irregular (PAC)
Rate: 63 beats/minute (basic rhythm)
P waves: Sinus (basic rhythm); premature and abnormal (PAC)
PR interval: 0.12 to 0.14 second (basic rhythm); 0.14 second (PAC)
QRS complex: 0.06 to 0.08 second (basic rhythm); 0.08 second (PAC)
Rhythm interpretation: Normal sinus rhythm with one PAC (fourth complex); a small U wave is present.

Strip 7-75
Rhythm: Regular
Rate: 150 beats/minute
P waves: Hidden in T waves
PR interval: Not measurable
QRS complex: 0.06 to 0.08 second
Rhythm interpretation: Paroxysmal atrial tachycardia; ST-segment depression is present.

Strip 7-76
Rhythm: Irregular
Rate: 80 beats/minute (ventricular); atrial not measurable
P waves: Fibrillatory waves present
PR interval: Not measurable
QRS complex: 0.04 second
Rhythm interpretation: Atrial fibrillation; ST-segment depression and T-wave inversion are present.

Strip 7-77
Rhythm: Regular
Rate: 88 beats/minute
P waves: Vary in size, shape, and position
PR interval: 0.12 to 0.14 second
QRS complex: 0.06 to 0.08 second
Rhythm interpretation: Wandering atrial pacemaker; T-wave inversion is present.

Strip 7-78
Rhythm: Irregular
Rate: 50 beats/minute
P waves: Vary in size, shape, and position
PR interval: 0.12 to 0.16 second
QRS complex: 0.08 second
Rhythm interpretation: Wandering atrial pacemaker; ST-segment depression is present.

Strip 7-79
Rhythm: Regular
Rate: 232 beats/minute (atrial); 58 beats/minute (ventricular)
P waves: Four flutter waves to each QRS complex
PR interval: Not measurable
QRS complex: 0.08 second
Rhythm interpretation: Atrial flutter with 4:1 AV conduction

Strip 7-80
Rhythm: Regular (basic rhythm); irregular (nonconducted PACs)
Rate: 107 beats/minute (basic rhythm)
P waves: Sinus (basic rhythm); premature and abnormal (nonconducted PACs)
PR interval: 0.16 to 0.18 second
QRS complex: 0.06 to 0.08 second
Rhythm interpretation: Sinus tachycardia with two nonconducted PACs (after the third and eighth QRS complex)

Strip 7-81
Rhythm: Regular
Rate: 68 beats/minute
P waves: Vary in size, shape, and direction
PR interval: 0.12 to 0.16 second
QRS complex: 0.08 second
Rhythm interpretation: Wandering atrial pacemaker; a U wave is present.

Strip 7-82
Rhythm: Regular
Rate: 240 beats/minute (atrial); 60 beats/minute (ventricular)
P waves: Four flutter waves to each QRS complex
PR interval: Not measurable
QRS complex: 0.06 second
Rhythm interpretation: Atrial flutter with 4:1 AV conduction

Strip 7-83
Rhythm: Regular
Rate: 167 beats/minute
P waves: Hidden in preceding T wave
PR interval: Not measurable
QRS complex: 0.08 to 0.10 second
Rhythm interpretation: Paroxysmal atrial tachycardia

Strip 7-84
Rhythm: Irregular
Rate: 50 beats/minute
P waves: Fibrillatory waves
PR interval: Not measurable
QRS complex: 0.08 to 0.10 second
Rhythm interpretation: Atrial fibrillation

Strip 7-85
Rhythm: Irregular
Rate: 40 beats/minute
P waves: Vary in size, shape, and direction
PR interval: 0.14 to 0.16 second
QRS complex: 0.08 second
Rhythm interpretation: Wandering atrial pacemaker

Strip 7-86
Rhythm: Regular (basic rhythm); irregular (PACs)
Rate: 107 beats/minute (basic rhythm)
P waves: Sinus (basic rhythm); premature and pointed (PACs)
PR interval: 0.16 second (basic rhythm)
QRS complex: 0.06 second
Rhythm interpretation: Sinus tachycardia with three PACs (fourth, ninth, and eleventh complexes)

Strip 7-87
Rhythm: Irregular
Rate: 250 beats/minute (atrial); 40 beats/minute (ventricular)
P waves: Flutter waves before each QRS complex (varying ratios)
PR interval: Not measurable
QRS complex: 0.06 to 0.08 second
Rhythm interpretation: Atrial flutter with variable AV conduction

Strip 7-88
Rhythm: Irregular
Rate: 40 beats/minute (ventricular); atrial not measurable
P waves: Fibrillatory waves present
PR interval: Not measurable
QRS complex: 0.04 to 0.06 second
Rhythm interpretation: Atrial fibrillation; ST-segment depression is present.

Strip 7-89
Rhythm: Regular (basic rhythm); irregular (nonconducted PAC)
Rate: 84 beats/minute (basic rhythm)
P waves: Sinus (basic rhythm); premature and pointed (nonconducted PAC)
PR interval: 0.16 to 0.20 second
QRS complex: 0.06 to 0.08 second
Rhythm interpretation: Normal sinus rhythm with one nonconducted PAC (after the fifth QRS complex); ST-segment depression is present.

Strip 7-90
Rhythm: Regular (basic rhythm); irregular (PAC)
Rate: 54 beats/minute (basic rhythm)
P waves: Sinus (basic rhythm); premature and abnormal (PAC)
PR interval: 0.16 to 0.18 second
QRS complex: 0.06 second
Rhythm interpretation: Sinus bradycardia with one PAC (fourth complex)

Strip 7-91
Rhythm: Regular (basic rhythm); irregular (PAC)
Rate: 63 beats/minute (basic rhythm)
P waves: Sinus (basic rhythm); premature and abnormal (PAC)
PR interval: 0.14 to 0.16 second
QRS complex: 0.06 second
Rhythm interpretation: Normal sinus rhythm with one PAC (fifth complex); a U wave is present.

Strip 7-92
Rhythm: Regular
Rate: 235 beats/minute (atrial); 47 beats/minute (ventricular)
P waves: Five flutter waves to each QRS complex
PR interval: Not discernible
QRS complex: 0.08 second
Rhythm interpretation: Atrial flutter with 5:1 AV conduction; T-wave inversion is present.

Strip 7-93
Rhythm: Regular
Rate: 150 beats/minute
P waves: Pointed
PR interval: Not measurable
QRS complex: 0.06 to 0.08 second
Rhythm interpretation: Paroxysmal atrial tachycardia

Strip 7-94
Rhythm: Irregular
Rate: 50 beats/minute
P waves: Wavy
PR interval: Not measurable
QRS complex: 0.04 to 0.06 second
Rhythm interpretation: Atrial fibrillation

Strip 7-95
Rhythm: Regular (basic rhythm); irregular after a burst of PAT
Rate: 84 beats/minute (basic rhythm)
P waves: Sinus (basic rhythm); abnormal and premature with a run of PAT
PR interval: 0.16 to 0.18 second (basic rhythm); not measurable in PAT
QRS complex: 0.04 to 0.06 second (basic rhythm and PAT)
Rhythm interpretation: Normal sinus rhythm with burst of PAT (three PACs after the fourth QRS complex)

Strip 8-1
Rhythm: Regular (basic rhythm); irregular (PJC)
Rate: 58 beats/minute (basic rhythm)
P waves: Sinus (basic rhythm); premature and inverted (PJC)
PR interval: 0.14 to 0.16 (basic rhythm); 0.08 (PJC)
QRS complex: 0.06 second (basic rhythm and PJC)
Rhythm interpretation: Sinus bradycardia with one PJC (fifth complex); a U wave is present.

Strip 8-2
Rhythm: Regular
Rate: 60 beats/minute
P waves: Sinus
PR interval: 0.24 second
QRS complex: 0.06 to 0.08 second
Rhythm interpretation: Normal sinus rhythm with first-degree AV block; ST-segment elevation and T-wave inversion are present.

Strip 8-3
Rhythm: Regular (atrial and ventricular)
Rate: 46 beats/minute (atrial); 23 beats/minute (ventricular)
P waves: Two sinus P waves before each QRS complex
PR interval: 0.22 to 0.24 second (remains constant)
QRS complex: 0.08 to 0.10 second
Rhythm interpretation: Second-degree AV block, Mobitz II (clinical correlation is suggested to diagnose Mobitz II when 2:1 conduction is present); ST-segment elevation is present.

Strip 8-4
Rhythm: Regular (basic rhythm); irregular (junctional beat)
Rate: 58 beats/minute (basic rhythm)
P waves: Sinus (basic rhythm); hidden P wave (junctional beat)
PR interval: 0.16 to 0.18 second (basic rhythm)
QRS complex: 0.08 to 0.10 second (basic rhythm and junctional beat)
Rhythm interpretation: Sinus bradycardia with junctional escape beat (fourth complex) after pause in basic rhythm; ST-segment depression is present.

Strip 8-5
Rhythm: Regular
Rate: 115 beats/minute
P waves: Inverted
PR interval: 0.08 second
QRS complex: 0.04 to 0.06 second
Rhythm interpretation: Junctional tachycardia

Strip 8-6
Rhythm: Regular
Rate: 84 beats/minute
P waves: Sinus
PR interval: 0.22 to 0.24 second
QRS complex: 0.08 to 0.10 second
Rhythm interpretation: Normal sinus rhythm with first-degree AV block

Strip 8-7
Rhythm: Regular
Rate: 65 beats/minute
P waves: Inverted before each QRS complex
PR interval: 0.08 second
QRS complex: 0.06 to 0.08 second
Rhythm interpretation: Accelerated junctional rhythm;
ST-segment elevation and T-wave inversion are present.

Strip 8-8
Rhythm: Regular (atrial); irregular (ventricular)
Rate: 75 beats/minute (atrial); 70 beats/minute (ventricular)
P waves: Sinus; one P wave without a QRS complex
PR interval: Lengthens from 0.28 to 0.32 second
QRS complex: 0.04 to 0.08 second
Rhythm interpretation: Second-degree AV block, Mobitz I;
ST-segment depression and T-wave inversion are present.

Strip 8-9
Rhythm: Regular
Rate: 47 beats/minute
P waves: Hidden in QRS complex
PR interval: Not measurable
QRS complex: 0.08 second
Rhythm interpretation: Junctional rhythm; ST-segment
depression is present.

Strip 8-10
Rhythm: Regular (atrial); irregular (ventricular)
Rate: 75 beats/minute (atrial); 30 beats/minute (ventricular)
P waves: Two sinus P waves before each QRS complex
PR interval: 0.20 to 0.22 second
QRS complex: 0.08 to 0.10 second
Rhythm interpretation: Second-degree AV block, Mobitz II
(clinical correlation is suggested to diagnose Mobitz II
when 2:1 conduction is present); ST-segment depression
is present.

Strip 8-11
Rhythm: Regular (atrial and ventricular)
Rate: 63 beats/minute (atrial); 33 beats/minute (ventricular)
P waves: Sinus (bear no relationship to the QRS complex;
found hidden in the QRS complex and T waves)
PR interval: Varies greatly
QRS complex: 0.12 second
Rhythm interpretation: Third-degree AV block; ST-
segment depression and T-wave inversion are present.

Strip 8-12
Rhythm: Regular
Rate: 84 beats/minute
P waves: Hidden in the QRS complex
PR interval: Not measurable
QRS complex: 0.06 to 0.08 second
Rhythm interpretation: Accelerated junctional rhythm;
ST-segment depression is present.

Strip 8-13
Rhythm: Regular
Rate: 65 beats/minute
P waves: Sinus
PR interval: 0.44 to 0.48 second
QRS complex: 0.08 to 0.10 second
Rhythm interpretation: Normal sinus rhythm with first-
degree AV block; an elevated ST-segment is present.

Strip 8-14
Rhythm: Regular (basic rhythm); irregular (PJC)
Rate: 136 beats/minute (basic rhythm)
P waves: Sinus (basic rhythm); hidden P wave (PJC)
PR interval: 0.12 to 0.14 second
QRS complex: 0.04 to 0.06 second
Rhythm interpretation: Sinus tachycardia with one PJC
(thirteenth complex)

Strip 8-15
Rhythm: Regular
Rate: 94 beats/minute
P waves: Sinus
PR interval: 0.26 to 0.28 second
QRS complex: 0.06 second
Rhythm interpretation: Normal sinus rhythm with first-
degree AV block; ST-segment depression is present.

Strip 8-16
Rhythm: Regular (basic rhythm); irregular (premature beat)
Rate: 58 beats/minute (basic rhythm)
P waves: Sinus (basic rhythm); inverted (premature beat)
PR interval: 0.16 to 0.18 second (basic rhythm); 0.08 second (PJC)
QRS complex: 0.06 to 0.08 second
Rhythm interpretation: Sinus bradycardia with one PJC
(fourth complex); ST-segment depression is present.

Strip 8-17
Rhythm: Regular (atrial and ventricular)
Rate: 108 beats/minute (atrial); 54 beats/minute (ventricular)
P waves: Two P waves to each QRS complex
PR interval: 0.20 second and constant
QRS complex: 0.08 to 0.10 second
Rhythm interpretation: Second-degree AV block Mobitz II (clinical correlation is suggested to diagnose Mobitz II when 2:1 conduction is present); ST-segment elevation and T-wave inversion are present.

Strip 8-18
Rhythm: Regular (atrial); irregular (ventricular)
Rate: 65 beats/minute (atrial); 50 beats/minute (ventricular)
P waves: Sinus; one P wave without a QRS complex
PR interval: Lengthens from 0.20 to 0.48 second
QRS complex: 0.04 second
Rhythm interpretation: Second-degree AV block, Mobitz I

Strip 8-19
Rhythm: Regular
Rate: 125 beats/minute
P waves: Inverted before each QRS complex
PR interval: 0.08 to 0.10 second
QRS complex: 0.06 second
Rhythm interpretation: Junctional tachycardia

Strip 8-20
Rhythm: Regular (atrial and ventricular)
Rate: 100 beats/minute (atrial); 38 beats/minute (ventricular)
P waves: Sinus (bear no relationship to the QRS complex; found hidden in the QRS complex and T waves)
PR interval: Varies greatly
QRS complex: 0.06 to 0.08 second
Rhythm interpretation: Third-degree AV block; ST-segment depression is present.

Strip 8-21
Rhythm: Regular (basic rhythm); irregular (PJC)
Rate: 60 beats/minute (basic rhythm)
P waves: Sinus (basic rhythm); premature and inverted (PJC)
PR interval: 0.12 to 0.14 second (basic rhythm); 0.08 second (PJC)
QRS complex: 0.08 second (basic rhythm and PJC)
Rhythm interpretation: Normal sinus rhythm with one PJC (fourth complex)

Strip 8-22
Rhythm: Regular (atrial and ventricular)
Rate: 100 beats/minute (atrial); 50 beats/minute (ventricular)
P waves: Two sinus P waves before each QRS complex
PR interval: 0.16 second and constant
QRS complex: 0.08 second
Rhythm interpretation: Second-degree AV block, Mobitz II (clinical correlation is suggested to diagnose Mobitz II when 2:1 conduction is present)

Strip 8-23
Rhythm: Regular
Rate: 35 beats/minute
P waves: Sinus
PR interval: 0.60 to 0.62 second (remains constant)
QRS complex: 0.06 second
Rhythm interpretation: Sinus bradycardia with first-degree AV block

Strip 8-24
Rhythm: Regular (atrial); irregular (ventricular)
Rate: 68 beats/minute (atrial); 60 beats/minute (ventricular)
P waves: Sinus; one without a QRS complex
PR interval: 0.28 to 0.36 second
QRS complex: 0.08 second
Rhythm interpretation: Second-degree AV block, Mobitz I; a U wave is present.

Strip 8-25
Rhythm: Regular
Rate: 75 beats/minute
P waves: Sinus
PR interval: 0.28 second
QRS complex: 0.08 second
Rhythm interpretation: Sinus rhythm with first-degree AV block

Strip 8-26
Rhythm: Regular (basic rhythm); irregular (PJCs)
Rate: 100 beats/minute (basic rhythm)
P waves: Sinus (basic rhythm); premature and inverted (PJCs)
PR interval: 0.20 second (basic rhythm); 0.06 second (PJCs)
QRS complex: 0.06 to 0.08 second (basic rhythm and PJCs)
Rhythm interpretation: Normal sinus rhythm with paired PJCs (eighth and ninth complexes); ST-segment depression is present.

Strip 8-27
Rhythm: Regular
Rate: 65 beats/minute
P waves: Inverted before each QRS complex
PR interval: 0.08 second
QRS complex: 0.08 second
Rhythm interpretation: Accelerated junctional rhythm;
elevated ST segment is present.

Strip 8-28
Rhythm: Regular (basic rhythm); irregular (nonconduct-
ed PAC)
Rate: 56 beats/minute (basic rhythm)
P waves: Sinus (basic rhythm); premature, abnormal P
wave without a QRS complex
PR interval: 0.24 to 0.26 second (remains constant)
QRS complex: 0.08 second
Rhythm interpretation: Sinus bradycardia with first-
degree AV block and nonconducted PAC (follows the 4th
QRS complex); ST-segment depression is present.

Strip 8-29
Rhythm: Regular (atrial); irregular (ventricular)
Rate: 63 beats/minute (atrial); 50 beats/minute (ventricu-
lar)
P waves: Sinus
PR interval: Progressively lengthens from 0.28 to 0.32
second
QRS complex: 0.06 to 0.08 second
Rhythm interpretation: Second-degree AV block, Mobitz I;
ST-segment depression is present.

Strip 8-30
Rhythm: Regular (atrial and ventricular)
Rate: 79 beats/minute (atrial); 32 beats/minute (ventricu-
lar)
P waves: Sinus (bear no relationship to the QRS complex;
found hidden in the QRS complex and T waves)
PR interval: Varies greatly
QRS complex: 0.12 second
Rhythm interpretation: Third-degree AV block

Strip 8-31
Rhythm: Regular (atrial and ventricular)
Rate: 84 beats/minute (atrial); 28 beats/minute (ventricu-
lar)
P waves: Three sinus P waves to each QRS complex
PR interval: 0.28 to 0.32 (remains constant)
QRS complex: 0.08 second
Rhythm interpretation: Second-degree AV block, Mobitz II

Strip 8-32
Rhythm: Regular (atrial and ventricular)
Rate: 75 beats/minute (atrial); 34 beats/minute (ventricu-
lar)
P waves: Sinus (bear no relationship to the QRS complex;
found hidden in the QRS complex and T waves)
PR interval: Varies greatly
QRS complex: 0.12 to 0.14 second
Rhythm interpretation: Third-degree AV block; ST-
segment elevation is present.

Strip 8-33
Rhythm: Regular (basic rhythm); irregular (PAC)
Rate: 100 beats/minute (basic rhythm)
P waves: Inverted before the QRS complex (basic rhythm);
upright and pointed (PAC)
PR interval: 0.08 second (basic rhythm); 0.12 second
(PAC)
QRS complex: 0.08 second (basic rhythm and PAC)
Rhythm interpretation: Accelerated junctional rhythm
with one PAC (sixth complex); ST-segment depression is
present.

Strip 8-34
Rhythm: Regular (atrial); irregular (ventricular)
Rate: 75 beats/minute (atrial); 50 beats/minute (ventricu-
lar)
P waves: Sinus; two P waves without a QRS complex
PR interval: 0.28 to 0.40 second
QRS complex: 0.08 to 0.10 second
Rhythm interpretation: Second-degree AV block, Mobitz I

Strip 8-35
Rhythm: Regular
Rate: 60 beats/minute
P waves: Sinus
PR interval: 0.24 to 0.26 second
QRS complex: 0.06 to 0.08 second
Rhythm interpretation: Normal sinus rhythm with first-
degree AV block

Strip 8-36
Rhythm: Regular
Rate: 41 beats/minute
P waves: Inverted after the QRS complex
PR interval: 0.04 to 0.06 second
QRS complex: 0.06 to 0.08 second
Rhythm interpretation: Junctional rhythm

Strip 8-37
Rhythm: Regular (basic rhythm); irregular (PJCs)
Rate: 58 beats/minute (basic rhythm)
P waves: Sinus (basic rhythm); premature and inverted (PJCs)
PR interval: 0.16 second (basic rhythm); 0.08 to 0.10 second (PJCs)
QRS complex: 0.08 second (basic rhythm and PJCs)
Rhythm interpretation: Sinus bradycardia with two PJCs (fourth and sixth complexes); a U wave is present.

Strip 8-38
Rhythm: Regular (atrial and ventricular)
Rate: 66 beats/minute (atrial); 33 beats/minute (ventricular)
P waves: Two sinus P waves to each QRS complex
PR interval: 0.44 second (remains constant)
QRS complex: 0.14 to 0.16 second
Rhythm interpretation: Second-degree AV block, Mobitz II (clinical correlation is suggested to diagnose Mobitz II when 2:1 conduction is present)

Strip 8-39
Rhythm: Regular (atrial and ventricular)
Rate: 52 beats/minute (atrial); 26 beats/minute (ventricular)
P waves: Two sinus P waves before each QRS complex
PR interval: 0.22 (remains constant)
QRS complex: 0.12 second
Rhythm interpretation: Second-degree AV block, Mobitz II (clinical correlation is suggested to diagnose Mobitz II when 2:1 conduction is present)

Strip 8-40
Rhythm: Regular (atrial); irregular (ventricular)
Rate: 107 beats/minute (atrial); 50 beats/minute (ventricular)
P waves: Sinus (bear no relationship to QRS complex; found hidden in the QRS complex and T waves)
PR interval: Varies greatly
QRS complex: 0.08 second
Rhythm interpretation: Third-degree AV block

Strip 8-41
Rhythm: Regular
Rate: 68 beats/minute
P waves: Inverted before each QRS complex
PR interval: 0.08 second
QRS complex: 0.06 to 0.08 second
Rhythm interpretation: Accelerated junctional rhythm

Strip 8-42
Rhythm: Regular (atrial and ventricular)
Rate: 104 beats/minute (atrial); 52 beats/minute (ventricular)
P waves: Two sinus P waves to each QRS complex
PR interval: 0.24 second and constant
QRS complex: 0.06 to 0.08 second
Rhythm interpretation: Second-degree AV block, Mobitz II (clinical correlation is suggested to diagnose Mobitz II when 2:1 conduction is present); ST-segment elevation and T-wave inversion are present.

Strip 8-43
Rhythm: Irregular (first rhythm); regular (second rhythm)
Rate: 80 beats/minute (first rhythm); 42 beats/minute (second rhythm)
P waves: Fibrillatory waves (first rhythm); hidden P waves (second rhythm)
PR interval: Not measurable in either rhythm
QRS complex: 0.06 to 0.08 second
Rhythm interpretation: Atrial fibrillation to junctional rhythm; ST-segment depression is present.

Strip 8-44
Rhythm: Regular (basic rhythm); irregular (premature beats)
Rate: 60 beats/minute (basic rhythm)
P waves: Sinus (basic rhythm); premature and abnormal (premature beats)
PR interval: 0.12 to 0.16 second (basic rhythm); 0.12 second (PAC); 0.08 second (PJC)
QRS complex: 0.06 to 0.08 second
Rhythm interpretation: Normal sinus rhythm with one PAC (fourth complex) and one PJC (fifth complex); ST-segment depression and T-wave inversion are present.

Strip 8-45
Rhythm: Regular (atrial and ventricular)
Rate: 72 beats/minute (atrial); 32 beats/minute (ventricular)
P waves: Sinus (bear no relationship to the QRS complex; hidden in the QRS complex and T waves)
PR interval: Varies greatly
QRS complex: 0.12 second
Rhythm interpretation: Third-degree AV block; ST-segment elevation is present.

Strip 8-46
Rhythm: Irregular
Rate: 40 beats/minute
P waves: Sinus
PR interval: 0.28 second (remains constant)
QRS complex: 0.08 to 0.10 second
Rhythm interpretation: Sinus arrhythmia with bradycardic rate and first-degree AV block; a U wave is present.

Strip 8-47
Rhythm: Regular (atrial); irregular (ventricular)
Rate: 79 beats/minute (atrial); 50 beats/minute (ventricular)
P waves: Sinus
PR interval: Lengthens from 0.24 to 0.40 second
QRS complex: 0.08 to 0.10 second
Rhythm interpretation: Second-degree AV block, Mobitz I

Strip 8-48
Rhythm: Regular (atrial and ventricular)
Rate: 108 beats/minute (atrial); 54 beats/minute (ventricular)
P waves: Two sinus P waves before each QRS complex
PR interval: 0.18 to 0.20 second (remains constant)
QRS complex: 0.08 second
Rhythm interpretation: Second-degree AV block, Mobitz II (clinical correlation is suggested to diagnose Mobitz II when 2:1 conduction is present); ST-segment elevation and T-wave inversion are present.

Strip 8-49
Rhythm: Irregular
Rate: 40 beats/minute
P waves: Inverted before each QRS complex
PR interval: 0.04 to 0.06 second
QRS complex: 0.08 to 0.10 second
Rhythm interpretation: Junctional rhythm; ST-segment depression is present.

Strip 8-50
Rhythm: Regular (basic rhythm); irregular (escape beat)
Rate: 84 beats/minute (basic rhythm); slows to 75 beats/minute after escape beat (temporary rate suppression can occur after premature or escape beats; after several cycles rate will return to basic rate)
P waves: Sinus; P wave hidden with escape beat
PR interval: 0.14 to 0.16 second
QRS complex: 0.06 to 0.08 second
Rhythm interpretation: Normal sinus rhythm with junctional escape beat (fifth complex) after a pause in the basic rhythm; a U wave is present.

Strip 8-51
Rhythm: Irregular (atrial); regular (ventricular)
Rate: 70 beats/minute (atrial); 25 beats/minute (ventricular)
P waves: Sinus (bear no relationship to the QRS complex)
PR interval: Varies greatly
QRS complex: 0.12 second
Rhythm interpretation: Third-degree AV block

Strip 8-52
Rhythm: Regular
Rate: 63 beats/minute
P waves: Hidden in the QRS complex
PR interval: Not measurable
QRS complex: 0.08 second
Rhythm interpretation: Accelerated junctional rhythm

Strip 8-53
Rhythm: Regular (atrial and ventricular)
Rate: 76 beats/minute (atrial); 38 beats/minute (ventricular)
P waves: Two sinus P waves before each QRS complex
PR interval: 0.24 to 0.26 second
QRS complex: 0.12 to 0.14 second
Rhythm interpretation: Second-degree AV block, Mobitz II (clinical correlation is suggested to diagnose Mobitz II when 2:1 conduction is present)

Strip 8-54
Rhythm: Regular
Rate: 94 beats/minute
P waves: Inverted before the QRS complex
PR interval: 0.08 second
QRS complex: 0.06 to 0.08 second
Rhythm interpretation: Accelerated junctional rhythm

Strip 8-55
Rhythm: Regular (basic rhythm)
Rate: 55 beats/minute (basic rhythm)
P waves: Sinus (basic rhythm); notched P waves usually indicate left atrial hypertrophy; no P wave seen with fourth complex; fifth complex has a P wave on top of the preceding T wave
PR interval: 0.20 second (basic rhythm)
QRS complex: 0.06 to 0.08 second
Rhythm interpretation: Sinus bradycardia with one junctional escape beat (fourth complex) and one PAC (fifth complex); both follow a pause in the basic rhythm.

Strip 8-56
Rhythm: Regular (first and second rhythms)
Rate: 72 beats/minute (first rhythm); about 140 beats/minute (second rhythm)
P waves: Sinus (first rhythm); inverted (second rhythm)
PR interval: 0.12 second (first rhythm); 0.08 to 0.10 second (second rhythm)
QRS complex: 0.08 second
Rhythm interpretation: Normal sinus rhythm changing to junctional tachycardia; ST-segment depression is present.

Strip 8-57
Rhythm: Regular
Rate: 84 beats/minute
P waves: Sinus
PR interval: 0.30 to 0.32 second (remains constant)
QRS complex: 0.04 to 0.06 second
Rhythm interpretation: Normal sinus rhythm with first-degree AV block; ST-segment elevation is present.

Strip 8-58
Rhythm: Regular (atrial and ventricular)
Rate: 75 beats/minute (atrial); 30 beats/minute (ventricular)
P waves: Sinus (bear no relationship to the QRS complex)
PR interval: Varies greatly
QRS complex: 0.12 to 0.14 second
Rhythm interpretation: Third-degree AV block

Strip 8-59
Rhythm: Regular (atrial and ventricular)
Rate: 93 beats/minute (atrial); 31 beats/minute (ventricular)
P waves: Three sinus waves to each QRS complex (one hidden in T wave)
PR interval: 0.32 to 0.36 second
QRS complex: 0.08 second
Rhythm interpretation: Second-degree AV block, Mobitz II; ST-segment depression is present.

Strip 8-60
Rhythm: Regular (basic rhythm); irregular (premature beats)
Rate: 60 beats/minute (basic rhythm)
P waves: Sinus (basic rhythm); premature and abnormal (premature beats)
PR interval: 0.12 second (basic rhythm); 0.12 second (PAC); 0.08 to 0.10 second (PJCs)
QRS complex: 0.08 second
Rhythm interpretation: Normal sinus rhythm with one PAC (third complex) and paired PJCs (sixth and seventh complexes)

Strip 8-61
Rhythm: Regular
Rate: 47 beats/minute
P waves: Hidden in the QRS complex
PR interval: Not measurable
QRS complex: 0.08 second
Rhythm interpretation: Junctional rhythm

Strip 8-62
Rhythm: Regular (basic rhythm); irregular (nonconducted PAC)
Rate: 79 beats/minute (basic rhythm); slows to 63 beats/minute after a pause (temporary rate suppression is common after a pause in the basic rhythm)
P waves: Sinus (basic rhythm); premature, pointed P wave distorting T wave after the sixth QRS complex
PR interval: 0.24 second (remains constant)
QRS complex: 0.08 second
Rhythm interpretation: Normal sinus rhythm with first-degree AV block; a nonconducted PAC is present after the sixth QRS complex

Strip 8-63
Rhythm: Regular (atrial); irregular (ventricular)
Rate: 75 beats/minute (atrial); 50 beats/minute (ventricular)
P waves: Sinus
PR interval: Lengthens from 0.24 to 0.32 second
QRS complex: 0.08 second
Rhythm interpretation: Second-degree AV block, Mobitz I

Strip 8-64
Rhythm: Regular (atrial and ventricular)
Rate: 72 beats/minute (atrial); 31 beats/minute (ventricular)
P waves: Sinus (bear no relationship to the QRS complex; hidden in the QRS complex and T waves)
PR interval: Varies greatly
QRS complex: 0.12 second
Rhythm interpretation: Third-degree AV block

Strip 8-65
Rhythm: Regular (atrial and ventricular)
Rate: 90 beats/minute (atrial); 45 beats/minute (ventricular)
P waves: Two sinus waves to each QRS complex
PR interval: 0.26 to 0.28 second (remains constant)
QRS complex: 0.12 second
Rhythm interpretation: Second-degree AV block, Mobitz II (clinical correlation is suggested to diagnose Mobitz II when 2:1 conduction is present); ST-segment elevation is present.

Strip 8-66
Rhythm: Regular
Rate: 79 beats/minute
P waves: Inverted before each QRS complex
PR interval: 0.08 to 0.10 second
QRS complex: 0.06 to 0.08 second
Rhythm interpretation: Accelerated junctional rhythm

Strip 8-67
Rhythm: Regular
Rate: 94 beats/minute
P waves: Sinus
PR interval: 0.24 second
QRS complex: 0.08 second
Rhythm interpretation: Normal sinus rhythm with first-degree AV block

Strip 8-68
Rhythm: Regular (basic rhythm); irregular (premature beats)
Rate: 72 beats/minute (basic rhythm)
P waves: Sinus (basic rhythm); premature and abnormal (premature beats)
PR interval: 0.14 to 0.16 second (basic rhythm); 0.12 second (PACs); 0.10 second (PJC)
QRS complex: 0.06 to 0.08 second
Rhythm interpretation: Normal sinus rhythm with two PACs (third and eighth complex) and one PJC (fifth complex); a U wave is present.

Strip 8-69
Rhythm: Regular (basic rhythm); irregular (premature beats)
Rate: 52 beats/minute (basic rhythm)
P waves: Hidden (basic rhythm); premature and abnormal (premature beats)
PR interval: Not measurable (basic rhythm); 0.12 to 0.14 second (PACs)
QRS complex: 0.06 to 0.08 second
Rhythm interpretation: Junctional rhythm with two PACs (second and fifth complex); ST-segment depression is present.

Strip 8-70
Rhythm: Regular (atrial); irregular (ventricular)
Rate: 79 beats/minute (atrial); 70 beats/minute (ventricular)
P waves: Sinus
PR interval: Lengthens from 0.24 to 0.28 second
QRS complex: 0.08 second
Rhythm interpretation: Second-degree AV block, Mobitz I

Strip 8-71
Rhythm: Regular (atrial and ventricular)
Rate: 80 beats/minute (atrial); 40 beats/minute (ventricular)
P waves: Two sinus P waves to each QRS complex
PR interval: 0.24 second (remains constant)
QRS complex: 0.04 to 0.06 second
Rhythm interpretation: Second-degree AV block, Mobitz II (clinical correlation is suggested to diagnose Mobitz II when 2:1 conduction is present); ST-segment depression is present.

Strip 8-72
Rhythm: Regular (atrial and ventricular)
Rate: 94 beats/minute (atrial); 40 beats/minute (ventricular)
P waves: Sinus (bear no relationship to the QRS complex; hidden in the QRS complex and T waves)
PR interval: Varies greatly
QRS complex: 0.10 second
Rhythm interpretation: Third-degree AV block

Strip 8-73
Rhythm: Regular
Rate: 84 beats/minute
P waves: Hidden in QRS complexes
PR interval: Not measurable
QRS complex: 0.06 second
Rhythm interpretation: Accelerated junctional rhythm; ST-segment depression and T-wave inversion are present.

Strip 8-74
Rhythm: Regular (atrial); irregular (ventricular)
Rate: 54 beats/minute (atrial); 50 beats/minute (ventricular)
P waves: Sinus
PR interval: Lengthens from 0.34 to 0.44 second
QRS complex: 0.08 second
Rhythm interpretation: Second-degree AV block, Mobitz I

Strip 8-75
Rhythm: Regular (basic rhythm); irregular (escape beat)
Rate: 58 beats/minute (basic rhythm)
P waves: Sinus (basic rhythm); hidden P wave (escape beat)
PR interval: 0.16 to 0.18 second
QRS complex: 0.08 to 0.10 second
Rhythm interpretation: Sinus bradycardia with junctional escape beat (fourth complex) after a pause in the basic rhythm

Strip 8-76
Rhythm: Regular
Rate: 47 beats/minute
P waves: Hidden in the QRS complex
PR interval: Not measurable
QRS complex: 0.06 to 0.08 second
Rhythm interpretation: Junctional rhythm; ST-segment depression is present.

Strip 8-77
Rhythm: Regular (atrial and ventricular)
Rate: 94 beats/minute (atrial); 44 beats/minute (ventricular)
P waves: Sinus (bear no relationship to the QRS complex; found hidden in the QRS complex and T waves)
PR interval: Varies greatly
QRS complex: 0.14 to 0.16 second
Rhythm interpretation: Third-degree AV block; ST-segment elevation is present.

Strip 8-78
Rhythm: Regular (basic rhythm); irregular (premature beats)
Rate: 68 beats/minute (basic rhythm)
P waves: Sinus (basic rhythm); premature, abnormal P waves (premature beats)
PR interval: 0.12 to 0.14 second (basic rhythm); 0.14 second (PAC); 0.10 second (PJC)
QRS complex: 0.06 to 0.08 second
Rhythm interpretation: Normal sinus rhythm with one PAC (third complex) and one PJC (seventh complex); a U wave is present.

Strip 8-79
Rhythm: Regular (atrial and ventricular)
Rate: 80 beats/minute (atrial); 40 beats/minute (ventricular)
P waves: Two P waves to each QRS complex
PR interval: 0.12 to 0.14 second (remain constant)
QRS complex: 0.06 to 0.08 second
Rhythm interpretation: Second-degree AV block, Mobitz II (clinical correlation is suggested to diagnose Mobitz II when 2:1 conduction is present)

Strip 8-80
Rhythm: Regular (basic rhythm); irregular (nonconducted PAC)
Rate: 72 beats/minute (basic rhythm)
P waves: Sinus (basic rhythm); premature, pointed P wave without a QRS complex after the sixth QRS complex
PR interval: 0.22 to 0.24 second (remains constant)
QRS complex: 0.04 to 0.06 second
Rhythm interpretation: Normal sinus rhythm with first-degree AV block and one nonconducted PAC (after the sixth QRS complex); ST-segment depression and T-wave inversion are present.

Strip 8-81
Rhythm: Regular
Rate: 88 beats/minute
P waves: Inverted before each QRS complex
PR interval: 0.08 second
QRS complex: 0.06 to 0.08 second
Rhythm interpretation: Accelerated junctional rhythm

Strip 8-82
Rhythm: regular (atrial); irregular (ventricular)
Rate: 75 beats/minute (atrial); 50 beats/minute (ventricular)
P waves: Sinus P waves present
PR interval: Lengthens from 0.26 to 0.40 second
QRS complex: 0.06 to 0.08 second
Rhythm interpretation: Second-degree AV block, Mobitz I; ST-depression is present.

Strip 8-83
Rhythm: Regular
Rate: 107 beats/minute
P waves: Inverted before each QRS complex
PR interval: 0.08 second
QRS complex: 0.08 to 0.10 second
Rhythm interpretation: Junctional tachycardia

Strip 8-84
Rhythm: Two separate rhythms, both regular
Rate: 79 beats/minute (first rhythm); 84 beats/minute (second rhythm)
P waves: Sinus (first rhythm); inverted (second rhythm)
PR interval: 0.14 to 0.16 second (first rhythm); 0.08 second (second rhythm)
QRS complex: 0.06 to 0.08 second (both rhythms)
Rhythm interpretation: Normal sinus rhythm changing to accelerated junctional rhythm

Strip 8-85
Rhythm: Regular (atrial and ventricular)
Rate: 79 beats/minute (atrial); 31 beats/minute (ventricular)
P waves: Sinus (bear no relationship to the QRS complex; hidden in QRS complexes and T waves)
PR interval: Varies greatly
QRS complex: 0.12 second
Rhythm interpretation: Third-degree AV block

Strip 8-86
Rhythm: Regular
Rate: 60 beats/minute
P waves: Sinus P waves present
PR interval: 0.24 second
QRS complex: 0.08 second
Rhythm interpretation: Normal sinus rhythm with first-degree AV block; ST-segment depression and T-wave inversion are present.

Strip 8-87
Rhythm: Regular (atrial and ventricular)
Rate: 88 beats/minute (atrial); 33 beats/minute (ventricular)
P waves: Sinus (bear no relationship to the QRS complex; found hidden in the QRS complex and T waves)
PR interval: Varies greatly
QRS complex: 0.12 to 0.14 second
Rhythm interpretation: Third-degree AV block

Strip 8-88
Rhythm: Regular (basic rhythm); irregular (premature and escape beats)
Rate: 60 beats/minute (basic rhythm)
P waves: Sinus (basic rhythm); pointed (atrial beat); inverted (junctional beats)
PR interval: 0.12 to 0.14 second (basic rhythm); 0.14 second (atrial beat); 0.08 to 0.10 second (junctional beat)
QRS complex: 0.06 to 0.08 second
Rhythm interpretation: Normal sinus rhythm with one PJC (third complex), one atrial escape beat (fourth complex), and one junctional escape beat (fifth complex)

Strip 8-89
Rhythm: Regular (atrial); irregular (ventricular)
Rate: 65 beats/minute (atrial); 50 beats/minute (ventricular)
P waves: Sinus
PR interval: Lengthens from 0.32 to 0.40 second
QRS complex: 0.08 to 0.10 second
Rhythm interpretation: Second-degree AV block, Mobitz I

Strip 8-90
Rhythm: Regular
Rate: 107 beats/minute
P waves: Inverted before each QRS complex
PR interval: 0.08 to 0.10 second
QRS complex: 0.06 second
Rhythm interpretation: Junctional tachycardia

Strip 8-91
Rhythm: Regular (basic rhythm); irregular (nonconducted PAC)
Rate: 88 beats/minute (basic rhythm)
P waves: Sinus (basic rhythm); premature pointed P wave deforming T wave after the sixth QRS complex; pointed, abnormal P wave with the seventh QRS complex
PR interval: 0.22 to 0.24 second (remains constant)
QRS complex: 0.06 to 0.08 second
Rhythm interpretation: Normal sinus rhythm with first-degree AV block; nonconducted PAC (after the sixth QRS complex); an atrial escape beat (seventh complex) occurs during the pause after the nonconducted PAC (note different P wave when compared with that of underlying rhythm).

Strip 8-92
Rhythm: Regular (atrial); irregular (ventricular)
Rate: 75 beats/minute (atrial); 30 beats/minute (ventricular)
P waves: Sinus (two to three before each QRS complex)
PR interval: 0.16 second (remains constant)
QRS complex: 0.12 second
Rhythm interpretation: Second-degree AV block, Mobitz II; ST-segment depression is present.

Strip 8-93
Rhythm: Regular
Rate: 65 beats/minute
P waves: Inverted before each QRS complex
PR interval: 0.08 to 0.10 second
QRS complex: 0.06 second
Rhythm interpretation: Accelerated junctional rhythm; ST-segment elevation is present.

Strip 8-94
Rhythm: Regular (basic rhythm); irregular (PJCs)
Rate: 72 beats/minute (basic rhythm)
P waves: Sinus (basic rhythm); inverted (PJCs)
PR interval: 0.14 second (basic rhythm); 0.08 second (PJCs)
QRS complex: 0.08 second
Rhythm interpretation: Normal sinus rhythm with two PJCs (fourth and sixth complex)

Strip 8-95
Rhythm: Regular (atrial and ventricular)
Rate: 90 beats/minute (atrial); 45 beats/minute (ventricular)
P waves: Two sinus P waves before each QRS complex
PR interval: 0.16 second (remains constant)
QRS complex: 0.12 second
Rhythm interpretation: Second-degree AV block, Mobitz II (clinical correlation is suggested to diagnose Mobitz II when 2:1 conduction is present); T-wave inversion is present.

Strip 8-96
Rhythm: Regular (atrial); irregular (ventricular)
Rate: 75 beats/minute (atrial); 70 beats/minute (ventricular)
P waves: Sinus
PR interval: Lengthens from 0.32 to 0.40 second
QRS complex: 0.04 to 0.06 second
Rhythm interpretation: Second-degree AV block, Mobitz I

Strip 8-97
Rhythm: Regular
Rate: 40 beats/minute
P waves: Hidden in the QRS complex
PR interval: Not measurable
QRS complex: 0.10 second
Rhythm interpretation: Junctional rhythm; ST-segment elevation is present.

Strip 8-98
Rhythm: Regular (atrial and ventricular)
Rate: 80 beats/minute (atrial); 40 beats/minute (ventricular)
P waves: Two sinus P waves to each QRS complex
PR interval: 0.22 to 0.24 second (remains constant)
QRS complex: 0.10 second
Rhythm interpretation: Second-degree AV block, Mobitz II (clinical correlation is suggested to diagnose Mobitz II when 2:1 conduction is present); ST-segment elevation is present.

Strip 8-99
Rhythm: Regular (basic rhythm); irregular (PJC)
Rate: 84 beats/minute (basic rhythm)
P waves: Sinus (basic rhythm); inverted (PJC)
PR interval: 0.12 second (basic rhythm); 0.08 second (PJC)
QRS complex: 0.06 to 0.08 second
Rhythm interpretation: Normal sinus rhythm with one PJC

Strip 8-100
Rhythm: Regular (basic rhythm); irregular after PJC and run of PJT
Rate: 100 beats/minute (basic rhythm); 136 beats/minute (PJT)
P waves: Sinus (basic rhythm); inverted (PJC and PJT)
PR interval: 0.12 to 0.14 second (basic rhythm); 0.08 second (PJC and PJT)
QRS complex: 0.06 to 0.08 second (basic rhythm); 0.08 to 0.10 second (PJC and PJT)
Rhythm interpretation: Normal sinus rhythm with one PJC (fifth complex) and a three-beat run of PJT (eighth, ninth, and tenth complexes)

Strip 8-101
Rhythm: Regular
Rate: 44 beats/minute
P waves: Hidden in the QRS complex
PR interval: Not measurable
QRS complex: 0.08 to 0.10 second
Rhythm interpretation: Junctional rhythm

Strip 9-1
Rhythm: Regular
Rate: 167 beats/minute
P waves: Absent
PR interval: Not measurable
QRS complex: 0.12 to 0.14 second
Rhythm interpretation: Ventricular tachycardia

Strip 9-2
Rhythm: Regular
Rate: 65 beats/minute
P waves: Sinus; notched P waves usually indicate left atrial hypertrophy
PR interval: 0.14 to 0.16 second
QRS complex: 0.12 to 0.14 second
Rhythm interpretation: Normal sinus rhythm with bundle-branch block; an elevated ST-segment is present.

Strip 9-3
Rhythm: Regular (basic rhythm); irregular (PVCs)
Rate: 75 beats/minute (basic rhythm)
P waves: Sinus (basic rhythm); no P waves associated with PVCs; sinus P waves can be seen after the PVCs
PR interval: 0.18 to 0.20 second
QRS complex: 0.08 second (basic rhythm); 0.12 second (PVCs)
Rhythm interpretation: Normal sinus rhythm with two unifocal PVCs (fifth complex and eighth complex)

Strip 9-4
Rhythm: Irregular
Rate: 30 beats/minute
P waves: Absent
PR interval: Not measurable
QRS complex: 0.16 second
Rhythm interpretation: Idioventricular rhythm

Strip 9-5
Rhythm: 0
Rate: Not measurable
P waves: Chaotic wave deflection of varying height, size, and shape
PR interval: Not measurable
QRS complex: Absent
Rhythm interpretation: Ventricular fibrillation

Strip 9-6
Rhythm: Regular (basic rhythm); irregular (PVCs)
Rate: 100 beats/minute (basic rhythm)
P waves: Sinus (basic rhythm)
PR interval: 0.14 to 0.16 second (basic rhythm)
QRS complex: 0.08 second (basic rhythm); 0.12 second (PVCs)
Rhythm interpretation: Normal sinus rhythm with unifocal PVCs in a bigeminal pattern (second, fourth, sixth, and eighth complexes)

**Strip 9-7**
Rhythm: First rhythm can't be determined (only one cardiac cycle); second rhythm irregular
Rate: 54 beats/minute (first rhythm); 80 beats/minute (second rhythm)
P waves: Sinus P waves (basic rhythm)
PR interval: 0.16 second (basic rhythm)
QRS complex: 0.08 second (basic rhythm); 0.12 second (ventricular beats)
Rhythm interpretation: Sinus bradycardia changing to accelerated idioventricular rhythm; ST-segment depression is present (basic rhythm).

**Strip 9-8**
Rhythm: Irregular (first and second rhythms)
Rate: 60 beats/minute (first rhythm); about 200 beats/minute (second rhythm)
P waves: Fibrillation waves (first rhythm); none identified in the second rhythm
PR interval: Not measurable
QRS complex: 0.06 to 0.08 second (first rhythm); 0.12 to 0.14 second (second rhythm)
Rhythm interpretation: Atrial fibrillation with burst of ventricular tachycardia; ST-segment depression with basic rhythm

**Strip 9-9**
Rhythm: Slightly irregular (atrial); regular (ventricular)
Rate: 40 beats/minute (atrial); 38 beats/minute (ventricular)
P waves: Sinus (bear no consistent relationship to the QRS complex)
PR interval: Varies (first, 0.92 second; second, 0.84 second)
QRS complex: 0.12 second
Rhythm interpretation: Third-degree AV block changing to ventricular standstill; ST-segment elevation is present.

**Strip 9-10**
Rhythm: Regular (basic rhythm); irregular (PVCs)
Rate: 79 beats/minute (basic rhythm)
P waves: Sinus (basic rhythm)
PR interval: 0.16 second
QRS complex: 0.06 second (basic rhythm); 0.14 to 0.16 second (PVCs)
Rhythm interpretation: Normal sinus rhythm with paired unifocal PVCs (sixth and seventh complex)

**Strip 9-11**
Rhythm: Regular
Rate: 42 beats/minute
P waves: Absent
PR interval: Not measurable
QRS complex: 0.12 to 0.14 second
Rhythm interpretation: Idioventricular rhythm

**Strip 9-12**
Rhythm: Regular
Rate: 125 beats/minute
P waves: Sinus
PR interval: 0.12 second
QRS complex: 0.12 second
Rhythm interpretation: Sinus tachycardia with bundle-branch block; an elevated ST-segment is present.

**Strip 9-13**
Rhythm: 0
Rate: 0
P waves: None identified
PR interval: Not measurable
QRS complex: None identified
Rhythm interpretation: Ventricular standstill (asystole)

**Strip 9-14**
Rhythm: Regular
Rate: 214 beats/minute
P waves: None identified
PR interval: Not measurable
QRS complex: 0.16 second
Rhythm interpretation: Ventricular tachycardia

**Strip 9-15**
Rhythm: Regular (basic rhythm)
Rate: 50 beats/minute (basic rhythm)
P waves: Sinus (basic rhythm)
PR interval: 0.16 to 0.18 second
QRS complex: 0.08 second (basic rhythm); 0.14 second (PVC)
Rhythm interpretation: Sinus bradycardia with one PVC (third complex); ST-segment depression is present.

**Strip 9-16**
Rhythm: Chaotic
Rate: 0
P waves: Absent; wave deflections are irregular and vary in height, size, and shape
PR interval: Not measurable
QRS complex: Absent
Rhythm interpretation: Ventricular fibrillation

**Strip 9-17**
Rhythm: Chaotic
Rate: 0
P waves: Wave deflections are chaotic and vary in height, size, and shape
PR interval: Not measurable
QRS complex: Absent
Rhythm interpretation: Ventricular fibrillation is followed by electrical shock and a return to ventricular fibrillation.

Strip 9-18
Rhythm: Regular
Rate: 107 beats/minute
P waves: Sinus
PR interval: 0.16 to 0.18 second
QRS complex: 0.12 second
Rhythm interpretation: Sinus tachycardia with bundle-branch block

Strip 9-19
Rhythm: Irregular
Rate: 300 beats/minute (atrial); 50 beats/minute (ventricular)
P waves: Flutter waves before each QRS complex
PR interval: Not measurable
QRS complex: 0.06 to 0.08 second (basic rhythm); 0.12 second (PVC)
Rhythm interpretation: Atrial flutter with variable AV conduction and one PVC (fifth complex)

Strip 9-20
Rhythm: Regular (atrial)
Rate: 136 beats/minute (atrial); 0 (ventricular; no QRS complexes)
P waves: Sinus
PR interval: Not measurable
QRS complex: Absent
Rhythm interpretation: Ventricular standstill

Strip 9-21
Rhythm: Irregular
Rate: 40 beats/minute
P waves: Absent
PR interval: Not measurable
QRS complex: 0.16 second
Rhythm interpretation: Idioventricular rhythm

Strip 9-22
Rhythm: Chaotic
Rate: 0 (no QRS complexes)
P waves: None identified
PR interval: Not measurable
QRS complex: Absent
Rhythm interpretation: Ventricular fibrillation

Strip 9-23
Rhythm: Regular
Rate: 100 beats/minute
P waves: Absent
PR interval: Not measurable
QRS complex: 0.12 second
Rhythm interpretation: Accelerated idioventricular rhythm

Strip 9-24
Rhythm: Irregular
Rate: 60 beats/minute
P waves: Fibrillation waves present
PR interval: Not measurable
QRS complex: 0.12 second
Rhythm interpretation: Atrial fibrillation with bundle-branch block; ST-segment depression and T-wave inversion are present.

Strip 9-25
Rhythm: Regular (basic rhythm)
Rate: 100 beats/minute (first rhythm); 188 beats/minute (second rhythm)
P waves: Sinus (basic rhythm)
PR interval: 0.14 to 0.16 second
QRS complex: 0.08 second (basic rhythm); 0.12 to 0.16 second (ventricular beats)
Rhythm interpretation: Normal sinus rhythm with burst of ventricular tachycardia and paired PVCs

Strip 9-26
Rhythm: Regular (basic rhythm); irregular (PVC)
Rate: 107 beats/minute (basic rhythm)
P waves: Sinus (basic rhythm)
PR interval: 0.18 to 0.20 second
QRS complex: 0.08 to 0.10 second (basic rhythm); 0.16 second (PVC)
Rhythm interpretation: Sinus tachycardia with one PVC (R-on-T pattern); an elevated ST-segment is present.

Strip 9-27
Rhythm: Regular
Rate: 43 beats/minute
P waves: Absent
PR interval: Not measurable
QRS complex: 0.16 to 0.18 second
Rhythm interpretation: Idioventricular rhythm

Strip 9-28
Rhythm: Regular
Rate: 250 beats/minute
P waves: None identified
PR interval: Not measurable
QRS complex: 0.12 to 0.16 second (QRS complexes change in polarity from negative to positive across the strip)
Rhythm interpretation: Ventricular tachycardia (torsades de pointes)

**Strip 9-29**
Rhythm: Regular
Rate: 84 beats/minute
P waves: None identified
PR interval: Not measurable
QRS complex: 0.14 to 0.16 second
Rhythm interpretation: Accelerated idioventricular rhythm

**Strip 9-30**
Rhythm: Chaotic
Rate: 0
P waves: Absent; wave deflections are irregular and vary in height, size, and shape
PR interval: Not measurable
QRS complex: Absent
Rhythm interpretation: Ventricular fibrillation

**Strip 9-31**
Rhythm: Regular (basic rhythm); irregular (PVCs)
Rate: 115 beats/minute (basic rhythm)
P waves: Sinus (basic rhythm)
PR interval: 0.14 to 0.16 second
QRS complex: 0.04 to 0.06 second (basic rhythm); 0.12 second (PVCs)
Rhythm interpretation: Sinus tachycardia with two unifocal PVCs (fourth complex and twelfth complex)

**Strip 9-32**
Rhythm: Regular (basic rhythm); irregular (PVCs)
Rate: 125 beats/minute (basic rhythm)
P waves: Sinus (basic rhythm)
PR interval: 0.14 to 0.16 second
QRS complex: 0.08 to 0.10 second (basic rhythm); 0.12 second (PVCs)
Rhythm interpretation: Sinus tachycardia with multifocal paired PVCs (eighth and ninth complex)

**Strip 9-33**
Rhythm: Regular (basic rhythm)
Rate: 37 beats/minute (basic rhythm)
P waves: Sinus (basic rhythm)
PR interval: 0.14 to 0.16 second
QRS complex: 0.06 to 0.08 second (basic rhythm); 0.12 second (escape beat)
Rhythm interpretation: Sinus bradycardia with one ventricular escape beat (third complex)

**Strip 9-34**
Rhythm: Regular (first and second rhythms)
Rate: 72 beats/minute (first rhythm); 150 beats/minute (second rhythm)
P waves: Sinus (basic rhythm)
PR interval: 0.18 to 0.20 second
QRS complex: 0.08 second (basic rhythm); 0.12 second (ventricular beats)
Rhythm interpretation: Normal sinus rhythm with a burst of ventricular tachycardia; an inverted T wave is present in basic rhythm.

**Strip 9-35**
Rhythm: Chaotic
Rate: 0
P waves: Absent; wave deflections vary in height, size, and shape
PR interval: Not measurable
QRS complex: Absent
Rhythm interpretation: Ventricular fibrillation

**Strip 9-36**
Rhythm: Irregular
Rate: About 30 beats/minute
P waves: Absent
PR interval: Not measurable
QRS complex: 0.12 second
Rhythm interpretation: Idioventricular rhythm; ST-segment elevation is present.

**Strip 9-37**
Rhythm: Not measurable
Rate: Not measurable (one complex present)
P waves: None identified
PR interval: Not measurable
QRS complex: 0.28 second or wider
Rhythm interpretation: One ventricular complex followed by ventricular standstill

**Strip 9-38**
Rhythm: Regular
Rate: 84 beats/minute
P waves: None identified
PR interval: Not measurable
QRS complex: 0.14 to 0.16 second
Rhythm interpretation: Accelerated idioventricular rhythm

Strip 9-39
Rhythm: Regular (basic rhythm)
Rate: 115 beats/minute (basic rhythm)
P waves: Inverted before each QRS complex in basic rhythm
PR interval: 0.08 second (basic rhythm)
QRS complex: 0.06 to 0.08 second (basic rhythm); 0.12 second (PVC)
Rhythm interpretation: Junctional tachycardia with one PVC (tenth complex)

Strip 9-40
Rhythm: Regular (atrial)
Rate: 30 beats/minute (atrial); 0 (ventricular; no QRS complexes)
P waves: Sinus
PR interval: Not measurable
QRS complex: Absent
Rhythm interpretation: Ventricular standstill

Strip 9-41
Rhythm: Regular (basic rhythm); irregular (PVCs)
Rate: 65 beats/minute (basic rhythm)
P waves: Sinus (basic rhythm)
PR interval: 0.16 second
QRS complex: 0.06 to 0.08 second (basic rhythm); 0.12 second (PVCs)
Rhythm interpretation: Normal sinus rhythm with two unifocal PVCs (third and sixth complex); ST-segment depression is present.

Strip 9-42
Rhythm: Irregular (first rhythm); regular (second rhythm)
Rate: 100 beats/minute (first rhythm); 167 beats/minute (second rhythm)
P waves: Fibrillation waves (basic rhythm)
PR interval: Not measurable
QRS complex: 0.08 second (basic rhythm); 0.12 second (VT)
Rhythm interpretation: Atrial fibrillation with a burst of ventricular tachycardia

Strip 9-43
Rhythm: Regular (first rhythm); irregular (second rhythm)
Rate: 100 beats/minute (first rhythm); 100 beats/minute (second rhythm)
P waves: Sinus (basic rhythm)
PR interval: 0.12 second
QRS complex: 0.12 to 0.14 second (first rhythm); 0.12 second (second rhythm)
Rhythm interpretation: Normal sinus rhythm with bundle-branch block with transient episode of accelerated idioventricular rhythm

Strip 9-44
Rhythm: First rhythm can't be determined (only one cardiac cycle present); second rhythm regular
Rate: 50 beats/minute (first rhythm); 41 beats/minute (second rhythm)
P waves: Sinus (first rhythm)
PR interval: 0.12 second (first rhythm)
QRS complex: 0.06 to 0.08 second (first rhythm); 0.12 to 0.14 second (second rhythm)
Rhythm interpretation: Sinus bradycardia changing to idioventricular rhythm; a U wave is present.

Strip 9-45
Rhythm: Regular
Rate: 214 beats/minute
P waves: Not identified
PR interval: Not measurable
QRS complex: 0.16 to 0.18 second or wider
Rhythm interpretation: Ventricular tachycardia

Strip 9-46
Rhythm: Regular (basic rhythm); irregular (ventricular beats)
Rate: About 58 beats/minute (basic rhythm)
P waves: Sinus (basic rhythm)
PR interval: 0.20 second
QRS complex: 0.06 second (basic rhythm); 0.16 second (first ventricular beat); 0.12 second (second ventricular beat)
Rhythm interpretation: Sinus bradycardia with one PVC (fourth complex) and one ventricular escape beat (fifth complex); ST-segment depression is present.

Strip 9-47
Rhythm: Regular (basic rhythm); irregular (PVC)
Rate: 94 beats/minute (basic rhythm)
P waves: Sinus (basic rhythm)
PR interval: 0.20 second
QRS complex: 0.08 second (basic rhythm); 0.12 second (PVC)
Rhythm interpretation: Normal sinus rhythm with one PVC (fifth complex)

Strip 9-48
Rhythm: Not measurable
Rate: Not measurable (one complex present)
P waves: None identified
PR interval: Not measurable
QRS complex: 0.12 second
Rhythm interpretation: One ventricular complex followed by ventricular standstill

Strip 9-49
Rhythm: Regular
Rate: 56 beats/minute
P waves: Sinus
PR interval: 0.12 to 0.16 second
QRS complex: 0.12 second
Rhythm interpretation: Sinus bradycardia with bundle-branch block; ST-segment depression is present.

Strip 9-50
Rhythm: Regular
Rate: 188 beats/minute
P waves: Not identified
PR interval: Not measurable
QRS complex: 0.12 second
Rhythm interpretation: Ventricular tachycardia

Strip 9-51
Rhythm: Regular (atrial); irregular (ventricular)
Rate: 58 beats/minute (atrial); about 40 beats/minute (ventricular)
P waves: Sinus
PR interval: Lengthens from 0.30 to 0.36 second
QRS complex: 0.08 second (basic rhythm); 0.12 second (escape beat)
Rhythm interpretation: Second-degree AV block, Mobitz I with one ventricular escape beat (third complex)

Strip 9-52
Rhythm: Regular (first and second rhythms)
Rate: 72 beats/minute (first rhythm); 72 beats/minute (second rhythm)
P waves: Sinus in first rhythm
PR interval: 0.12 to 0.14 second (first rhythm)
QRS complex: 0.08 second (first rhythm); 0.12 to 0.14 second (2nd rhythm)
Rhythm interpretation: Normal sinus rhythm with a transient episode of accelerated idioventricular rhythm

Strip 9-53
Rhythm: Slightly irregular (atrial)
Rate: About 40 beats/minute (atrial); 0 (ventricular; no QRS complexes)
P waves: Sinus
PR interval: Not measurable
QRS complex: Absent
Rhythm interpretation: Ventricular standstill

Strip 9-54
Rhythm: Regular
Rate: 84 beats/minute
P waves: Sinus
PR interval: 0.16 second
QRS complex: 0.12 to 0.14 second
Rhythm interpretation: Normal sinus rhythm with bundle-branch block; a depressed ST-segment is present.

Strip 9-55
Rhythm: Regular
Rate: 41 beats/minute
P waves: Absent
PR interval: Not measurable
QRS complex: 0.16 second
Rhythm interpretation: Idioventricular rhythm

Strip 9-56
Rhythm: Regular
Rate: 75 beats/minute
P waves: Sinus
PR interval: 0.12 second
QRS complex: 0.16 to 0.18 second
Rhythm interpretation: Normal sinus rhythm with bundle-branch block; T-wave inversion is present

Strip 9-57
Rhythm: Regular (basic rhythm); irregular (PVCs)
Rate: 72 beats/minute (basic rhythm)
P waves: Sinus (basic rhythm)
PR interval: 0.12 second
QRS complex: 0.08 second (basic rhythm); 0.12 to 0.14 second (PVCs)
Rhythm interpretation: Normal sinus rhythm with unifocal PVCs (fourth and eighth complexes) in a quadrigeminal pattern

Strip 9-58
Rhythm: Regular (atrial); ventricular not measurable (only one QRS complex present)
Rate: 29 beats/minute (atrial); ventricular not measurable (only one QRS complex present)
P waves: Sinus
PR interval: Not measurable
QRS complex: 0.08 second
Rhythm interpretation: One QRS complex followed by ventricular standstill

Strip 9-59
Rhythm: Chaotic
Rate: 0
P waves: Absent; wave deflections are irregular and chaotic and vary in size, shape, and height
PR interval: Not measurable
QRS complex: Absent
Rhythm interpretation: Ventricular fibrillation

Strip 9-60
Rhythm: Not measurable (only one QRS complex)
Rate: Not measurable (only one QRS complex)
P waves: None identified
PR interval: Not measurable
QRS complex: 0.12 second or greater
Rhythm interpretation: One QRS complex followed by ventricular standstill

Strip 9-61
Rhythm: Regular (first and second rhythms)
Rate: 100 beats/minute (first rhythm); 100 beats/minute (second rhythm)
P waves: Sinus (first rhythm); none (second rhythm)
PR interval: 0.14 to 0.16 second (first rhythm)
QRS complex: 0.06 to 0.08 second (first rhythm); 0.12 second (second rhythm)
Rhythm interpretation: Normal sinus rhythm changing to accelerated idioventricular rhythm

Strip 9-62
Rhythm: Regular
Rate: 40 beats/minute
P waves: Absent
PR interval: Not measurable
QRS complex: 0.16 second
Rhythm interpretation: Idioventricular rhythm

Strip 9-63
Rhythm: Regular
Rate: 167 beats/minute
P waves: Not identified
PR interval: Not measurable
QRS complex: 0.16 to 0.18 second
Rhythm interpretation: Ventricular tachycardia

Strip 9-64
Rhythm: Regular
Rate: 88
P waves: Sinus
PR interval: 0.22 to 0.24 second
QRS complex: 0.12 second
Rhythm interpretation: Normal sinus rhythm with bundle-branch block and first-degree AV block

Strip 9-65
Rhythm: Irregular
Rate: 80 beats/minute (basic rhythm)
P waves: Fibrillation waves
PR interval: Not measurable
QRS complex: 0.06 to 0.08 second (basic rhythm); 0.12 second (PVCs)
Rhythm interpretation: Atrial fibrillation with paired PVCs

Strip 9-66
Rhythm: Regular (basic rhythm)
Rate: 84 beats/minute (basic rhythm)
P waves: Sinus
PR interval: 0.24 second
QRS complex: 0.08 second
Rhythm interpretation: Normal sinus rhythm with first-degree AV block changing to ventricular standstill

Strip 9-67
Rhythm: Chaotic
Rate: 0
P waves: None identified
PR interval: Not measurable
QRS complex: Absent
Rhythm interpretation: Ventricular fibrillation

Strip 9-68
Rhythm: Regular
Rate: 167 beats/minute
P waves: None identified
PR interval: Not measurable
QRS complex: 0.14 to 0.16 second
Rhythm interpretation: Ventricular tachycardia

Strip 9-69
Rhythm: Regular (first rhythm); slightly irregular (second rhythm)
Rate: 115 beats/minute (first rhythm); about 214 beats/minute (second rhythm)
P waves: Sinus (first rhythm); none identified in the second rhythm
PR interval: 0.12 to 0.14 second (first rhythm)
QRS complex: 0.10 second (first rhythm); 0.12 to 0.16 second (second rhythm)
Rhythm interpretation: Sinus tachycardia with a burst of ventricular tachycardia returning to sinus tachycardia; an inverted T wave is present.

Strip 9-70
Rhythm: Regular
Rate: 40 beats/minute
P waves: Absent
PR interval: Not measurable
QRS complex: 0.16 second
Rhythm interpretation: Idioventricular rhythm

Strip 9-71
Rhythm: Regular
Rate: 100 beats/minute
P waves: Absent
PR interval: Not measurable
QRS complex: 0.12 second
Rhythm interpretation: Accelerated idioventricular rhythm

Strip 9-72
Rhythm: 0 (only one QRS complex present)
Rate: 0 (only one QRS complex present)
P waves: None identified
PR interval: Not measurable
QRS complex: 0.24 to 0.26 second
Rhythm interpretation: One QRS complex followed by ventricular standstill

Strip 9-73
Rhythm: Regular
Rate: 188 beats/minute
P waves: Not identified
PR interval: Not measurable
QRS complex: 0.16 to 0.20 second or wider
Rhythm interpretation: Ventricular tachycardia followed by electrical shock and return to ventricular tachycardia

Strip 9-74
Rhythm: Regular (basic rhythm); irregular (PVC)
Rate: 100 beats/minute (basic rhythm)
P waves: Sinus (basic rhythm)
PR interval: 0.14 to 0.16 second
QRS complex: 0.08 second (basic rhythm); 0.12 second (PVC)
Rhythm interpretation: Normal sinus rhythm with one PVC (fifth complex)

Strip 9-75
Rhythm: Regular
Rate: 50 beats/minute
P waves: Sinus
PR interval: 0.16 to 0.18 second
QRS complex: 0.12 to 0.14 second
Rhythm interpretation: Sinus bradycardia with bundle-branch block

Strip 9-76
Rhythm: 0
Rate: 0 (no QRS complexes)
P waves: Sinus
PR interval: Not measurable
QRS complex: Absent
Rhythm interpretation: Ventricular standstill

Strip 9-77
Rhythm: Regular
Rate: 41 beats/minute
P waves: Absent
PR interval: Not measurable
QRS complex: 0.12 second
Rhythm interpretation: Idioventricular rhythm

Strip 9-78
Rhythm: 0 (only one QRS complex)
Rate: 0 (only one QRS complex)
P waves: None identified
PR interval: Not measurable
QRS complex: 0.14 second
Rhythm interpretation: One ventricular complex followed by ventricular standstill

Strip 9-79
Rhythm: 0
Rate: 0
P waves: Absent; wave deflections are chaotic and vary in height, size, and shape
PR interval: Not measurable
QRS complex: Absent
Rhythm interpretation: Ventricular fibrillation changing to ventricular standstill

Strip 9-80
Rhythm: Regular (first and second rhythms)
Rate: 94 beats/minute (first rhythm); 75 beats/minute (second rhythm)
P waves: Sinus (first rhythm)
PR interval: 0.16 second
QRS complex: 0.12 second (first rhythm); 0.12 second (second rhythm)
Rhythm interpretation: Normal sinus rhythm with bundle-branch block changing to accelerated idioventricular rhythm and back to normal sinus rhythm with bundle-branch block; T-wave inversion is present.

Strip 9-81
Rhythm: Regular (atrial); ventricular rhythm can't be determined (only one cardiac cycle)
Rate: 94 beats/minute (atrial); 40 beats/minute (ventricular)
P waves: Sinus (bear no relationship to the QRS complex)
PR interval: Varies greatly
QRS complex: 0.14 second
Rhythm interpretation: Third-degree AV block changing to ventricular standstill

Strip 9-82
Rhythm: Regular
Rate: 72 beats/minute
P waves: Sinus
PR interval: 0.16 second
QRS complex: 0.12 second
Rhythm interpretation: Normal sinus rhythm with bundle-branch block

Strip 9-83
Rhythm: Regular (first rhythm); irregular and chaotic (second rhythm)
Rate: 214 beats/minute (first rhythm)
P waves: None identified
PR interval: Not measurable
QRS complex: 0.16 to 0.18 second (first rhythm)
Rhythm interpretation: Ventricular tachycardia changing to ventricular fibrillation

**Strip 9-84**
Rhythm: Regular
Rate: 32 beats/minute
P waves: Absent
PR interval: Not measurable
QRS complex: 0.20 second
Rhythm interpretation: Idioventricular rhythm

**Strip 9-85**
Rhythm: Regular (basic rhythm); irregular (PVCs)
Rate: 125 beats/minute (basic rhythm)
P waves: Sinus (basic rhythm)
PR interval: 0.12 second
QRS complex: 0.06 to 0.08 second (basic rhythm); 0.12
second (PVCs)
Rhythm interpretation: Sinus tachycardia with multifocal
paired PVCs (eighth and ninth complexes)

**Strip 9-86**
Rhythm: Regular (atrial)
Rate: 52 beats/minute (atrial); 0 (ventricular)
P waves: Sinus
PR interval: Not measurable
QRS complex: Absent
Rhythm interpretation: Ventricular standstill

**Strip 9-87**
Rhythm: Regular (first rhythm); irregular (second
rhythm)
Rate: 68 beats/minute (first rhythm); about 80 beats/
minute (second rhythm)
P waves: Sinus (first rhythm)
PR interval: 0.12 to 0.14 second
QRS complex: 0.08 second (first rhythm); 0.12 second
(second rhythm)
Rhythm interpretation: Normal sinus rhythm changing to
accelerated idioventricular rhythm

**Strip 9-88**
Rhythm: Regular
Rate: 167 beats/minute
P waves: Not identified
PR interval: Not measurable
QRS complex: 0.16 to 0.20 second
Rhythm interpretation: Ventricular tachycardia (torsades
de pointes)

**Strip 9-89**
Rhythm: Regular (basic rhythm); irregular (PVCs)
Rate: 125 beats/minute (basic rhythm)
P waves: Sinus (basic rhythm)
PR interval: 0.12 second
QRS complex: 0.06 to 0.08 second (basic rhythm); 0.12
second (PVC)
Rhythm interpretation: Sinus tachycardia with paired
PVCs (seventh and eighth complexes)

**Strip 9-90**
Rhythm: Regular (atrial)
Rate: 72 beats/minute (atrial); 0 (ventricular)
P waves: Sinus
PR interval: Not measurable
QRS complex: Absent
Rhythm interpretation: Ventricular standstill

**Strip 9-91**
Rhythm: Regular
Rate: 188 beats/minute
P waves: None identified
PR interval: Not measurable
QRS complex: 0.18 to 0.20 second or wider
Rhythm interpretation: Ventricular tachycardia

**Strip 9-92**
Rhythm: Chaotic
Rate: 0
P waves: Wave deflections chaotic; vary in size, shape, and
direction
PR interval: Not measurable
QRS complex: Absent
Rhythm interpretation: Ventricular fibrillation; 60-cycle
(electrical) interference noted on baseline

**Strip 9-93**
Rhythm: Regular
Rate: 28 beats/minute
P waves: None
PR interval: Not measurable
QRS complex: 0.20 second or wider
Rhythm interpretation: Idioventricular rhythm

**Strip 9-94**
Rhythm: Regular
Rate: 79 beats/minute
P waves: Sinus
PR interval: 0.18 to 0.20 second
QRS complex: 0.12 second
Rhythm interpretation: Normal sinus rhythm with
bundle-branch block

**Strip 9-95**
Rhythm: Regular (basic rhythm)
Rate: 68 beats/minute (basic rhythm)
P waves: Sinus (basic rhythm)
PR interval: 0.16 to 0.18 second
QRS complex: 0.06 to 0.08 second (basic rhythm); 0.12
second (PVC)
Rhythm interpretation: Normal sinus rhythm with one in-
terpolated PVC (seventh complex). Interpolated PVCs are
sandwiched between two sinus beats and have no compen-
satory pause. ST-segment depression and T-wave inversion
are present.

**Strip 9-96**
Rhythm: Regular (basic rhythm); irregular (PVCs)
Rate: 72 beats/minute (basic rhythm)
P waves: Sinus (basic rhythm)
PR interval: 0.12 to 0.14 second
QRS complex: 0.08 second (basic rhythm); 0.12 to 0.14 second (PVCs)
Rhythm interpretation: Normal sinus rhythm with PVCs in a trigeminal pattern

**Strip 9-97**
Rhythm: Irregular
Rate: 80 beats/minute
P waves: Wavy fibrillatory waves
PR interval: Not measurable
QRS complex: 0.14 to 0.16 second
Rhythm interpretation: Atrial fibrillation with bundle-branch block

**Strip 9-98**
Rhythm: Regular (first rhythm); regular but off by two squares (second rhythm)
Rate: 43 beats/minute (first rhythm); 45 beats/minute (second rhythm)
P waves: Sinus (first rhythm); no associated P waves (second rhythm)
PR interval: 0.14 to 0.16 second (basic rhythm)
QRS complex: 0.10 second (basic rhythm); 0.14 to 0.16 second (second rhythm)
Rhythm interpretation: Sinus bradycardia with three-beat run of idioventricular rhythm

**Strip 9-99**
Rhythm: Regular (basic rhythm); irregular during pause
Rate: 79 beats/minute (basic rhythm)
P waves: Sinus (basic rhythm); absent during pause
PR interval: 0.20 second
QRS complex: 0.14 to 0.16 second
Rhythm interpretation: Normal sinus rhythm with bundle-branch block and sinus exit block

**Strip 9-100**
Rhythm: None
Rate: 0
P waves: None identified; wavy baseline
PR interval: Not measurable
QRS complex: Absent
Rhythm interpretation: Ventricular fibrillation changing to ventricular standstill

**Strip 10-1**
Automatic interval rate: 72 beats/minute
Analysis: The first four beats are paced beats, followed by one patient beat and three paced beats.
Interpretation: Normal pacemaker function

**Strip 10-2**
Automatic interval rate: 84 beats/minute
Analysis: The first three beats are paced beats, followed by two patient beats, a pacer spike occurring too early, a patient beat, a fusion beat, and two paced beats.
Interpretation: Undersensing malfunction

**Strip 10-3**
Automatic interval rate: 72 beats/minute
Analysis: All beats are pacemaker induced.
Interpretation: Pacemaker rhythm (normal pacemaker function)

**Strip 10-4**
Automatic interval rate: 68 beats/minute
Analysis: First two beats are paced, followed by a failure to capture spike, paced beat, failure to capture spike, patient beat, paced beat, failure to capture spike, and patient beat.
Interpretation: Frequent failure to capture

**Strip 10-5**
Automatic interval rate: 72 beats/minute
Analysis: No patient or paced beats are seen.
Interpretation: Failure to capture in the presence of ventricular standstill (asystole)

**Strip 10-6**
Automatic interval rate: 72 beats/minute
Analysis: First five beats are patient beats followed by two paced beats, two patient beats, and one paced beat.
Interpretation: Normal pacemaker function; underlying rhythm is normal sinus rhythm with frequent PVCs (multifocal)

**Strip 10-7**
Automatic interval rate: 50 beats/minute
Analysis: The first two beats are pacemaker induced, followed by a pseudofusion beat, two patient beats, and one paced beat.
Interpretation: Normal pacemaker function

**Strip 10-8**
Automatic interval rate: 72 beats/minute
Analysis: All beats are pacemaker induced.
Interpretation: Pacemaker rhythm (normal pacemaker function)

**Strip 10-9**
Automatic interval rate: 63 beats/minute
Analysis: The first two beats are paced beats, followed by a pacing spike that occurs on time but doesn't capture, a native beat, three paced beats, and a native beat.
Interpretation: Failure to capture

Strip 10-10
Automatic interval rate: 72 beats/minute
Analysis: All beats are pacemaker induced.
Interpretation: Pacemaker rhythm (normal pacemaker function)

Strip 10-11
Automatic interval rate: 72 beats/minute
Analysis: First three beats are paced beats, followed by one patient beat, a pacing spike that occurs too early, one patient beat, a paced beat that occurs too early, and three paced beats.
Interpretation: Undersensing malfunction

Strip 10-12
Automatic interval rate: 72 beats/minute
Analysis: First six beats are patient beats, followed by two paced beats and two patient beats.
Interpretation: Normal pacemaker function; underlying rhythm is atrial fibrillation

Strip 10-13
Automatic interval rate: 60 beats/minute
Analysis: All beats are pacemaker induced.
Interpretation: Pacemaker rhythm (normal pacemaker function)

Strip 10-14
Automatic interval rate: 72 beats/minute
Analysis: The first three beats are paced beats, followed by two patient beats, two paced beats, one patient beat, and one paced beat.
Interpretation: Normal pacemaker function

Strip 10-15
Automatic interval rate: 84 beats/minute
Analysis: The first three beats are paced beats; when the pacemaker is turned off the underlying rhythm is ventricular standstill. Two paced beats are seen when the pacemaker is turned back on.
Interpretation: This strip shows an indication for permanent pacemaker implantation, if the underlying rhythm doesn't resolve.

Strip 10-16
Automatic interval rate: 72 beats/minute
Analysis: First two beats are paced beats, followed by one patient beat, a pacing spike that occurs on time but doesn't capture, two paced beats, two patient beats, and one paced beat.
Interpretation: Failure to capture

Strip 10-17
Automatic interval rate: 72 beats/minute
Analysis: The first two beats are paced, followed by a fusion beat (note the spike in the native QRS complex with a decrease in height), two native beats, a spike that occurs too early, a native beat, a spike that occurs too early, a native beat, a paced beat that occurs too early, and a paced beat.
Interpretation: Undersensing malfunction (spikes too early after the fifth and sixth complexes and a paced beat too early after the seventh complex)

Strip 10-18
Automatic interval rate: 72 beats/minute
Analysis: The first two beats are patient beats, followed by a spike that occurs on time but doesn't capture, a patient beat, and five paced beats.
Interpretation: Failure to capture

Strip 10-19
Automatic interval rate: 60 beats/minute
Analysis: First four beats are paced beats, followed by one patient beat (PVC) and three paced beats.
Interpretation: Normal pacemaker function

Strip 10-20
Automatic interval rate: 72 beats/minute
Analysis: All beats are pacemaker induced.
Interpretation: Pacemaker rhythm (normal pacemaker function)

Strip 10-21
Automatic interval rate: 72 beats/minute
Analysis: All beats are pacemaker induced.
Interpretation: Pacemaker rhythm (normal pacemaker function)

Strip 10-22
Automatic interval rate: Can't be determined (only one paced beat)
Analysis: One paced beat with rhythm changing to ventricular tachycardia
Interpretation: One paced beat changing to ventricular tachycardia (torsades de pointes)

Strip 10-23
Automatic interval rate: 63 beats/minute
Analysis: The first four beats are paced beats, followed by a patient beat (PVC), a pacing spike that occurs too early, a fusion beat, and a paced beat.
Interpretation: Undersensing malfunction (pacing spike occurs too early after the fifth complex)

Strip 10-24
Automatic interval rate: 72 beats/minute
Analysis: The first beat is paced, followed by one failure to capture spike, one patient beat, one failure to capture spike, one patient beat, one paced beat, one failure to capture spike, one patient beat, one failure to capture spike, and one patient beat.
Interpretation: Frequent failure to capture

Strip 10-25
Automatic interval rate: 63 beats/minute
Analysis: All beats are pacemaker induced.
Interpretation: Pacemaker rhythm (normal pacemaker function)

Strip 10-26
Automatic interval rate: 72 beats/minute
Analysis: The first two beats are paced beats, followed by one PVC, two paced beats, one pseudofusion beat, one patient beat, and two paced beats.
Interpretation: Normal pacemaker function

Strip 10-27
Automatic interval rate: 72 beats/minute
Analysis: The first two beats are paced beats, followed by a spike, which occurs on time but doesn't capture, a patient beat, a spike that occurs on time but doesn't capture, a patient beat, a spike that occurs on time but doesn't capture, a patient beat, a spike that occurs on time but doesn't capture, and a patient beat.
Interpretation: Loss of capture malfunction (loss of capture spikes occur after second, third, fourth, and fifth complexes)

Strip 10-28
Automatic interval rate: 72 beats/minute
Analysis: The first three beats are paced beats, followed by one patient beat, two paced beats, one pseudofusion beat (spike superimposed on R wave), and two paced beats.
Interpretation: Normal pacemaker function

Strip 10-29
Automatic interval rate: 72 beats/minute
Analysis: The first two beats are paced beats, followed by three patient beats (second a PVC), and three paced beats.
Interpretation: Normal pacemaker function; underlying rhythm is atrial fibrillation.

Strip 10-30
Automatic interval rate: 65 beats/minute
Analysis: The first two beats are patient beats, followed by three pseudofusion beats and four patient beats.
Interpretation: Normal pacemaker function

Strip 10-31
Automatic interval rate: Can't be determined because there aren't two consecutively paced beats present.
Analysis: Strip shows six patient beats and five failure-to-capture spikes. No paced beats are seen.
Interpretation: Complete failure to capture

Strip 10-32
Automatic interval rate: 68 beats/minute
Analysis: The first beat is a patient beat, followed by a pacing spike that occurs too early, a patient beat, a paced beat that occurs too early, three paced beats that sense and capture appropriately, a pseudofusion beat, a patient beat, a pacing spike that occurs too early, and two patient beats.
Interpretation: Undersensing malfunction (pacing spikes occur too early after the first and eighth complex; paced beat occurs too early after the second complex)

Strip 10-33
Automatic interval rate: 65 beats/minute
Analysis: First two beats are paced beats followed by two patient beats, one fusion beat, and two paced beats.
Interpretation: Normal pacemaker function

Strip 10-34
Automatic interval rate: 72 beats/minute
Analysis: All beats are pacemaker induced.
Interpretation: Pacemaker rhythm (normal pacemaker function)

Strip 10-35
Automatic interval rate: 56 beats/minute
Analysis: The first two beats are paced beats, followed by one patient beat, one paced beat, one patient beat, one paced beat that occurs too early, two paced beats, and one patient beat.
Interpretation: Undersensing malfunction

Strip 10-36
Automatic interval rate: 72 beats/minute
Analysis: The first two beats are patient beats, followed by a pacing spike that occurs too early, three patient beats, a pacing spike that occurs too early, a patient beat, a paced beat that occurs too early, two paced beats, and a patient beat.
Interpretation: Frequent undersensing malfunction (pacing spikes occur too early after the second and fifth complexes; a paced beat that occurs too early after the sixth complex)

Strip 10-37
Automatic interval rate: 72 beats/minute
Analysis: All beats are pacemaker induced.
Interpretation: Pacemaker rhythm (normal pacemaker function)

**Strip 10-38**
Automatic interval rate: 72 beats/minute
Analysis: No patient beats or paced beats are seen.
Interpretation: Failure to capture in the presence of ventricular standstill (asystole)

**Strip 10-39**
Automatic interval rate: 60 beats/minute
Analysis: All beats are pacemaker produced.
Interpretation: Pacemaker rhythm (normal pacemaker function)

**Strip 10-40**
Automatic interval rate: 72 beats/minute
Analysis: The first four beats are patient beats, followed by a ventricular capture beat that occurs too early, three ventricular capture beats that occur on time and sense appropriately, and two patient beats.
Interpretation: Undersensing malfunction (ventricular capture beat occurs too early after the fourth complex)

**Strip 11-1**
Rhythm: Regular
Rate: 107 beats/minute
P waves: Sinus
PR interval: 0.12 second
QRS complex: 0.06 to 0.08 second
Rhythm interpretation: Sinus tachycardia

**Strip 11-2**
Rhythm: Regular
Rate: 58 beats/minute
P waves: Sinus
PR interval: 0.12 to 0.14 second
QRS complex: 0.12 second
Rhythm interpretation: Sinus bradycardia with bundle-branch block; ST-segment depression is present.

**Strip 11-3**
Rhythm: Regular (atrial and ventricular)
Rate: 42 beats/minute (atrial); 21 beats/minute (ventricular)
P waves: Two sinus P waves to each QRS complex
PR interval: 0.32 to 0.36 second (remain constant)
QRS complex: 0.12 second
Rhythm interpretation: Second-degree AV block, Mobitz II (clinical correlation is suggested to diagnose Mobitz II when 2:1 conduction is present); ST-segment elevation is present.

**Strip 11-4**
Rhythm: Irregular
Rate: 100 beats/minute
P waves: Fibrillatory waves present; some flutter waves mixed with the fibrillatory waves
PR interval: Not measurable
QRS complex: 0.04 second
Rhythm interpretation: Atrial fibrillation; ST-segment depression is present.

**Strip 11-5**
Rhythm: Regular
Rate: 48 beats/minute
P waves: Hidden in the QRS complex
PR interval: Not measurable
QRS complex: 0.08 second
Rhythm interpretation: Junctional rhythm; ST-segment depression is present.

**Strip 11-6**
Rhythm: Regular
Rate: 188 beats/minute
P waves: Hidden in preceding T waves
PR interval: Not measurable
QRS complex: 0.10 second
Rhythm interpretation: Paroxysmal atrial tachycardia

**Strip 11-7**
Automtic interval rate: 72 beats/minute
Analysis: First four beats are paced, followed by two patient beats, one paced beat, and two patient beats.
Rhythm interpretation: Normal pacemaker function

**Strip 11-8**
Rhythm: Regular (atrial and ventricular)
Rate: 75 beats/minute (atrial); 26 beats/minute (ventricular)
P waves: Sinus (bear no constant relationship to the QRS complex)
PR interval: Varies
QRS complex: 0.14 to 0.16 second
Rhythm interpretation: Third-degree AV block; ST-segment elevation is present.

**Strip 11-9**
Rhythm: Regular
Rate: 188 beats/minute
P waves: Not discernible
PR interval: Not discernible
QRS complex: 0.16 to 0.20 second
Rhythm interpretation: Ventricular tachycardia

**Strip 11-10**
Rhythm: Regular
Rate: 42 beats/minute
P waves: Absent
PR interval: Not measurable
QRS complex: 0.16 second
Rhythm interpretation: Idioventricular rhythm

**Strip 11-11**
Rhythm: Regular (basic rhythm)
Rate: 56 beats/minute (basic rhythm)
P waves: Sinus (appear notched, which may indicate left atrial hypertrophy)
PR interval: 0.16 second
QRS complex: 0.06 second (basic rhythm); 0.16 second (PVC)
Rhythm interpretation: Sinus bradycardia with one interpolated PVC; ST-segment depression is present.

**Strip 11-12**
Rhythm: Regular
Rate: 84 beats/minute
P waves: Inverted before each QRS complex
PR interval: 0.10 second
QRS complex: 0.06 to 0.08 second
Rhythm interpretation: Accelerated junctional rhythm

**Strip 11-13**
Rhythm: Regular
Rate: 232 beats/minute (atrial); 58 beats/minute (ventricular)
P waves: Four flutter waves before each QRS complex
PR interval: Not measurable
QRS complex: 0.06 to 0.08 second
Rhythm interpretation: Atrial flutter with 4:1 AV conduction

**Strip 11-14**
Rhythm: Regular
Rate: 88 beats/minute
P waves: Sinus
PR interval: 0.20 second
QRS complex: 0.08 to 0.10 second
Rhythm interpretation: Normal sinus rhythm

**Strip 11-15**
Rhythm: Regular
Rate: 88 beats/minute
P waves: Absent
PR interval: Not measurable
QRS complex: 0.14 to 0.16 second
Rhythm interpretation: Accelerated idioventricular rhythm

**Strip 11-16**
Rhythm: Regular (basic rhythm); irregular with pause
Rate: 75 beats/minute (basic rhythm)
P waves: Sinus (basic rhythm); one premature, abnormal P wave without a QRS complex (after the fifth QRS complex)
PR interval: 0.24 to 0.28 second
QRS complex: 0.06 to 0.08 second
Rhythm interpretation: Normal sinus rhythm with first-degree AV block and one nonconducted PAC (follows the fifth QRS complex)

**Strip 11-17**
Rhythm: Regular
Rate: 115 beats/minute
P waves: Sinus
PR interval: 0.14 to 0.16 second
QRS complex: 0.06 second
Rhythm interpretation: Sinus tachycardia

**Strip 11-18**
Rhythm: Regular
Rate: 48 beats/minute
P waves: Sinus
PR interval: 0.12 second
QRS complex: 0.08 to 0.10 second
Rhythm interpretation: Sinus bradycardia; ST-segment elevation is present.

**Strip 11-19**
Rhythm: Regular (basic rhythm); irregular (premature beats)
Rate: 72 beats/minute (basic rhythm)
P waves: Sinus (basic rhythm); inverted (premature beats)
PR interval: 0.12 to 0.14 second (basic rhythm); 0.08 second (premature beats)
QRS complex: 0.08 second
Rhythm interpretation: Normal sinus rhythm with two premature junctional contractions (fourth and sixth complexes)

**Strip 11-20**
Rhythm: Regular
Rate: 63 beats/minute
P waves: Vary in size, shape, and position
PR interval: 0.12 to 0.14 second
QRS complex: 0.06 to 0.08 second
Rhythm interpretation: Wandering atrial pacemaker; ST-segment depression is present.

Strip 11-21
Rhythm: Chaotic
Rate: 0 (no QRS complexes)
P waves: No P waves; wave deflections are chaotic and ir-
regular and vary in height, size, and shape
PR interval: Not measurable
QRS complex: Absent
Rhythm interpretation: Ventricular fibrillation

Strip 11-22
Rhythm: Regular
Rate: 107 beats/minute
P waves: Inverted before each QRS complex
PR interval: 0.08 second
QRS complex: 0.04 to 0.06 second
Rhythm interpretation: Junctional tachycardia

Strip 11-23
Rhythm: Irregular atrial rhythm
Rate: 40 beats/minute (atrial); 0 (ventricular)
P waves: Sinus
PR interval: Not measurable
QRS complex: Absent
Rhythm interpretation: Ventricular standstill

Strip 11-24
Rhythm: Irregular
Rate: 70 beats/minute
P waves: Sinus
PR interval: 0.44 to 0.48 second
QRS complex: 0.08 to 0.10 second
Rhythm interpretation: Sinus arrhythmia with first-
degree AV block; ST-segment elevation is present.

Strip 11-25
Rhythm: Regular
Rate: 188 beats/minute
P waves: Not discernible
PR interval: Unmeasurable
QRS complex: 0.16 to 0.20 second
Rhythm interpretation: Ventricular tachycardia; ST-
segment elevation is present.

Strip 11-26
Rhythm: Regular (atrial); irregular (ventricular)
Rate: 72 beats/minute (atrial); 40 beats/minute (ventricu-
lar)
P waves: Sinus
PR interval: Lengthens from 0.20 to 0.28 second
QRS complex: 0.04 to 0.06 second
Rhythm interpretation: Second-degree AV block, Mobitz I;
ST-segment depression is present.

Strip 11-27
Rhythm: Regular
Rate: 72 beats/minute
P waves: Sinus
PR interval: 0.20 second
QRS complex: 0.08 to 0.10 second
Rhythm interpretation: Normal sinus rhythm; ST-
segment depression and T-wave inversion is present.

Strip 11-28
Rhythm: Regular (basic rhythm); irregular with pause
Rate: 72 beats/minute (basic rhythm); slows to 63 beats/
minute during first cycle after a pause; rate suppression
can occur for several cycles after an interruption in the
basic rhythm
P waves: Sinus
PR interval: 0.16 to 0.18 second
QRS complex: 0.04 to 0.06 second
Rhythm interpretation: Normal sinus rhythm with sinus
arrest

Strip 11-29
Rhythm: Regular (basic rhythm); irregular (premature
beat)
Rate: 63 beats/minute (basic rhythm)
P waves: Sinus (basic rhythm); premature and pointed
(premature beat)
PR interval: 0.14 to 0.16 second (basic rhythm); 0.12 sec-
ond (premature beat)
QRS complex: 0.08 second
Rhythm interpretation: Normal sinus rhythm with one
PAC (fifth complex)

Strip 11-30
Rhythm: Regular (basic rhythm); irregular (PVCs)
Rate: 72 beats/minute (basic rhythm)
P waves: Sinus
PR interval: 0.12 to 0.14 second
QRS complex: 0.12 second (basic rhythm and PVCs)
Rhythm interpretation: Normal sinus rhythm with
bundle-branch block and paired PVCs; a U wave is present.

Strip 11-31
Rhythm: Regular (atrial and ventricular)
Rate: 240 beats/minute (atrial); 60 beats/minute (ventric-
ular)
P waves: Four flutter waves to each QRS complex
PR interval: Not measurable
QRS complex: 0.04 to 0.06 second
Rhythm interpretation: Atrial flutter with 4:1 AV conduc-
tion

**Strip 11-32**
Rhythm: Regular (basic rhythm); irregular with pause
Rate: 54 beats/minute (basic rhythm)
P waves: Sinus (basic rhythm); none (fourth and fifth complexes)
PR interval: 0.18 to 0.20 second (basic rhythm)
QRS complex: 0.06 to 0.08 second
Rhythm interpretation: Sinus bradycardia with sinus arrest and two junctional escape beats during pause

**Strip 11-33**
Rhythm: Regular
Rate: 25 beats/minute
P waves: None identified
PR interval: Not measurable
QRS complex: 0.24 second or greater
Rhythm interpretation: Idioventricular rhythm

**Strip 11-34**
Automatic interval rate: 63 beats/minute
Analysis: The first three beats are paced beats, followed by a pacing spike that doesn't capture, one patient beat, and two paced beats.
Rhythm interpretation: Failure to capture

**Strip 11-35**
Rhythm: Regular
Rate: 84 beats/minute
P waves: Not identified
PR interval: Not measurable
QRS complex: 0.12 to 0.14 second
Rhythm interpretation: Accelerated idioventricular rhythm

**Strip 11-36**
Rhythm: Chaotic
Rate: 0
P waves: Absent; wave deflections are chaotic and irregular and vary in size, shape, and height
PR interval: Not measurable
QRS complex: Absent
Rhythm interpretation: Ventricular fibrillation, followed by electrical shock and return to ventricular fibrillation

**Strip 11-37**
Rhythm: Regular
Rate: 52 beats/minute
P waves: Sinus
PR interval: 0.18 to 0.20 second
QRS complex: 0.06 to 0.08 second
Rhythm interpretation: Sinus bradycardia; a U wave is present.

**Strip 11-38**
Rhythm: Regular
Rate: 94 beats/minute
P waves: Inverted before each QRS complex
PR interval: 0.08 to 0.10 second
QRS complex: 0.08 second
Rhythm interpretation: Accelerated junctional rhythm; baseline artifact is present.

**Strip 11-39**
Rhythm: Irregular
Rate: 60 beats/minute
P waves: Fibrillatory waves
PR interval: Not measurable
QRS complex: 0.12 second
Rhythm interpretation: Atrial fibrillation with bundle-branch block; ST-segment depression and T-wave inversion are present.

**Strip 11-40**
Automatic interval rate: 72 beats/minute
Analysis: All beats are pacemaker induced.
Rhythm interpretation: Pacemaker rhythm (normal pacemaker function)

**Strip 11-41**
Rhythm: P waves occur regularly
Rate: 88 beats/minute (atrial); 0 (ventricular)
P waves: Sinus
PR interval: Not measurable
QRS complex: Absent
Rhythm interpretation: Ventricular standstill

**Strip 11-42**
Rhythm: Regular (basic rhythm); irregular (premature beats)
Rate: 63 beats/minute (basic rhythm)
P waves: Sinus (basic rhythm)
PR interval: 0.12 to 0.14 second
QRS complex: 0.08 second (basic rhythm); 0.12 to 0.16 second (PVC)
Rhythm interpretation: Normal sinus rhythm with paired multifocal PVCs (fourth and fifth complexes)

**Strip 11-43**
Rhythm: Regular (basic rhythm); irregular (PACs)
Rate: 136 beats/minute (basic rhythm)
P waves: Sinus (basic rhythm); premature and pointed (premature beats)
PR interval: 0.16 to 0.20 second
QRS complex: 0.06 to 0.08 second
Rhythm interpretation: Sinus tachycardia with two PACs (fourth and eighth complexes)

**Strip 11-44**
Rhythm: Regular (basic rhythm); irregular with pause
Rate: 84 beats/minute (basic rhythm); slows after pause but returns to basic rate after four cycles
P waves: Sinus
PR interval: 0.20 second
QRS complex: 0.08 second
Rhythm interpretation: Normal sinus rhythm with sinus arrest; ST-segment depression and T-wave inversion are present.

**Strip 11-45**
Automatic interval rate: 75 beats/minute
Analysis: Pacing spikes without ventricular capture are seen.
Interpretation: Failure to capture in presence of ventricular standstill

**Strip 11-46**
Automatic interval rate: 72 beats/minute
Analysis: First four beats are paced beats, followed by one patient beat, a pacing spike that occurs too early, a patient beat, a fusion beat, and two paced beats.
Rhythm interpretation: Sensing malfunction

**Strip 11-47**
Rhythm: Regular
Rate: 42 beats/minute
P waves: Hidden in QRS complex
PR interval: Not measurable
QRS complex: 0.08 to 0.10 second
Rhythm interpretation: Junctional rhythm

**Strip 11-48**
Rhythm: Regular (atrial); irregular (ventricular)
Rate: 79 beats/minute (atrial); 50 beats/minute (ventricular)
P waves: Sinus
PR interval: Lengthens from 0.20 to 0.32 second
QRS complex: 0.08 to 0.10 second
Rhythm interpretation: Second-degree AV block, Mobitz I

**Strip 11-49**
Rhythm: Regular (basic rhythm); irregular (premature beat)
Rate: 107 beats/minute
P waves: Inverted before each QRS complex (except the ninth QRS complex, which has a premature, pointed P wave)
PR interval: 0.08 to 0.10 second (basic rhythm); 0.10 second (premature beat)
QRS complex: 0.08 to 0.10 second
Rhythm interpretation: Junctional tachycardia with one PAC (ninth complex)

**Strip 11-50**
Rhythm: Regular (atrial and ventricular)
Rate: 84 beats/minute (atrial); 28 beats/minute (ventricular)
P waves: Sinus (bear no relationship to the QRS complex)
PR interval: Varies greatly
QRS complex: 0.12 second
Rhythm interpretation: Third-degree AV block; ST-segment depression is present.

**Strip 11-51**
Rhythm: Irregular
Rate: 50 beats/minute
P waves: Sinus
PR interval: 0.12 to 0.14 second
QRS complex: 0.08 second
Rhythm interpretation: Sinus arrhythmia with a bradycardic rate; a U wave is present.

**Strip 11-52**
Rhythm: Regular (basic rhythm); irregular (premature beats)
Rate: 72 beats/minute (basic rhythm)
P waves: Sinus (basic rhythm)
PR interval: 0.16 second
QRS complex: 0.10 second
Rhythm interpretation: Normal sinus rhythm with unifocal PVCs in a trigeminal pattern. ST-segment depression and T-wave inversion are present.

**Strip 11-53**
Rhythm: Regular
Rate: 93 beats/minute (atrial); 31 beats/minute (ventricular)
P waves: Three sinus P waves to each QRS complex (one hidden in the T wave)
PR interval: 0.36 second (remains constant)
QRS complex: 0.08 second
Rhythm interpretation: Second-degree AV block, Mobitz II

**Strip 11-54**
Rhythm: Regular (basic rhythm); irregular (PVCs)
Rate: 72 beats/minute (basic rhythm)
P waves: Sinus (basic rhythm)
PR interval: 0.12 to 0.14 second
QRS complex: 0.08 second (basic rhythm); 0.14 to 0.16 second (PVCs)
Rhythm interpretation: Normal sinus rhythm with multifocal PVCs

**Strip 11-55**
Rhythm: Regular (atrial and ventricular)
Rate: 62 beats/minute (atrial); 31 beats/minute (ventricular)
P waves: Two sinus P waves before each QRS complex
PR interval: 0.44 second (remains constant)
QRS complex: 0.14 to 0.16 second
Rhythm interpretation: Second-degree AV block, Mobitz II

**Strip 11-56**
Rhythm: Regular
Rate: 65 beats/minute
P waves: Inverted before each QRS complex
PR interval: 0.10 second
QRS complex: 0.04 second
Rhythm interpretation: Accelerated junctional rhythm; ST-segment elevation is present.

**Strip 11-57**
Rhythm: Regular (basic rhythm); irregular with pause
Rate: 68 beats/minute (basic rhythm)
P waves: Sinus
PR interval: 0.22 to 0.24 second
QRS complex: 0.08 to 0.10 second
Rhythm interpretation: Normal sinus rhythm with first-degree AV block and sinus arrest; ST-segment elevation is present.

**Strip 11-58**
Automatic interval rate: Can't be determined because there are no two consecutive paced beats or two consecutive pacing spikes (estimated to be 75 beats/minute when measured from beat immediately preceding each spike)
Analysis: All beats are patient beats; four pacing spikes appear at appropriate intervals for capture to occur, but capture doesn't occur.
Rhythm interpretation: Complete failure to capture

**Strip 11-59**
Rhythm: Regular
Rate: 188 beats/minute
P waves: Not identified
PR interval: Not measurable
QRS complex: 0.06 to 0.08 second
Rhythm interpretation: Paroxysmal atrial tachycardia

**Strip 11-60**
Rhythm: Irregular
Rate: 30 beats/minute
P waves: None present
PR interval: Not measurable
QRS complex: 0.16 second
Rhythm interpretation: Idioventricular rhythm; ST-segment depression is present.

**Strip 11-61**
Rhythm: Regular (atrial); irregular (ventricular)
Rate: 125 beats/minute (atrial); 80 beats/minute (ventricular)
P waves: Sinus
PR interval: Lengthens from 0.12 to 0.24 second
QRS complex: 0.06 to 0.08 second
Rhythm interpretation: Second-degree AV block, Mobitz I; T-wave inversion is present.

**Strip 11-62**
Rhythm: Regular (basic rhythm); irregular (nonconducted PACs)
Rate: 100 beats/minute (basic rhythm)
P waves: Sinus; two premature abnormal P waves without QRS complex (after the fourth and eighth complexes)
PR interval: 0.12 second
QRS complex: 0.06 to 0.08 second
Rhythm interpretation: Normal sinus rhythm with two nonconducted PACs; T-wave inversion is present.

**Strip 11-63**
Rhythm: Regular
Rate: 75 beats/minute
P waves: Sinus
PR interval: 0.16 to 0.18 second
QRS complex: 0.12 to 0.14 second
Rhythm interpretation: Normal sinus rhythm with bundle-branch block; ST-segment elevation is present.

**Strip 11-64**
Rhythm: Regular
Rate: 50 beats/minute
P waves: Sinus
PR interval: 0.16 second
QRS complex: 0.06 to 0.08 second
Rhythm interpretation: Sinus bradycardia; a U wave is present.

**Strip 11-65**
Automatic interval rate: 72 beats/minute
Analysis: All beats are pacemaker induced.
Rhythm interpretation: Pacemaker rhythm (normal pacemaker function)

**Strip 11-66**
Rhythm: Regular
Rate: 78 beats/minute (atrial); 39 beats/minute (ventricular)
P waves: Two sinus P waves to each QRS complex
PR interval: 0.24 second with a constant relationship to the QRS complex
QRS complex: 0.12 to 0.14 second
Rhythm interpretation: Second-degree AV block, Mobitz II (clinical correlation is suggested to diagnose Mobitz II when 2:1 conduction is present)

**Strip 11-67**
Rhythm: Regular (basic rhythm)
Rate: 54 beats/minute (basic rhythm)
P waves: Sinus (basic rhythm); none (third and fourth complexes)
PR interval: 0.20 second
QRS complex: 0.06 to 0.08 second
Rhythm interpretation: Sinus bradycardia with two junctional escape beats (third and fourth beat)

**Strip 11-68**
Automatic interval rate: 68 beats/minute
Analysis: Pacing spikes without ventricular capture are seen.
Interpretation: Failure to capture in presence of ventricular fibrillation

**Strip 11-69**
Rhythm: Regular
Rate: 115 beats/minute
P waves: Inverted before each QRS complex
PR interval: 0.08 to 0.10 second
QRS complex: 0.06 to 0.08 second
Rhythm interpretation: Junctional tachycardia

**Strip 11-70**
Rhythm: Regular (basic rhythm); irregular (PJC)
Rate: 58 beats/minute (basic rhythm)
P waves: Sinus (basic rhythm); inverted (PJC)
PR interval: 0.14 to 0.16 second (basic rhythm); 0.10 second (PJC)
QRS complex: 0.08 second
Rhythm interpretation: Sinus bradycardia with one PJC

**Strip 11-71**
Rhythm: Regular (basic rhythm); irregular (nonconducted PAC)
Rate: 63 beats/minute (basic rhythm)
P waves: Sinus (basic rhythm); one premature, abnormal P wave without a QRS complex (after the fourth complex)
PR interval: 0.28 to 0.32 second
QRS complex: 0.12 second
Rhythm interpretation: Normal sinus rhythm with first-degree AV block and bundle-branch block with one nonconducted PAC after the fourth QRS complex; ST-segment elevation and T-wave inversion are present.

**Strip 11-72**
Rhythm: Regular (basic rhythm); irregular (PVC)
Rate: 50 beats/minute (basic rhythm)
P waves: Sinus (basic rhythm)
PR interval: 0.12 to 0.14 second
QRS complex: 0.08 second (basic rhythm); 0.18 second (PVC)
Rhythm interpretation: Sinus bradycardia with one PVC (after the third QRS complex); ST-segment elevation is present.

**Strip 11-73**
Automatic interval rate: 79 beats/minute
Analysis: First two beats are paced beats, followed by one fusion beat, one pseudofusion beat (note spike at the beginning of the R wave), three patient beats, pacing spike that occurs too early, a patient beat followed by a pacing spike that occurs too early, and another patient beat followed by an early pacing spike.
Rhythm interpretation: Sensing malfunction

**Strip 11-74**
Rhythm: Regular
Rate: 50 beats/minute
P waves: None identified
PR interval: Not measurable
QRS complex: 0.04 to 0.06 second
Rhythm interpretation: Junctional rhythm; ST-segment depression and T-wave inversion are present.

**Strip 11-75**
Rhythm: Irregular atrial rhythm
Rate: 40 beats/minute (atrial); 0 (ventricular)
P waves: Sinus
PR interval: Not measurable
QRS complex: Absent
Rhythm interpretation: Ventricular standstill

**Strip 11-76**
Rhythm: Irregular
Rate: 60 beats/minute
P waves: Sinus
PR interval: 0.12 to 0.14 second
QRS complex: 0.08 to 0.10 second
Rhythm interpretation: Sinus arrhythmia; ST-segment elevation is present.

**Strip 11-77**
Rhythm: Regular
Rate: 68 beats/minute
P waves: P waves vary in size, shape, and position
PR interval: 0.14 to 0.16 second
QRS complex: 0.06 to 0.08 second
Rhythm interpretation: Wandering atrial pacemaker; T-wave inversion is present.

Strip 11-78
Rhythm: Regular
Rate: 214 beats/minute
P waves: Hidden
PR interval: Not measurable
QRS complex: 0.06 to 0.08 second
Rhythm interpretation: Paroxysmal atrial tachycardia

Strip 11-79
Rhythm: Regular (first and second rhythms)
Rate: 94 beats/minute (first rhythm); 136 beats/minute
(second rhythm)
P waves: Sinus (first rhythm)
PR interval: 0.18 to 0.20 second (first rhythm)
QRS complex: 0.06 to 0.08 second (first rhythm); 0.12 second (second rhythm)
Rhythm interpretation: Normal sinus rhythm changing to ventricular tachycardia

Strip 11-80
Rhythm: Regular (basic rhythm)
Rate: 107 beats/minute (basic rhythm)
P waves: Sinus (basic rhythm)
PR interval: 0.14 to 0.16 second
QRS complex: 0.06 to 0.08 second (basic rhythm); 0.12
second (ventricular beats)
Rhythm interpretation: Sinus tachycardia with a four-beat
burst of ventricular tachycardia and paired, unifocal PVCs

Strip 11-81
Rhythm: Irregular
Rate: 260 beats/minute (atrial); 70 beats/minute (ventricular)
P waves: Flutter waves
PR interval: Not measurable
QRS complex: 0.06 to 0.08 second
Rhythm interpretation: Atrial flutter with variable block

Strip 11-82
Rhythm: Regular
Rate: 88 beats/minute
P waves: Sinus
PR interval: 0.12 second
QRS complex: 0.04 to 0.06 second
Rhythm interpretation: Normal sinus rhythm

Strip 11-83
Automatic interval rate: 63 beats/minute
Analysis: First two beats are paced beats followed by one
patient beat, two paced beats, one patient beat, and two
paced beats.
Rhythm interpretation: Normal pacemaker function

Strip 11-84
Rhythm: Regular
Rate: 136 beats/minute
P waves: Sinus
PR interval: 0.12 to 0.14 second
QRS complex: 0.06 to 0.08 second
Rhythm interpretation: Sinus tachycardia

Strip 11-85
Rhythm: Regular
Rate: 54 beats/minute
P waves: Sinus
PR interval: 0.24 to 0.26 second
QRS complex: 0.04 to 0.06 second
Rhythm interpretation: Sinus bradycardia with first-
degree AV block

Strip 11-86
Rhythm: Regular (atrial and ventricular)
Rate: 94 beats/minute (atrial); 37 beats/minute (ventricular)
P waves: Sinus (bear no relationship to the QRS complex)
PR interval: Varies
QRS complex: 0.12 to 0.14 second
Rhythm interpretation: Third-degree AV block

Strip 11-87
Rhythm: Regular
Rate: 150 beats/minute
P waves: None identified
PR interval: Not measurable
QRS complex: 0.12 to 0.14 second
Rhythm interpretation: Ventricular tachycardia

Strip 11-88
Rhythm: Regular (basic rhythm); irregular with pause
Rate: 56 beats/minute (basic rhythm)
P waves: Sinus (basic rhythm); absent during pause
PR interval: 0.16 to 0.18 second
QRS complex: 0.08 to 0.10 second
Rhythm interpretation: Sinus bradycardia with sinus arrest; ST-segment depression and T-wave inversion are
present.

Strip 11-89
Rhythm: 0
Rate: 0
P waves: Absent
PR interval: Not measurable
QRS complex: Absent
Rhythm interpretation: Ventricular standstill

Strip 11-90
Rhythm: Regular
Rate: 88 beats/minute
P waves: Sinus
PR interval: 0.16 second
QRS complex: 0.06 to 0.08 second
Rhythm interpretation: Normal sinus rhythm; ST-segment depression and T-wave inversion are present.

Strip 11-91
Rhythm: Regular (basic rhythm); irregular (PVC)
Rate: 115 beats/minute (basic rhythm)
P waves: Inverted before each QRS complex
PR interval: 0.08 to 0.10 second
QRS complex: 0.04 to 0.06 second (basic rhythm); 0.12 second (premature beat)
Rhythm interpretation: Junctional tachycardia with one PVC

Strip 11-92
Rhythm: Regular
Rate: 188 beats/minute
P waves: Hidden in T waves
PR interval: Not measurable
QRS complex: 0.06 to 0.08 second
Rhythm interpretation: Paroxysmal atrial tachycardia; ST-segment depression is present.

Strip 11-93
Rhythm: Chaotic
Rate: 0
P waves: Absent; fibrillatory waves present
PR interval: Not measurable
QRS complex: Absent
Rhythm interpretation: Ventricular fibrillation

Strip 11-94
Rhythm: Irregular
Rate: 80 beats/minute
P waves: Vary in size, shape, and position
PR interval: 0.14 to 0.16 second
QRS complex: 0.06 to 0.08 second
Rhythm interpretation: Wandering atrial pacemaker; T-wave inversion is present.

Strip 11-95
Rhythm: Regular
Rate: 100 beats/minute
P waves: Inverted before each QRS complex
PR interval: 0.08 second
QRS complex: 0.06 to 0.08 second
Rhythm interpretation: Accelerated junctional rhythm

Strip 11-96
Rhythm: Regular (atrial); irregular (ventricular)
Rate: 84 beats/minute (atrial); 70 beats/minute (ventricular)
P waves: Sinus
PR interval: Lengthens from 0.20 to 0.36 second
QRS complex: 0.08 to 0.10 second
Rhythm interpretation: Second-degree AV block, Mobitz I; ST-segment depression is present.

Strip 11-97
Rhythm: Irregular
Rate: 100 beats/minute
P waves: Fibrillatory waves
PR interval: Not measurable
QRS complex: 0.06 to 0.08 second (basic rhythm); 0.12 second (PVC)
Rhythm interpretation: Atrial fibrillation with one PVC

Strip 11-98
Automatic interval rate: 63 beats/minute
Analysis: First two beats are paced beats followed by one patient beat, two paced beats, loss of capture spike, one patient beat, and one paced beat.
Rhythm interpretation: Loss of capture

Strip 11-99
Rhythm: Regular (basic rhythm); irregular (premature beat)
Rate: 125 beats/minute (basic rhythm)
P waves: Sinus
PR interval: 0.12 second
QRS complex: 0.04 to 0.06 second
Rhythm interpretation: Sinus tachycardia with one PAC (twelfth complex)

Strip 11-100
Rhythm: Regular
Rate: 272 beats/minute (atrial); 136 beats/minute (ventricular)
P waves: Two flutter waves to each QRS complex
PR interval: Not measurable
QRS complex: 0.04 second
Rhythm interpretation: Atrial flutter with 2:1 AV conduction

Strip 11-101
Rhythm: Irregular
Rate: 60 beats/minute
P waves: Sinus
PR interval: 0.14 to 0.16 second
QRS complex: 0.08 second
Rhythm interpretation: Sinus arrhythmia

**Strip 11-102**
Rhythm: Regular
Rate: 48 beats/minute
P waves: Sinus
PR interval: 0.14 to 0.16 second
QRS complex: 0.08 second
Rhythm interpretation: Sinus bradycardia; a U wave is
present.

**Strip 11-103**
Rhythm: Regular
Rate: 214 beats/minute
P waves: None identified
PR interval: Not measurable
QRS complex: 0.16 second or greater
Rhythm interpretation: Ventricular tachycardia

**Strip 11-104**
Rhythm: Irregular
Rate: 60 beats/minute
P waves: Fibrillatory waves
PR interval: Not measurable
QRS complex: 0.06 to 0.08 second
Rhythm interpretation: Atrial fibrillation

**Strip 11-105**
Rhythm: Regular (basic rhythm)
Rate: 72 beats/minute (basic rhythm)
P waves: Sinus
PR interval: 0.16 to 0.18 second
QRS complex: 0.06 to 0.08 second (basic rhythm); 0.12
second (PVC)
Rhythm interpretation: Normal sinus rhythm with one in-
terpolated PVC; ST-segment depression is present.

**Strip 11-106**
Rhythm: Regular (basic rhythm); irregular (PJC)
Rate: 65 beats/minute (basic rhythm)
P waves: Sinus (basic rhythm); inverted (PJC)
PR interval: 0.12 to 0.16 second (basic rhythm); 0.10 sec-
ond (PJC)
QRS complex: 0.06 to 0.08 second
Rhythm interpretation: Normal sinus rhythm with one
PJC; a U wave is present.

**Strip 11-107**
Rhythm: Regular (basic rhythm); irregular (PVCs)
Rate: 88 beats/minute (basic rhythm)
P waves: Sinus
PR interval: 0.12 to 0.14 second
QRS complex: 0.04 to 0.06 second
Rhythm interpretation: Normal sinus rhythm with three
PVCs

# Glossary

**Aberrant**  Abnormal

**Aberrant ventricular conduction**  An electrical impulse originating in the sinoatrial node, atria, or atrioventricular junction that's abnormally conducted through the bundle branches and ventricles. This usually occurs when the impulse arrives at the bundle branches prematurely, before the bundle branches (usually the right) have been sufficiently repolarized. The impulse is conducted down the fully recovered branch (usually the left) to depolarize one ventricle in a normal fashion and then spreads abnormally through adjacent muscle cells to depolarize the other ventricle (sequential depolarization). Because total ventricular depolarization takes longer than normal, the resulting QRS complex will be wider than normal or aberrant. Also known as *aberrancy*.

**Absolute refractory period**  The period of time during ventricular depolarization and most of repolarization when cells absolutely cannot respond to a stimulus. This period begins with the onset of the QRS and ends at the peak of the T wave.

**Accelerated idioventricular rhythm**  An arrhythmia originating in an ectopic site in the ventricles characterized by a regular rhythm, an absence of P waves, and wide QRS complexes at a rate of 50 to 100 beats/minute. The rate is faster than the inherent firing rate of the ventricles, but is slower than ventricular tachycardia.

**Accelerated junctional rhythm**  An arrhythmia originating in the atrioventricular (AV) junction characterized by a regular rhythm; inverted P waves immediately before the QRS, immediately after the QRS, or hidden within the QRS complex with a short PR interval of 0.10 second or less; a normal duration QRS complex; and a rate between 60 and 100 beats/minute. The rate is faster than the inherent firing rate of the AV junction, but slower than junctional tachycardia.

**Accessory conduction pathways**  Several abnormal electrical conduction pathways within the heart that bypass the atrioventricular node, allowing the electrical impulses to travel from the atria to the ventricles more rapidly than usual.

**Acetylcholine**  The chemical neurotransmitter for the parasympathetic nervous system.

**Acidosis**  A disturbance in the acid-base balance of the body. Acidosis is caused by an excess of carbon dioxide (respiratory acidosis), an excess of lactic acid (metabolic acidosis), or both.

**Actin**  One of the contractile protein filaments that give myocardial cells the property of contractility.

**Acute myocardial infarction**  Necrosis of the myocardium caused by prolonged and complete interruption of blood flow to an area of the myocardial muscle mass.

**Agonal rhythm**  A rhythm seen in a dying heart in which the QRS complexes deteriorate into irregular, wide, indistinguishable waveforms just prior to ventricular standstill.

**AIVR**  *abbr* accelerated idioventricular rhythm

**Amplitude**  The height or depth of a wave or complex on the ECG measured in millimeters. Also known as *voltage*.

**Angina**  Pain that results from a reduction in blood supply to the myocardium. The pain is typically described as chest heaviness, pressure, squeezing, or constriction. Associated symptoms include nausea and diaphoresis.

**Angioplasty**  The insertion of a balloon-tipped catheter into an occluded or narrowed coronary artery to reopen the artery by inflating the balloon, compressing the atherosclerotic plaque, and dilating the lumen of the artery. Often followed by insertion of a coronary artery stent. Also known as *percutaneous transluminal coronary angioplasty*.

**Anion**  An ion with a negative charge.

**Antegrade conduction**  Conduction of the electrical impulse in a forward direction.

**Aortic valve**  One of two semilunar valves. Located between the left ventricle and the aorta.

**Apex of the heart**  The pointed lower end of the heart formed by the tip of the left ventricle.

**Arrhythmia**  A general term referring to any cardiac rhythm other than a sinus rhythm. Often used interchangeably with *dysrhythmia,* a more appropriate term that's used less often.

**Artifacts**  Distortion of the ECG tracing by activity that is noncardiac in origin, such as patient movement, electrical interference, and muscle tremors. Also known as *interference* or *noise.*

**Asystole**  Absence of ventricular electrical activity. Tracing will show P waves only or a straight line. Also called *ventricular standstill.*

**Atria**  The two thin-walled upper chambers of the heart. The right and left atria are separated from the ventricles by the mitral and tricuspid valves.

**Atrial fibrillation**  An arrhythmia originating in an ectopic site (or numerous sites) in the atria characterized by an atrial rate of 400 beats/minute or more; atrial waveforms appearing as an irregular, wavy baseline; and a normal QRS duration with a grossly irregular ventricular rate.

**Atrial flutter**  An arrhythmia originating in an ectopic site in the atria characterized by an atrial rate between 250 and 400 beats/minute, atrial waveforms appearing in a sawtooth pattern, a normal QRS duration, and a ventricular response, which may be regular or irregular depending on the atrioventricular conduction ratio.

**Atrial kick**  Blood pushed into the ventricles due to atrial contraction during the last part of ventricular filling, just before the ventricles contract.

**Atrioventricular block**  A delay or failure of conduction of electrical impulses through the atrioventricular junction.

**Atrioventricular block, first-degree**  An arrhythmia in which there is a delay in the conduction of electrical impulses through the atrioventricular node. It's characterized by normal sinus P waves, a consistent PR interval that is abnormally prolonged (greater than 0.20 second), and a normal QRS duration.

**Atrioventricular block, second-degree, Mobitz I (Wenckenbach)**  An arrhythmia in which there is a progressive delay in the conduction of electrical impulses through the atrioventricular node until an impulse is completely blocked. Characterized by normal sinus P waves and progressive lengthening of the PR interval until a P wave appears not accompanied by a QRS, but followed by a pause, an irregular ventricular rhythm, a QRS of normal duration, and a pattern that is cyclic.

**Atrioventricular block, second-degree, Mobitz II**  An arrhythmia in which some electrical impulses are conducted to the ventricles, but most are blocked. Characterized by normal sinus P waves; consistent PR intervals with two, three, four or more P waves before each QRS; a ventricular rhythm that may be regular or irregular depending on atrioventricular conduction ratios; and a QRS complex that may be normal or wide depending on the site of the conduction disturbance.

**Atrioventricular block, third-degree**  An arrhythmia in which there is no conduction of electrical impulses through the atrioventricular (AV) node. There is independent beating of the atria and ventricles. The atria are paced by the sinoatrial node at a rate of 60 to 100 beats/minute, and the ventricles are paced either by the AV junction at 40 to 60 beats/minute or by the ventricles at a rate of 40 beats/minute or less. Characterized by normal sinus P waves with no consistent relationship to the QRS complex (variable PR intervals), P waves found hidden in QRS complexes and T waves, a regular atrial and ventricular rhythm, and a QRS that's normal if paced from the AV junction or wide if paced from the ventricles. Also known as *complete AV block.*

**Atrioventricular junction**  Consists of the atrioventricular (AV) node and the bundle of His. The AV junction includes three regions: the atrionodal or upper junctional region, the nodal or middle junctional region, and the nodal-His region or lower junctional region. The upper and lower junctional regions possess cells that demonstrate automaticity and are responsible for pacemaker function.

**Atrioventricular node**  Located in the lower portion of the right atrium near the interatrial septum. Only normal pathway for conduction of atrial impulses to the ventricles. Primary function is to slow conduction of electrical impulses through the atrioventricular node to allow for atrial contraction and complete filling of the ventricles (atrial kick).

**Atrioventricular valves**  The two valves located between the atria and the ventricles. The tricuspid valve separates the right atrium from the right ventricle; the mitral valve separates the left atrium from the left ventricle.

**Automaticity**  Ability of a cell to spontaneously generate an impulse.

**Autonomic nervous system**  Regulates functions of the body that are involuntary (not under conscious control). Includes the sympathetic and parasympathetic nervous systems, each producing opposite effects when stimulated.

**AV**  *abbr* atrioventricular

**Bachmann's bundle**  A branch of the internodal atrial conduction tracts. Conducts the electrical impulses from the sinoatrial node to the left atria.

**Baseline**  The straight line between ECG waveforms when no electrical activity is detected.

**Base of the heart**  Top of the heart located at approximately the level of the second intercostal space.

**Beta blockers**  A group of drugs that block sympathetic activity. Used to treat tachyarrhythmias, myocardial infarction, angina, and hypertension.

**Bigeminy**  An arrhythmia in which every other beat is a premature ectopic beat.

**Biphasic deflection**  A waveform that is part positive and part negative.

**Bradycardia**  An arrhythmia with a rate of less than 60 beats/minute.

**Bundle-branch block**  A block of conduction of the electrical impulses through either the right or left bundle branch, resulting in a right or left bundle-branch block.

**Bundle branches**  A part of the electrical conduction system consisting of the right and left bundle branches that conducts the electrical impulses from the bundle of His to the Purkinje network.

**Bundle of His**  A part of the electrical conduction system that connects the atrioventricular node to the bundle branches.

**Bursts**  Three or more consecutive premature ectopic beats (atrial, junctional, or ventricular). Also known as *salvo* and *run.*

**Calcium channel blockers**  A group of drugs that block entry of calcium ions into cells, especially those of cardiac and vascular smooth muscle. Used as an antiarrhythmic and to treat hypertension and angina.

**Cardiac cells**  Cells of the heart consisting of the myocardial (working or mechanical) cells, which are responsible for contraction of the heart muscle, and the pacemaker cells of the electrical conduction system, which spontaneously generate electrical impulses.

**Cardiac cycle**  Consists of one heartbeat or one PQRST sequence. Represents atrial contraction and relaxation followed by ventricular contraction and relaxation.

**Cardiac tamponade**  Compression of the heart due to the effusion of fluid into the pericardial cavity (as occurs in pericarditis) or the accumulation of blood in the pericardium (as occurs in heart rupture or penetrating trauma).

**Cardioaccelerator center**  One of the nerve centers of the sympathetic nervous system. Responsible for accelerated responses, such as increased speed of conduction and increased heart rate. Innervates the heart by way of the sympathetic nerve fibers located in the thoracic segment of the spinal cord.

**Cardioinhibitor center**  One of the nerve centers of the parasympathetic nervous system. Responsible for inhibitory responses, such as decreased speed of conduction and decreased heart rate. Innervates the heart by way of the vagal nerve fibers located in the medulla oblongata.

**Cardiomyopathy**  A disease of the heart muscle. Characterized by chamber dilation, wall thickening, decreased contractility, and conduction disturbances. End result is usually severe dysfunction of the heart muscle, resulting in terminal heart failure.

**Cardioversion**  A direct current electrical shock synchronized with the QRS complex used to terminate the following: atrial fibrillation, atrial flutter, paroxysmal atrial tachycardia, ventricular tachycardia, and wide QRS complex tachycardia of unknown origin. Also known as *synchronized countershock.*

**Cation**  An ion with a positive charge.

**CHF**  *abbr* congestive heart failure

**Chordae tendineae**  Thin strands of fibrous connective tissue that extend from the cusps of the atrioventricular (AV) valves to the papillary muscles and prevent the AV valves from bulging back into the atria during ventricular contraction.

**Chronic obstructive pulmonary disease**  A chronic disease of the lungs characterized by diffuse airway obstruction with varying degrees of chronic bronchitis and emphysema. Associated symptoms include a chronic productive cough and dyspnea on exertion.

**Circulatory system** A closed system consisting of two separate circuits: the systemic circuit and the pulmonary circuit. The *systemic circuit* consists of the left heart and blood vessels that carry blood from the left heart to the body and back to the right heart. The *pulmonary circuit* consists of the right heart and blood vessels that carry blood to the lungs and back to the left heart.

**Compensatory pause** A pause following a premature beat. A compensatory pause occurs when the sinoatrial (SA) node is not depolarized by the ectopic beat and the timing of the SA node discharge is unaffected. Because the timing of the SA node discharge is unaffected by the premature beat, the cadence of the underlying rhythm is unchanged and will resume on time following the pause. A compensatory pause is identified on the ECG by measuring from the R wave before the premature beat to the R wave following the premature beat—if that measurement equals two cardiac cycles (the sum of two R-R intervals), the pause is considered compensatory. A compensatory pause cannot be identified if the underlying rhythm is irregular. Also known as *complete pause*.

**Conductivity** The ability of a cardiac cell to receive an electrical impulse and conduct that impulse to an adjacent cardiac cell.

**Congestive heart failure** An overload of fluid in the lungs or body caused by inefficient pumping of the ventricles.

**Contractility** The ability of cardiac cells to shorten and cause cardiac muscle contraction in response to an electrical stimulus.

**Couplet** Two consecutive premature beats.

**Cyanosis** A purplish discoloration of the skin caused by the presence of unoxygenated blood.

**Defibrillation** An unsynchronized direct current electrical shock used to terminate ventricular fibrillation and pulseless ventricular tachycardia. Also known as *unsynchronized countershock*.

**Deflection** Refers to the waveforms in the ECG tracing (P wave, QRS complex, T wave, and U wave). A deflection may be positive (upright), negative (inverted), biphasic (having both positive and negative components), or equiphasic (equally positive and negative).

**Depolarization** Electrical activation of a cardiac cell due to movement of ions across a cell membrane, causing the inside of the cell to become more positive. Depolarization is an electrical event expected to result in muscle contraction, a mechanical event.

**Diaphoresis** Profuse sweating.

**Diastole** The period of atrial or ventricular relaxation.

**Dying heart** See *agonal rhythm*.

**Dyspnea** Shortness of breath.

**Dysrhythmia** Any rhythm other than a sinus rhythm. Used interchangeably with arrhythmia.

**ECG** *abbr* electrocardiogram

**Ectopic** A beat or rhythm originating from a source other than the sinoatrial node.

**Electrocardiogram** A graphic recording of the electrical activity of the heart generated by the depolarization and repolarization of the atria and ventricles.

**Electrocardiograph** A machine used to record the electrocardiogram.

**Electrolyte** A substance whose molecules dissociate into charged components when placed in water, producing positively and negatively charged ions.

**Endocardium** The innermost layer of the heart composed of thin, smooth connective tissue.

**Enhanced automaticity** An abnormal condition of latent pacemaker cells in which their firing rate is increased beyond the inherent rate.

**Equiphasic deflection** A biphasic deflection in which the sum of the positive deflection or deflections is equal to the sum of the negative deflection or deflections (equally positive and negative).

**Escape beats or rhythms** A term used when the sinus node slows down or fails to initiate an impulse and a lower pacemaker site spontaneously produces electrical impulses, assuming responsibility for pacing the heart.

**Excitability** The ability of a cardiac cell to respond to an electrical stimulus.

**Fascicle** A bundle of muscle or nerve fibers. The left anterior fascicle and the left posterior fascicle extend from the left main bundle branch to form the two major divisions of the left bundle branch before it divides into the Purkinje fibers, forming the Purkinje network.

**Fibrillation** Chaotic disorganized beating of the myocardium from multiple ectopic foci in which each muscle cell contracts and relaxes independently, producing ineffectual contractions. Fibrillation may occur in both the atria and the ventricles.

Heart rate  The number of heart beats or QRS complexes per minute.

His-Purkinje system  The part of the electrical conduction system consisting of the bundle of His, the bundle branches, and the Purkinje fibers.

Hypertrophy  An increase in the thickness of a heart chamber because of a chronic increase in pressure or volume within the chamber. Hypertrophy may occur in both the atria and the ventricles.

Idioventricular rhythm  An arrhythmia arising in an ectopic site in the ventricles characterized by a regular rhythm, absence of P waves, wide QRS complexes, and a rate between 30 and 40 (sometimes less) beats per minute. It's the inherent rhythm of the ventricles.

Infarction  Death (necrosis) of tissue caused by an interruption of blood supply to the affected tissue.

Inferior vena cava  One of two large veins that empty venous blood into the right atrium.

Inherent firing rate  The normal rate at which electrical impulses are generated in a pacemaker, whether it is the sinoatrial node or an ectopic pacemaker. Also known as the *intrinsic firing rate.*

Interatrial septum  The wall separating the right and left atria.

Internodal atrial conduction tract  Part of the electrical conduction system. Consists of three pathways of specialized conducting tissue located in the walls of the right atrium. Conducts impulses from the sinoatrial node to the atrioventricular node.

Intraventricular septum  The wall separating the right and left ventricles.

Ion  Electrically charged particle.

Ischemia  Reduced blood flow to tissue caused by narrowing or occlusion of the artery supplying blood to it.

Isoelectric line  See Baseline.

IVR  *abbr* idioventricular rhythm

J point  The point where the QRS complex and ST segment meet.

Junctional rhythm  An arrhythmia arising in the atrioventricular junction characterized by a regular rhythm; inverted P waves immediately before the QRS, immediately after the QRS, or hidden within the QRS complex with a short PR interval of 0.10 second or less; a normal duration QRS complex; and a rate between 40 and 60 beats/minute. Junctional rhythm is the inherent rhythm of the atrioventricular node.

Junctional tachycardia  An arrhythmia arising in the atrioventricular junction characterized by a regular rhythm; inverted P waves immediately before the QRS, immediately after the QRS, or hidden within the QRS complex with a short PR interval of 0.10 second or less; a normal duration QRS complex; and a rate greater than 100 beats/minute.

Latent pacemaker cells  Cells in the electrical conduction system located below the sinoatrial (SA) node with the property of automaticity. These cells hold the property of automaticity in reserve in case the SA node fails to function properly or electrical impulses fail to be conducted. Also known as *subsidiary pacemaker cells.*

mA  *abbr* milliampere

Mediastinum  Located in the middle of the thoracic cavity. Contains the heart, trachea, esophagus, and great vessels (pulmonary arteries and veins, aorta, and the superior and inferior vena cava).

Medulla oblongata  Part of the brainstem containing specialized nerve centers for special senses, respiration, and circulation. Includes the sympathetic and parasympathetic nervous systems with their respective cardioaccelerator and cardioinhibitor centers.

MI  *abbr* myocardial infarction

Milliampere  Unit of measure of electrical current needed to cause depolarization of the myocardium.

Mitral valve  One of two atrioventricular valves. Located between the left atrium and left ventricle. Similar in structure to the tricuspid valve, but has only two cusps.

Monomorphic  Having the same shape.

Multifocal  Indicates an arrhythmia originating in multiple pacemaker sites.

**Multifocal premature ventricular contractions** Premature ventricular contractions that appear different (vary in size, shape, and direction) in the same tracing, originating from multiple ectopic pacemaker sites in the ventricles.

**Myocardium** The middle and thickest layer of the heart composed primarily of cardiac muscle cells and responsible for the heart's ability to contract.

**Myosin** One of the contractile protein filaments that give the myocardial cells the property of contractility.

**Noncompensatory pause** A pause following a premature beat. A noncompensatory pause occurs when the sinoatrial (SA) node is depolarized by the ectopic beat, resetting the timing of the SA node discharge. Due to resetting of the SA node discharge, the underlying rhythm will not resume on time following the pause. A noncompensatory pause is identified on the ECG by measuring from the R wave before the premature beat to the R wave following the premature beat. If that measurement is less than two cardiac cycles (less than the sum of two R-R intervals), the pause is considered noncompensatory. A noncompensatory pause cannot be identified if the underlying rhythm is irregular. Also known as *incomplete pause*.

**Nonconducted premature atrial contraction** A premature abnormal P wave not accompanied by a QRS complex, but followed by a pause.

**Normal sinus rhythm** The normal rhythm of the heart originating in the sinoatrial (SA) node characterized by a regular rhythm; normal P waves, PR interval, and QRS duration; and a rate between 60 and 100 beats/minute.

**PAC** *abbr* premature atrial contraction

**Pacemaker** A device that delivers an electric current to the heart to stimulate depolarization.

**Papillary muscles** Projections of myocardium arising from the ventricular walls, which are attached to the chordae tendineae. During ventricular contraction the papillary muscles contract and pull on the chordae tendineae, thus preventing inversion of the atrioventricular valves into the atria.

**Parasympathetic nervous system** A part of the autonomic nervous system involved in the control of involuntary bodily functions, such as control of cardiac and blood vessel activity. Stimulation of the parasympathetic nervous system depresses cardiac activity and produces effects opposite to those of the sympathetic nervous system. Some effects of parasympathetic stimulation include a decrease in heart rate, drop in blood pressure, nausea, vomiting, and faintness.

**Paroxysmal** The sudden onset or cessation of an arrhythmia.

**Paroxysmal atrial tachycardia** An arrhythmia originating in the atria characterized by abnormal, upright P waves that are usually hidden in the preceding T waves; a normal QRS duration; and a regular rhythm between 140 and 250 beats/minute.

**PAT** *abbr* paroxysmal atrial tachycardia

**Premature atrial contraction** An early beat originating in the atria characterized by a premature, abnormal P wave (usually upright), a PR interval that may vary (usually normal duration), and a normal duration QRS complex followed by a pause.

**Premature junctional contraction** An early beat originating in the atrioventricular junction characterized by a premature inverted P wave occurring immediately before the QRS, immediately after the QRS, or hidden within the QRS complex with a short PR interval of 0.10 second or less and a normal duration QRS complex followed by a pause.

**Premature ventricular contraction** An early beat originating in the ventricles characterized by a premature, wide, bizarre QRS complex with no associated P wave, followed by a pause.

**PR interval** The period of time from the beginning of atrial depolarization (P wave) to the beginning of ventricular depolarization (QRS complex). The normal PR interval duration is 0.12 to 0.20 second.

**Prinzmetal's angina** A type of angina occurring when the coronary arteries experience spasms and constrict.

**PR segment** The portion of the ECG between the end of the P wave and the beginning of the QRS complex.

**PTCA** *abbr* percutaneous transluminal coronary angioplasty

**Pulmonic valve** One of two semilunar valves. Located between the right ventricle and the pulmonary artery.

**Purkinje fibers** A network of fibers that carry electrical impulses directly to ventricular muscle cells.

**PVC** *abbr* premature ventricular contraction

**P wave** The waveform representing depolarization of the right and left atria. The P wave is upright when it originates in the sinus node and in most atrial ectopic sites. The P wave is negative when it originates from the atrioventricular junction.

**QT interval** Portion of the ECG between the onset of the QRS complex and the end of the T wave, representing ventricular depolarization and repolarization.

**Q wave** The negative deflection of the QRS complex that precedes the R wave.

**Relative refractory period** The period of time during ventricular repolarization during which the ventricles can be stimulated to depolarize by an electrical impulse stronger than usual. This period begins at the peak of the T wave and ends with the end of the T wave.

**Repolarization** An electrical process by which a depolarized cell returns to its resting state due to the movement of ions across a cell membrane, restoring the cell to its negative charge.

**Retrograde** Moving backward or in the opposite direction to that which is considered normal.

**R-on-T phenomenon** A premature ventricular contraction that falls on the T wave of the preceding beat. This phenomenon can cause ventricular tachycardia or ventricular fibrillation because it falls during the vulnerable period of ventricular repolarization.

**R-R interval** The period of time from one R wave to the next consecutive R wave.

**R wave** The positive wave in the QRS complex.

**SA** *abbr* sinoatrial

**Sinus arrest** An arrhythmia caused by a failure of the sinoatrial node to initiate an impulse (a disorder of automaticity). The ECG tracing will show a sudden pause in the sinus rhythm in which one or more beats is missing. The underlying rhythm does not resume on time following the pause.

**Sinus arrhythmia** An arrhythmia originating in the sinoatrial (SA) node that occurs when the SA node discharges impulses irregularly. Sinus arrhythmia is a normal phenomenon associated with the phases of respiration. This rhythm is characterized by an irregular rate, normal P waves, PR interval, and QRS duration, and may be associated with a normal or bradycardic rate.

**Sinus bradycardia** An arrhythmia originating in the sinus node characterized by a regular rhythm, normal P waves, PR interval, and QRS duration with a rate between 40 and 60 beats/minute.

**Sinus exit block** An arrhythmia caused by a block in the conduction of the electrical impulse from the sinoatrial node to the atria (a disorder of conduction). The ECG tracing will show a sudden pause in the sinus rhythm in which one or more beats is missing. The underlying rhythm resumes on time following the pause.

**Sinus node** The dominant pacemaker of the heart located in the wall of the right atrium close to the inlet of the superior vena cava.

**Sinus tachycardia** An arrhythmia originating in the sinus node characterized by a regular rhythm and normal P waves, PR interval, and QRS duration with a rate between 100 and 180 beats/minute.

**ST segment** The flat line between the QRS complex and the T wave that represents early ventricular repolarization. The ST segment is normally at baseline.

**Superior vena cava** One of two large veins that empty venous blood into the right atrium.

**Supernormal period** The last phase of repolarization during which the cell can be stimulated to depolarize by a weaker than normal electrical stimulus. This period occurs near the end of the T wave just before the cells have completely repolarized.

**Supraventricular** A general term used to describe arrhythmias that originate in sites above the bundle branches, such as the sinus node, atria, and atrioventricular junction.

**S wave** The negative deflection of the QRS complex that follows the R wave.

**Sympathetic nervous system** A part of the autonomic nervous system involved in the control of involuntary bodily functions, such as cardiac activity and blood vessel activity. Stimulation of the sympathetic nervous system increases cardiac activity and produces effects opposite to those of the parasympathetic nervous system. Some effects of sympathetic stimulation include an increase in heart rate and blood pressure.

**Syncope** Fainting, usually resulting from cardiac or neurologic events.

**TCP** *abbr* transcutaneous pacing

**Torsade de pointes** A form of ventricular tachycardia associated with a prolonged QT interval. The ECG tracing will show a QRS that changes in shape, width, and amplitude and seems to rotate or twist around the isoelectric line (pointing downward for a series of beats, then changing direction and pointing upward).

**Transcutaneous pacing** External cardiac pacing. Consists of two large electrode pads commonly placed in an anterior-posterior position on the patient's chest to conduct electrical impulses through the skin to the heart.

**Transvenous pacing** Cardiac pacing through a vein. A lead wire is inserted into a large vein and positioned in the right ventricle. Electrical impulses are conducted from an external power source (pacing generator) through the lead wire to the right ventricle.

**Tricuspid valve** One of two atrioventricular valves. Located between the right atrium and the right ventricle. Similar in structure to the mitral valve, but has three cusps.

**T wave** A wave that follows the ST segment. Represents the latter phase of ventricular repolarization.

**Unifocal premature ventricular contractions** Premature ventricular contractions (PVCs) originating in the same ventricular pacemaker site having the same appearance. Also known as *uniform PVCs*.

**U wave** A wave that sometimes follows the T wave. Represents the final phase of ventricular repolarization.

**Vagal maneuvers** Methods to increase vagal (parasympathetic) tone. Used to convert paroxysmal atrial tachycardia.

**Valsalva maneuver** Forceful act of expiration with mouth and nose closed producing a "bearing down" action. It's a vagal maneuver that increases parasympathetic tone and is used to convert paroxysmal atrial tachycardia.

**Vasovagal** Pertaining to a vascular as well as neurogenic cause.

**Ventricles** The two thick-walled lower chambers of the heart. They receive blood from the atria and pump it into the pulmonary and systemic circulation. The ventricles are separated from the atria by the mitral and tricuspid valves.

**Ventricular fibrillation** An arrhythmia arising from a disorganized, chaotic electrical focus in the ventricles in which the ventricles quiver instead of contract effectively. The ECG tracing shows an irregular, wavy baseline without QRS complexes.

**Ventricular standstill** An arrhythmia in which there is an absence of all ventricular activity. The ECG tracing will show either P waves without QRS complexes or a straight line. Also known as *ventricular asystole.*

**Ventricular tachycardia** An arrhythmia arising from an ectopic site in the ventricles. On the ECG, the rhythm appears as a series of wide QRS complexes with no associated P waves at a rate of 140 to 250 beats/minute.

**Vulnerable period** The period of time during ventricular repolarization in which a strong electrical stimulus can stimulate the ventricles to depolarize. This period corresponds to the downslope of the T wave (relative refractory period). Electrical stimuli occurring during the vulnerable period may lead to ventricular tachycardia or ventricular fibrillation.

**Wandering atrial pacemaker** An arrhythmia arising from multiple pacemaker sites in the atria. The ECG tracing will show a normal or slow rate; a regular (sometimes irregular) rhythm; P waves that vary in size, shape, and direction across the rhythm strip; PR intervals that may vary slightly; and normal QRS duration.

# Index

i refers to an illustration; t referes to a table.

i refers to an illustration; t referes to a table.

## Electrocardiographic conversion table for heart rate

| Number of small spaces | Rate per minute | Number of small spaces | Rate per minute | Number of small spaces | Rate per minute |
|---|---|---|---|---|---|
| 5 | 300 | 26 | 58 | 47 | 32 |
| 6 | 250 | 27 | 56 | 48 | 31 |
| 7 | 214 | 28 | 54 | 49 | 31 |
| 8 | 188 | 29 | 52 | 50 | 30 |
| 9 | 167 | 30 | 50 | 52 | 29 |
| 10 | 150 | 31 | 48 | 54 | 28 |
| 11 | 136 | 32 | 47 | 56 | 27 |
| 12 | 125 | 33 | 45 | 58 | 26 |
| 13 | 115 | 34 | 44 | 60 | 25 |
| 14 | 107 | 35 | 43 | 62 | 24 |
| 15 | 100 | 36 | 42 | 64 | 23 |
| 16 | 94 | 37 | 41 | 68 | 22 |
| 17 | 88 | 38 | 40 | 72 | 21 |
| 18 | 84 | 39 | 39 | 76 | 20 |
| 19 | 79 | 40 | 38 | 80 | 19 |
| 20 | 75 | 41 | 37 | 84 | 18 |
| 21 | 72 | 42 | 36 | 88 | 17 |
| 22 | 68 | 43 | 35 | 92 | 16 |
| 23 | 65 | 44 | 34 | 98 | 15 |
| 24 | 63 | 45 | 33 | 104 | 14 |
| 25 | 60 | 46 | 33 | 112 | 13 |

**1**

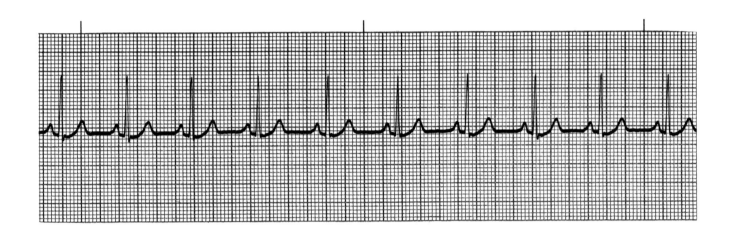

**2**

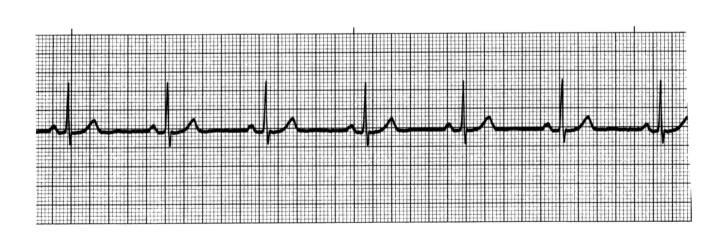

**Answer:** Normal sinus rhythm

## Normal sinus rhythm: Identifying ECG features

**Rhythm interpretation:** Regular

**Rate:** 60 to 100 beats/minute

**P waves:** Normal in size, shape, direction; positive in lead II; one P wave precedes each QRS complex

**PR interval:** Normal (0.12 to 0.20 second)

**QRS complex:** Normal (0.10 second or less)

## 2

**Answer:** Sinus bradycardia

## Sinus bradycardia: Identifying ECG features

**Rhythm interpretation:** Regular

**Rate:** 40 to 60 beats/minute

**P waves:** Normal in size, shape, direction; positive in lead II; one P wave precedes each QRS complex

**PR interval:** Normal (0.12 to 0.20 second)

**QRS complex:** Normal (0.10 second or less)

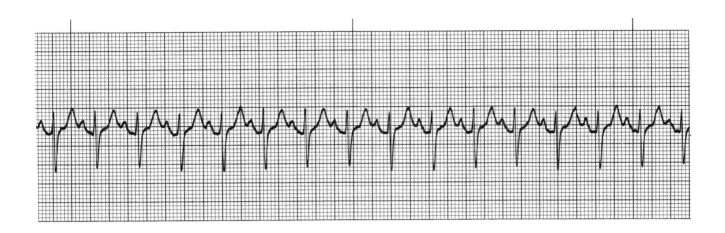

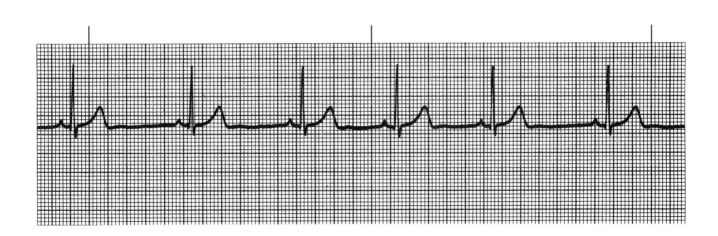

**Answer:** Sinus tachycardia

## Sinus tachycardia: Identifying ECG features

**Rhythm interpretation:** Regular

**Rate:** 100 to 180 beats/minute

**P waves:** Normal in size, shape, direction; positive in lead II; one P wave precedes each QRS complex

**PR interval:** Normal (0.12 to 0.20 second)

**QRS complex:** Normal (0.10 second or less)

**Answer:** Sinus arrhythmia with bradycardic rate

## Sinus arrhythmia: Identifying ECG features

**Rhythm interpretation:** Irregular

**Rate:** Normal (60 to 100 beats/minute) or slow (< 60 beats/minute; often seen with bradycardia)

**P waves:** Normal in size, shape, direction; positive in lead II; one P wave precedes each QRS complex

**PR interval:** Normal (0.12 to 0.20 second)

**QRS complex:** Normal (0.10 second or less)

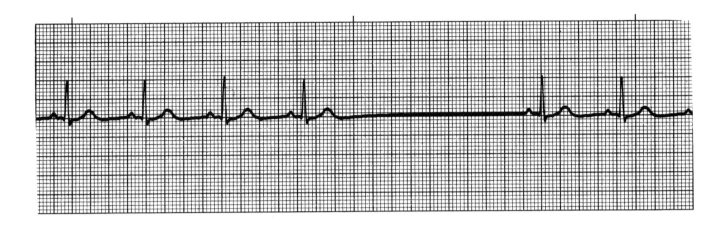

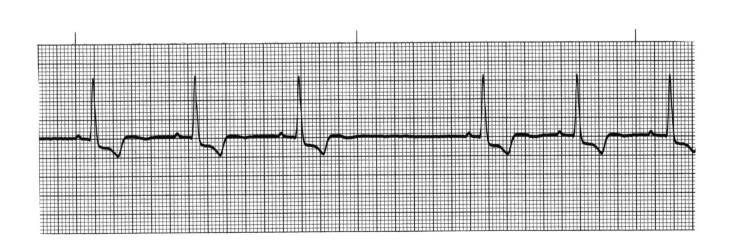

**Answer:** Normal sinus rhythm with sinus block

## Sinus block: Identifying ECG features

**Rhythm interpretation:** Basic rhythm usually regular; sudden pause in basic rhythm (causing irregularity) with one or more missing cardiac cycles; rhythm (R-R irregularity) resumes on time following pause; heart rate may slow for several beats following pause (temporary rate suppression) but returns to basic rate

**Rate:** Normal (60 to 100 beats/minute) or slow (< 60 beats/minute)

**P waves:** Normal with basic rhythm; absent during pause

**PR interval:** Normal with basic rhythm; absent during pause

**QRS complex:** Normal with basic rhythm; absent during pause

**Answer:** Normal sinus rhythm with sinus arrest

## Sinus arrest: Identifying ECG features

**Rhythm interpretation:** Basic rhythm usually regular; sudden pause in basic rhythm (causing irregularity) with one or more missing cardiac cycles; rhythm (R-R regularity) does not resume on time following pause; heart rate may slow for several beats following pause (temporary rate suppression) but returns to basic rate

**Rate:** Normal (60 to 100 beats/minute) or slow (< 60 beats/minute)

**P waves:** Normal with basic rhythm; absent during pause

**PR interval:** Normal with basic rhythm; absent during pause

**QRS complex:** Normal with basic rhythm; absent during pause

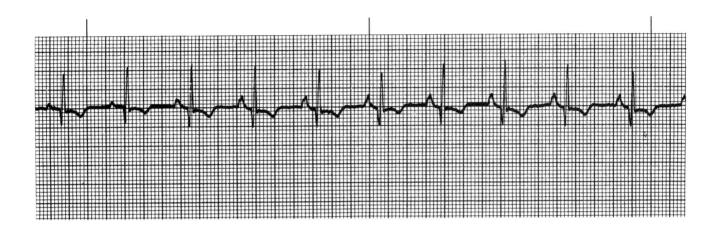

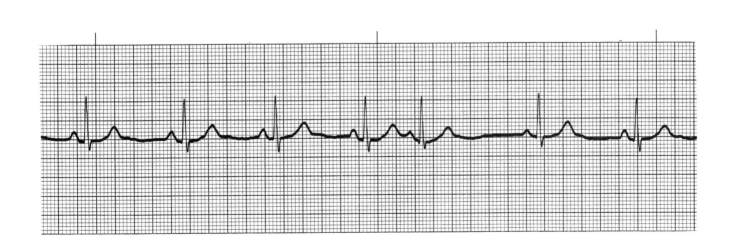

**Answer:** Wandering atrial pacemaker

## Wandering atrial pacemaker: Identifying ECG features

**Rhythm interpretation:** Regular or irregular

**Rate:** Normal (60 to 100 beats/minute) or slow (< 60 beats/minute)

**P waves:** Vary in size, shape, direction across rhythm strip; one P wave precedes each QRS complex

**PR interval:** Usually normal duration but may vary depending on changing pacemaker location

**QRS complex:** Normal (0.10 second or less)

**Answer:** Normal sinus rhythm with premature atrial contraction (PAC)

## Premature atrial contraction: Identifying ECG features

**Rhythm interpretation:** Underlying rhythm usually regular; irregular with PACs

**Rate:** That of underlying rhythm

**P waves:** P wave associated with PAC is premature and abnormal in size, shape, or direction; abnormal P wave is often found hidden in preceding T wave, distorting T wave contour

**PR interval:** Usually normal but can be prolonged; not measurable if hidden in preceding T wave

**QRS complex:** Premature with normal duration (0.10 second or less)

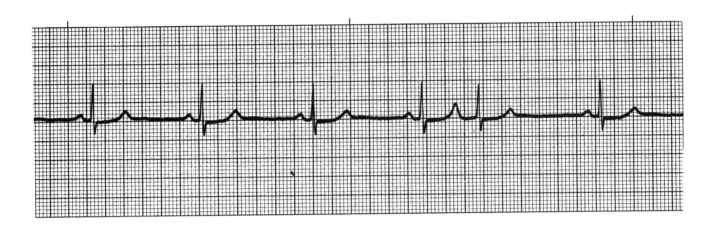

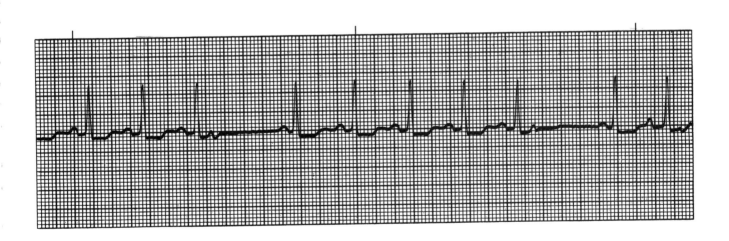

**Answer:** Sinus bradycardia with premature atrial contraction (PAC) (abnormal P wave associated with PAC is hidden in preceding T wave, distorting T wave contour)

## Premature atrial contraction: Identifying ECG features

**Rhythm interpretation:** Underlying rhythm usually regular; irregular with PACs

**Rate:** That of underlying rhythm

**P waves:** Premature and abnormal in size, shape or direction; abnormal P wave is often found hidden in preceding T wave, distorting T wave contour

**PR interval:** Usually normal but can be prolonged; not measurable if hidden in preceding T wave

**QRS complex:** Premature with normal duration (0.10 second or less)

**Answer:** Sinus tachycardia with two nonconducted premature atrial contractions (PACs)

## Nonconducted PACs: Identifying ECG features

**Rhythm interpretation:** Underlying rhythm usually regular; irregular with nonconducted PACs

**Rate:** That of underlying rhythm

**P waves:** Premature and abnormal in size, shape, or direction; often found hidden in preceding T wave, distorting T wave contour

**PR interval:** Absent with nonconducted PAC

**QRS complex:** Absent with nonconducted PAC

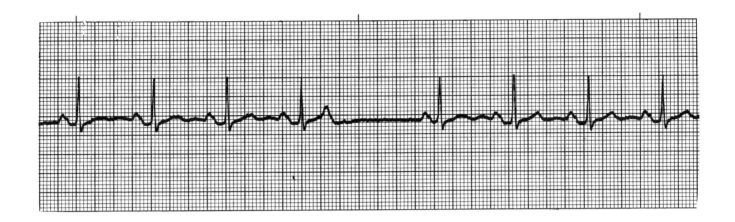

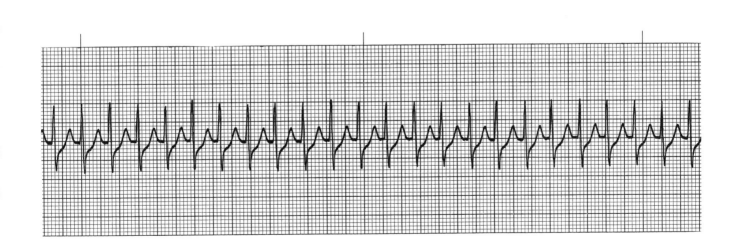

**Answer:** Normal sinus rhythm with one nonconducted premature atrial contraction (PAC) (abnormal P wave associated with nonconducted PAC is hidden in preceding T wave, distorting T wave contour)

## Nonconducted PACs: Identifying ECG features

**Rhythm interpretation:** Underlying rhythm usually regular; irregular with nonconducted PAC

**Rate:** That of underlying rhythm

**P waves:** Premature and abnormal in size, shape, or direction; often found hidden in preceding T wave, distorting T wave contour

**PR interval:** Absent with nonconducted PAC

**QRS complex:** Absent with nonconducted PAC

**Answer:** Paroxysmal atrial tachycardia

## Paroxysmal atrial tachycardia: Identifying ECG features

**Rhythm interpretation:** Regular

**Rate:** 140 to 250 beats/minute

**P waves:** Abnormal (often pointed); usually hidden in preceding T wave so that T wave and P wave appear as one wave deflection (T-P wave); one P wave to each QRS complex unless atrioventricular block is present

**PR interval:** Usually not measurable

**QRS complex:** Normal (0.10 second or less)

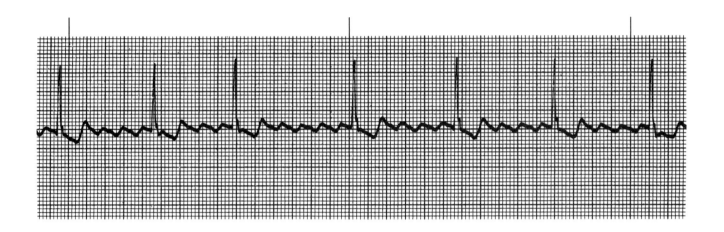

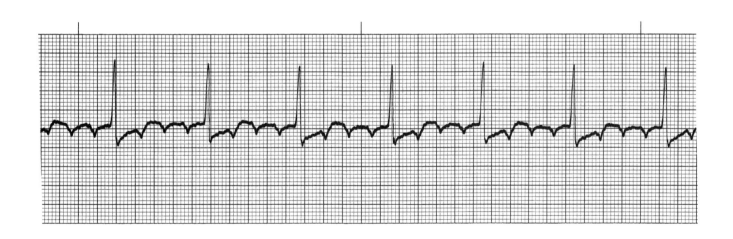

**Answer:** Atrial flutter with variable atrioventricular (AV) conduction

## Atrial flutter: Identifying ECG features

**Rhythm interpretation:** Regular or irregular (depends on AV conduction ratios)
**Rate:**
  **Atrial:** 250 to 400 beats/minute
  **Ventricular:** Varies with number of impulses conducted through AV node; will be less than atrial rate
**P waves:** Sawtooth wave deflection affecting the entire baseline
**PR interval:** Not measurable
**QRS complex:** Normal (0.10 second or less)

**Answer:** Atrial flutter with 4:1 atrioventricular (AV) conduction

## Atrial flutter: Identifying ECG features

**Rhythm interpretation:** Regular or irregular (depends on AV conduction ratios)
**Rate:**
  **Atrial:** 250 to 400 beats/minute
  **Ventricular:** Varies with number of impulses conducted through AV node; will be less than atrial rate
**P waves:** Sawtooth wave deflection affecting the entire baseline
**PR interval:** Not measurable
**QRS complex:** Normal (0.10 second or less)

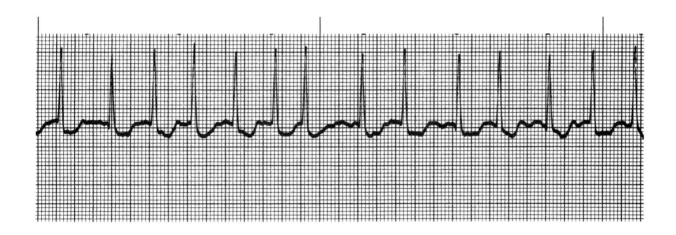

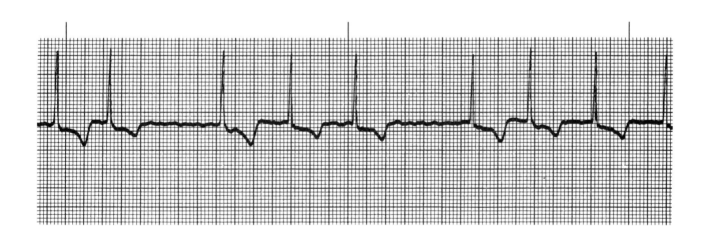

**Answer:** Atrial fibrillation with uncontrolled ventricular rate

## Atrial fibrillation: Identifying ECG features

**Rhythm interpretation:** Grossly irregular (unless ventricular rate is very rapid, in which case the rhythm becomes more regular)

**Rate:**

**Atrial:** 400 beats/minute or more; not measurable on surface ECG

**Ventricular:** Varies with number of impulses conducted through atrioventricular node to ventricles; ventricular rate is controlled if rate is less than 100 beats/minute, uncontrolled if it is greater than 100 beats/minute

**P waves:** Wave deflections that affect entire baseline

**PR interval:** Not measurable

**QRS complex:** Normal (0.10 second or less)

**Answer:** Atrial fibrillation with controlled ventricular rate

## Atrial fibrillation: Identifying ECG features

**Rhythm interpretation:** Grossly irregular (unless ventricular rate is very rapid, in which case the rhythm becomes more regular)

**Rate:**

**Atrial:** 400 beats/minute or more; not measurable on surface ECG

**Ventricular:** Varies with number of impulses conducted through atrioventricular node to ventricles; ventricular rate is controlled if rate is less than 100 beats/minute, uncontrolled if it is greater than 100 beats/minute

**P waves:** Wave deflections that affect entire baseline

**PR interval:** Not measurable

**QRS complex:** Normal (0.10 second or less)

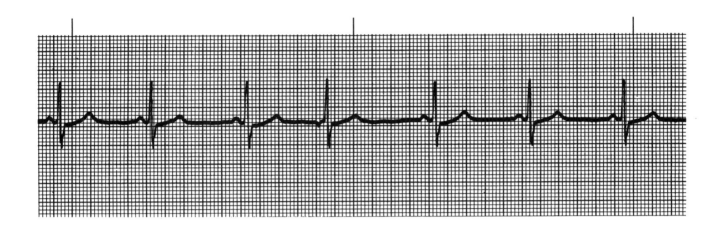

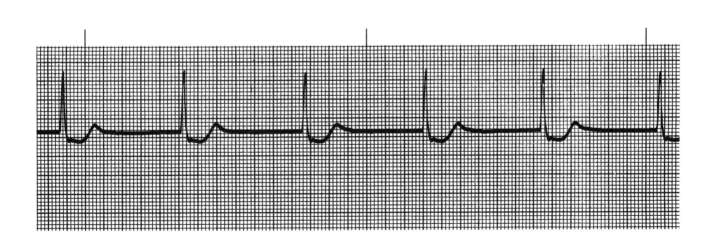

**Answer:** Normal sinus rhythm with premature junctional contraction (PJC)

## Premature junctional contraction: Identifying ECG features

**Rhythm interpretation:** Underlying rhythm usually regular; irregular with PJC

**Rate:** That of the underlying rhythm

**P waves:** Premature, inverted in lead II, and will occur immediately before the QRS complex, immediately after the QRS complex, or be hidden within the QRS complex

**PR interval:** 0.10 second or less

**QRS complex:** Premature with normal duration (0.10 second or less)

**Answer:** Junctional rhythm

## Junctional rhythm: Identifying ECG features

**Rhythm interpretation:** Regular

**Rate:** 40 to 60 beats/minute

**P waves:** Inverted in lead II and will occur immediately before the QRS complex, immediately after the QRS complex, or will be hidden within the QRS complex

**PR interval:** Short (0.10 second or less)

**QRS complex:** Normal (0.10 second or less)

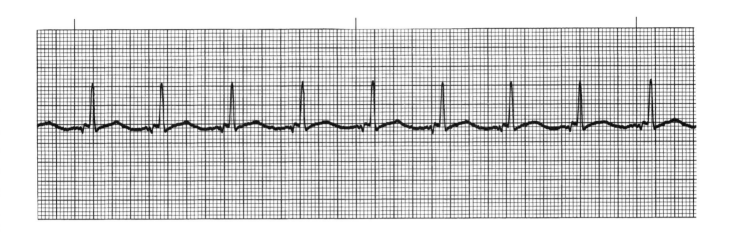

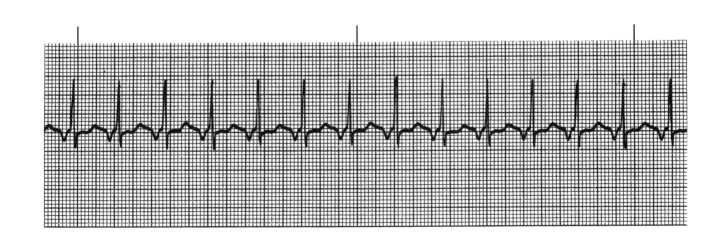

**Answer:** Accelerated junctional rhythm

## Accelerated junctional rhythm: Identifying ECG features

**Rhythm interpretation:** Regular

**Rate:** 60 to 100 beats/minute

**P waves:** Inverted in lead II and will occur immediately before the QRS complex, immediately after the QRS complex, or within the QRS complex

**PR interval:** Short (0.10 second or less)

**QRS complex:** Normal (0.10 second or less)

**Answer:** Junctional tachycardia

## Junctional tachycardia: Identifying ECG features

**Rhythm interpretation:** Regular

**Rate:** Greater than 100 beats/minute

**P waves:** Inverted in lead II and will occur immediately before the QRS complex, immediately after the QRS complex, or be hidden within the QRS complex

**PR interval:** Short (0.10 second or less)

**QRS complex:** Normal (0.10 second or less)

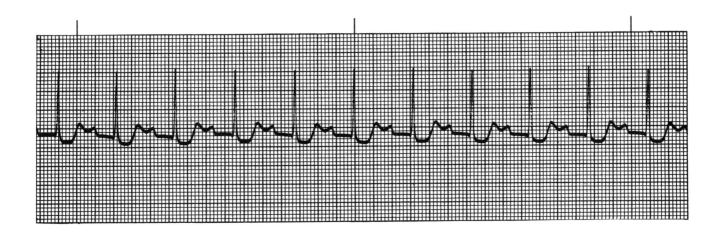

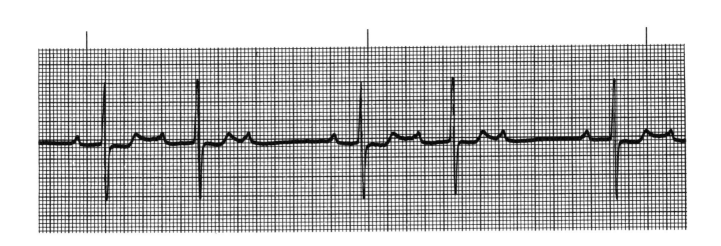

**Answer:** Normal sinus rhythm with first-degree atrioventricular (AV) block

## First-degree AV block: Identifying ECG features

**Rhythm interpretation:** Usually regular

**Rate:** That of underlying sinus rhythm; atrial and ventricular rates will be the same

**P waves:** Sinus; one P wave to each QRS complex

**PR interval:** Prolonged (greater than 0.20 second)

**QRS complex:** Normal (0.10 second or less)

**Answer:** Second-degree atrioventricular (AV) block (Mobitz I)

## Second-degree AV block: Identifying ECG features

**Rhythm interpretation:**
  **Atrial:** Regular
  **Ventricular:** Irregular

**Rate:**
  **Atrial:** That of underlying rhythm
  **Ventricular:** Depends on number of impulses conducted through AV node; less than atrial rate

**P waves:** Sinus origin

**PR interval:** Varies; progressively lengthens until a P wave is not conducted (P wave occurs without a QRS complex); a pause follows the dropped QRS complex

**QRS complex:** Normal (0.10 second or less)

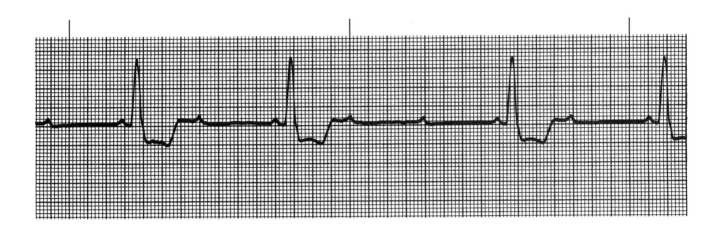

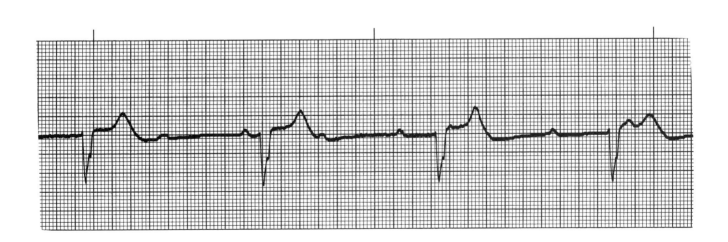

**Answer:** Second-degree atrioventricular (AV) block (Mobitz II)

## Second-degree AV block: Identifying ECG features

**Rhythm interpretation:**

  **Atrial:** Regular

  **Ventricular:** Usually regular but may be irregular if AV conduction ratios vary

**Rate:**

  **Atrial:** That of the underlying rhythm

  **Ventricular:** Depends on number of impulses conducted through AV node; less than the atrial rate

**P waves:** Sinus; two or three P waves (sometimes more) before each QRS complex

**PR interval:** May be normal or prolonged; remains constant

**QRS complex:** Normal if block at AV node or bundle of His; wide if block in bundle branches

**Answer:** Third-degree atrioventricular (AV) block (complete heart block)

## Third-degree AV block: Identifying ECG features

**Rhythm interpretation:**

  **Atrial:** Regular

  **Ventricular:** Regular

**Rate:**

  **Atrial:** That of underlying sinus rhythm

  **Ventricular:** 40 to 60 beats/minute if paced by AV junction; less than 40 beats/minute if paced by ventricles; ventricular rate less than atrial rate

**P waves:** Sinus P waves present with no constant relationship to QRS complex (P waves found marching through QRS complexes and T waves)

**PR interval:** Varies greatly

**QRS complex:** Normal if block at AV node or bundle of His; wide if block in bundle branches

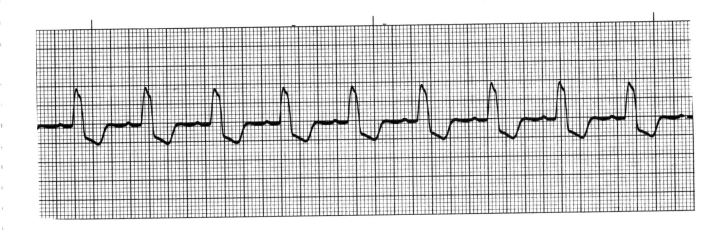

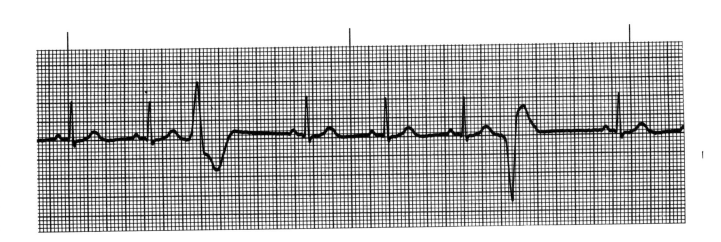

**Answer:** Normal sinus rhythm with bundle-branch block

## Bundle-branch block: Identifying ECG features

**Rhythm interpretation:** Usually regular
**Rate:** That of the underlying rhythm (usually sinus)
**P waves:** Sinus
**PR interval:** Normal (0.12 to 0.20 second)
**QRS complex:** Wide (0.12 second or greater)

**Answer:** Normal sinus rhythm with multifocal premature ventricular contractions (PVCs)

## Premature ventricular contractions: Identifying ECG features

**Rhythm interpretation:** Underlying rhythm usually regular; irregular with PVC
**Rate:** That of the underlying rhythm
**P waves:** None associated
**PR interval:** Not measurable
**QRS complex:** Premature and wide (0.12 second or greater)

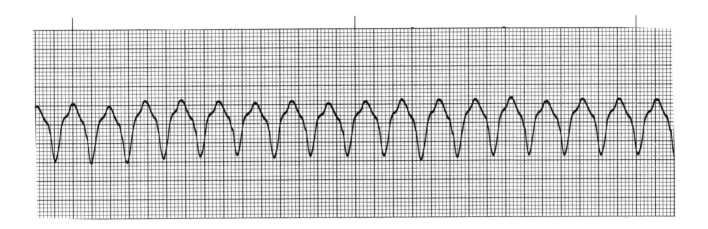

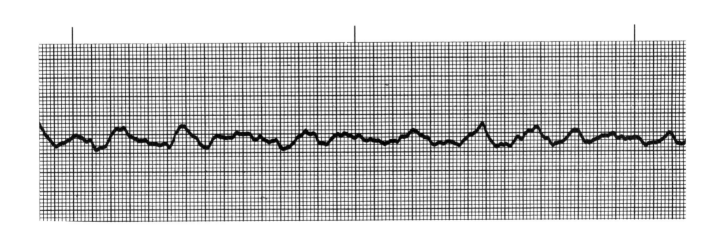

**Answer:** Ventricular tachycardia

## Ventricular tachycardia: Identifying ECG features

**Rhythm interpretation:** Regular
**Rate:** 140 to 250 beats/minute
**P waves:** None associated
**PR interval:** Not measurable
**QRS complex:** Wide (0.12 second or greater)

**Answer:** Ventricular fibrillation

## Ventricular fibrillation: Identifying ECG features

**Rhythm interpretation:** Chaotic, irregular deflections
**Rate:** 0 (P waves and QRS complexes absent)
**P waves:** Absent; wavy, irregular deflections are present that vary in size, height, and shape
**PR interval:** Not measurable
**QRS complex:** Absent

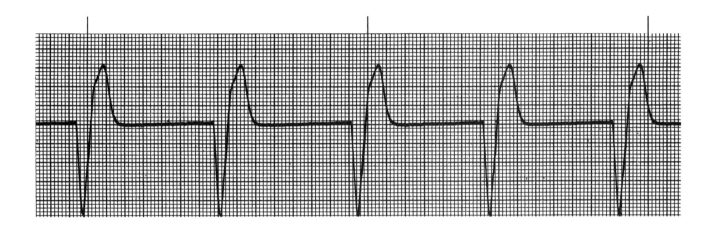

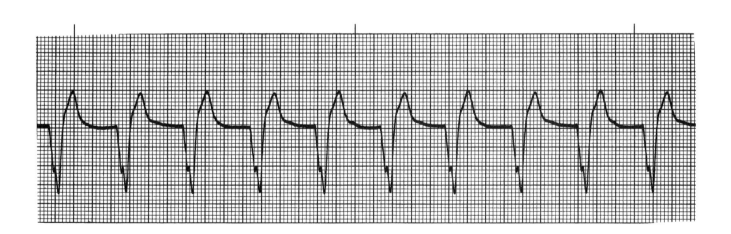

**Answer:** Idioventricular rhythm

## Idioventricular rhythm: Identifying ECG features

**Rhythm interpretation:** Regular
**Rate:** 30 to 40 beats/minute (sometimes less)
**P waves:** Absent
**PR interval:** Not measurable
**QRS complex:** Wide (0.12 second or greater)

**Answer:** Accelerated idioventricular rhythm

## Accelerated idioventricular rhythm: Identifying ECG features

**Rhythm interpretation:** Regular
**Rate:** 50 to 100 beats/minute
**P waves:** Absent
**PR interval:** Not measurable
**QRS complex:** 0.12 second or greater

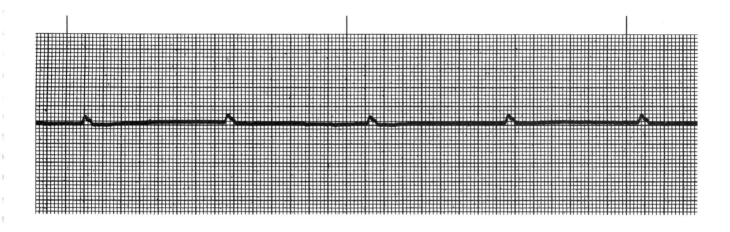

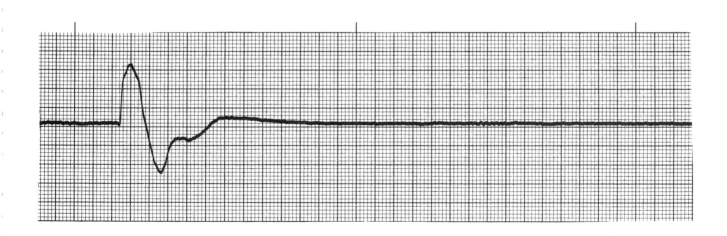

**Answer:** Ventricular standstill

## Ventricular standstill: Identifying ECG features

**Rhythm interpretation:** 0 (no QRS complexes present)

**Rate:** 0 (no QRS complexes present)

**P waves:** ECG will show either P waves without QRS complexes or a straight line

**PR interval:** Not measurable

**QRS complex:** Absent

**Answer:** One ventricular complex changing to ventricular standstill

## Ventricular standstill: Identifying ECG features

**Rhythm interpretation:** 0 (no QRS complexes present)

**Rate:** 0 (no QRS complexes present)

**P waves:** ECG will show either P waves without QRS complexes or a straight line

**PR interval:** Not measurable

**QRS complex:** Absent